Sports Cardiology

David J. Engel • Dermot M. Phelan

Editors

Sports Cardiology

Care of the Athletic Heart from the Clinic
to the Sidelines

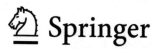 Springer

Editors
David J. Engel
Division of Cardiology
Columbia University Irving Medical Center
New York, NY
USA

Dermot M. Phelan
Sports Cardiology Center
Hypertrophic Cardiomyopathy Center
Atrium Health Sanger Heart &
Vascular Institute
Charlotte, NC
USA

ISBN 978-3-030-69386-2   ISBN 978-3-030-69384-8   (eBook)
https://doi.org/10.1007/978-3-030-69384-8

This Springer imprint is published by the registered company Springer Nature Switzerland AG
The registered company address is: Gewerbestrasse 11, 6330 Cham, Switzerland

Preface

Participation in organized sports across the globe has markedly increased over the past decade, and, in parallel, the clinical practice and research activity centered on the cardiac care for athletes within the field of sports cardiology has expanded exponentially. Recognizing the unique diagnostic and management challenges in optimizing the heart health of athletes and reflective of the increasing importance assigned to protecting the hearts of athletes, the American College of Cardiology (ACC) in 2011 launched the ACC Section of Sports and Exercise Cardiology.

A foundation in the growth of sports cardiology has been the development of a refined and enhanced understanding of the physiological manifestations of exercise on the heart. This improved characterization of exercise-induced cardiac remodeling, recognizing the relative influence of such modifiers as sport type, duration and intensity of training, age, gender, race, size, and genetics, has vastly improved our ability to screen for subclinical cardiac disease and differentiate normal physiology from pathology. It is essential for healthcare providers who screen and treat athletes at all skill levels to have a firm grasp of the tenets of sports cardiology and readily available reference data encompassing the key elements within this growing field.

The cumulative clinical experience gained from caring for athletes training and competing with existing cardiac conditions has resulted in the rapid evolution of recommendations guiding sporting participation and the recognition of the importance of shared decision-making. A contemporaneous challenge has been the devastation wrought by the COVID-19 pandemic. Sport and health organizations now confront significant challenges designing and implementing safe athlete return to play (RTP) strategies. In this textbook, we will review the critical issues and data surrounding concerns of potential cardiac sequelae of COVID-19, and their impact on athlete screening and RTP plans, as the newest element in the field of sports cardiology.

Finally, the field of sports cardiology has pushed the practicing cardiologist from the clinical facilities to the sports training facilities where they must participate in the acute evaluation and management of athletes in addition to provide guidance on effective emergence action plans.

Reflecting these challenges, this textbook is divided into three parts:

1. Pre-participation Cardiac screening of Athletes
2. Management and Recommendations for Athletes with Existing Cardiac Disorders
3. Sideline Management of Acute Cardiac Conditions in Athletes

The purpose of this textbook is to assist healthcare providers manage the cardiac care of athletes across the spectrum of these essential components. We will review best practices for using and interpreting diagnostic tests commonly employed in the cardiac evaluation of athletes, including the 12-lead electrocardiogram, advanced cardiac imaging, and genetic testing. Treatment of cardiac disorders, ranging from acute symptoms that develop suddenly during competition to chronic conditions that require longitudinal management and assessment, will be reviewed with incorporation of latest guideline recommendations. This textbook will provide a framework to aid in the provision of optimal care for athletic patients of all ages both on and off the playing field.

New York, NY, USA   David J. Engel
Charlotte, NC, USA   Dermot M. Phelan

Contents

Contributors

Hitesh Agrawal, MD, MBA, FSCAI Department of Pediatric Cardiology, University of Texas, Austin, TX, USA

D. Edmund Anstey, MD, MPH The Columbia Hypertension Center, Columbia University Irving Medical Center, New York, NY, USA

Chad Asplund, MD, MPH Department of Orthopedics and Sports Medicine, Mayo Clinic, Minneapolis, MN, USA

Peter F. Aziz, MD Cleveland Clinic Children's, Cleveland, OH, USA

Salima Bhimani, MD Cleveland Clinic Children's, Cleveland, OH, USA

George Chiampas, DO, CAQSM, FACEP Departments of Emergency Medicine and Orthopedic Surgery, Feinberg School of Medicine, Northwestern University, Chicago, IL, USA

Eugene H. Chung, MD Department of Medicine, University of Michigan, Ann Arbor, MI, USA

Brian J. Cross, MD Division of Cardiology, VA Pittsburgh Health System, Pittsburgh, PA, USA

Kara Denby, MD Department of Cardiovascular Medicine, Cleveland Clinic, Cleveland, OH, USA

John DiFiori, MD Sports Medicine Institute, Hospital for Special Surgery, New York, NY, USA

Christopher Drake, PhD Department of Sleep Medicine, Henry Ford Health System, Detroit, MI, USA

David J. Engel, MD, FACC Division of Cardiology, Columbia University Irving Medical Center, New York, NY, USA

Marc Estes, MD Heart and Vascular Institute, University of Pittsburgh, Pittsburgh, PA, USA

Benjamin H. Hammond, MD Division of Pediatric Cardiology, Cleveland Clinic Children's and Pediatric Institute, Cleveland, OH, USA

Jeffrey S. Hedley, MD Department of Cardiovascular Medicine, Section of Cardiac Pacing and Electrophysiology, Cleveland Clinic Foundation, Cleveland, OH, USA

Jeffrey J. Hsu, MD, PhD Department of Medicine (Cardiology), University of California, Los Angeles, CA, USA

Isha Kalia, MS, MPH Division of Cardiology, Columbia University Irving Medical Center, New York, NY, USA

Jonathan H. Kim, MD, MSc Emory Clinical Cardiovascular Research Institute, Atlanta, GA, USA

Jared Klein, MD, MPH Cleveland Clinic Children's, Cleveland, OH, USA

Justine S. Ko, MD Department of Emergency Medicine, Feinberg School of Medicine, Northwestern University, Chicago, IL, USA

Bradley Lander, MD Division of Cardiology, Columbia University Irving Medical Center, New York, NY, USA

Farhana Latif, MD Division of Cardiology, Columbia University Irving Medical Center, New York, NY, USA

Mark S. Link, MD Department of Medicine, Cardiology Division, Cardiac Electrophysiology, UT Southwestern Medical Center, Dallas, TX, USA

Kyle Mandsager, MD Centennial Heart, TriStar Centennial Heart and Vascular Center, Nashville, TN, USA

Matthew W. Martinez, MD, FACC Director of Sports Cardiology, Morristown Medical Center, Atlantic Health System, Morristown, NJ, USA

Silvana Molossi, MD, PhD Department of Pediatric Cardiology, Texas Children's Hospital, Baylor College of Medicine, Houston, TX, USA

David C. Peritz, MD Heart and Vascular Center, Dartmouth Hitchcock Medical Center, Lebanon, NH, USA

Dermot M. Phelan, MD, PhD, FASE, FACC Sports Cardiology Center, Hypertrophic Cardiomyopathy Center, Atrium Health Sanger Heart & Vascular Institute, Charlotte, NC, USA

James C. Puffer, MD Division of Sports Medicine, Department of Family Medicine, David Geffen School of Medicine at UCLA, Los Angeles, CA, USA

Prashant Rao, MBBS, MRCP(UK) Beth Israel Deaconess Medical Center, Harvard Medical School, Boston, MA, USA

Muredach P. Reilly, MBBCh, MSCE Division of Cardiology, Columbia University Irving Medical Center, New York, NY, USA

Thomas Roth, PhD Department of Sleep Medicine, Henry Ford Health System, Detroit, MI, USA

John J. Ryan, MD Division of Cardiovascular Medicine, Department of Internal Medicine, University of Utah, Salt Lake City, UT, USA

Elizabeth V. Saarel, MD Division of Pediatric Cardiology, St. Luke's Health System, Boise, ID, USA

Nishant P. Shah, MD Department of Cardiovascular Medicine, Cleveland Clinic, Cleveland, OH, USA

Daichi Shimbo, MD The Columbia Hypertension Center, Columbia University Irving Medical Center, New York, NY, USA

David Shipon, MD, FACC Thomas Jefferson University Hospital, Philadelphia, PA, USA

Meeta Singh, MD Department of Sleep Medicine, Thomas Roth Sleep Disorders Center, Henry Ford Health System, Detroit, MI, USA

Mohita Singh, MD Department of Medicine, Cardiology Division, Cardiac Electrophysiology, UT Southwestern Medical Center, Dallas, TX, USA

Tamanna K. Singh, MD, FAAC Sports Cardiology Center, Heart, Vascular and Thoracic Institute, Cleveland Clinic Foundation, Cleveland, OH, USA

John Symanski, MD Sports Cardiology Center, Hypertrophic Cardiomyopathy Center, Sanger Heart & Vascular Institute, Atrium Health, Charlotte, NC, USA

Marc P. Waase, MD, PhD Division of Cardiology, Columbia University Irving Medical Center, New York, NY, USA

Shayna Weinshel, BS, MS Department of Medicine, University of Central Florida, Orlando, FL, USA

Brad Witbrodt, MD Emory Clinical Cardiovascular Research Institute, Atlanta, GA, USA

Michael Workings, MD Department of Family Medicine, Henry Ford Health System, Detroit, MI, USA

Kenneth G. Zahka, MD Department of Pediatric Cardiology, Cardiovascular Medicine, Cleveland Clinic, Cleveland, OH, USA

Chapter 1
The Cardiovascular History and Examination

John DiFiori, Chad Asplund, and James C. Puffer

Introduction

A comprehensive preparticipation evaluation (PPE) is recommended prior to the initiation of training and competition for organized sports at the high school level, the NCAA, professional sports organizations, and most national and international sport governing bodies [1–6]. While the PPE is felt to be an important first step to ensuring athlete health and well-being, there is variation in how the PPE is performed among state scholastic programs and even among higher levels of sport competition [1, 7–10].

The Cardiovascular Component of the PPE

Given that the primary goal of the PPE is to promote the health and safety of the athlete [1], the cardiovascular (CV) screening portion of the PPE is perhaps the most essential piece of this assessment. The CV component aims to identify and evaluate symptoms or exam findings that may lead to the diagnosis of underlying

J. DiFiori (✉)
Sports Medicine Institute, Hospital for Special Surgery, New York, NY, USA
e-mail: difiorij@HSS.EDU

C. Asplund
Department of Orthopedics and Sports Medicine, Mayo Clinic, Minneapolis, MN, USA

J. C. Puffer
Division of Sports Medicine, Department of Family Medicine, David Geffen School of Medicine at UCLA, Los Angeles, CA, USA
e-mail: jpuffer@theabfm.org

© Springer Nature Switzerland AG 2021
D. J. Engel, D. M. Phelan (eds.), *Sports Cardiology*,
https://doi.org/10.1007/978-3-030-69384-8_1

cardiac conditions that could result in cardiac morbidity, sudden cardiac arrest, or sudden cardiac death. The American College of Cardiology and the American Heart Association state that "the principal objective of screening is to reduce the cardiovascular risks associated with organized sports and enhance the safety of athletic participation; however, raising the suspicion of a cardiac abnormality on a standard screening examination is only the first tier of recognition, after which subspecialty referral for further diagnostic testing is generally necessary" [11].

Consensus statements and recommendations for the PPE include specific details for the cardiac history and physical examination [1, 11–13]. Despite these published standards, there remains a lack of consistency in their implementation [7–10]. Further, it is important to understand that there is debate about the ability of the CV history and physical exam to detect significant CV conditions during PPEs. However, it is well recognized that no screening algorithm is capable of detecting all clinically relevant cardiac disorders [2, 12]. These important issues are beyond the scope of this chapter and are discussed in detail in other sections of this publication.

With these issues in mind, the goal of this chapter is to delineate the key features of the CV history and physical examination of the PPE.

Organization and Planning

A successful CV screening process is dependent upon planning. Organization should begin several months in advance. Planning meetings should include team physicians, team athletic training staff, coaching staff, and administrative staff (e.g., staff from the school, athletic department, and/or sport operations). Setting the date for the PPE with the key stakeholders is the first order of business. The date will need to consider the timing of the onset of the training and the travel schedules and availability of the athletes. For PPEs that are intended to be performed for a group of athletes at a set time, the availability of medical facilities should be confirmed. Key consultants in cardiology and radiology should be identified and informed of the dates of the screening, so that their availability for athletes potentially requiring further evaluation can be established, which will then help expedite the process for follow-up testing.

The organization process should also include the development of policies regarding issues such as liability coverage (for physicians, athletic trainers, and any other clinical staff), medical record documentation, and the use of chaperones. If an online medical history questionnaire is being used, information technology staff should ensure that the site is secure. Testing of the online process should be performed to identify any technical issues so that they can be resolved in advance.

The personnel needed to perform the CV screening should be identified. In many cases, especially at the collegiate and professional levels, the CV history and exam are performed by designated team physicians who are board certified in a primary specialty and also have completed fellowship training and are certified in sports medicine. In other situations, it may be ideal for an athlete who has an ongoing relationship with a personal physician to have that physician perform the screening examination [1]. This may be the best approach for children and adolescents who are participating in programs that do not have an identified team physician. Cardiologists may be used to perform the screening CV history and exam, but they are more commonly relied upon to evaluate concerning findings. In some cases, a nurse practitioner or a physician assistant may perform the screening [1]. Regardless of the certification of the clinician, *it is critical that the individual performing the CV history and exam has had clinical training in this component of the PPE, an intimate knowledge of the nuances of CV screening in athletes, and the necessary clinical experience to identify a potential concern in this population.*

Once the screening date is set, the athletes (and if minors, their families) should be notified well in advance. This will allow sufficient time to complete the CV history (especially if performed online) and obtain any pertinent documents related to prior screening and/or records involving CV diagnoses and treatment. In cases where athletes will have the PPE performed by a personal physician or provider, this provides ample time to arrange the examination.

Finally, the planning should occur with the understanding that the history and/or physical examination may raise suspicion for the presence of a cardiac condition that then requires additional evaluation. In such cases, screening events that occur immediately prior to the planned start of training could result in removal from participation while further investigations are performed. To lessen the likelihood of an athlete needing to be withheld from their training program for sports that have designated start periods (e.g., high school or collegiate sports), it is recommended that exams occur several weeks prior to the anticipated start date for that sport. As mentioned above, communication with consultants in cardiology and radiology should take place in advance so that they will be prepared to examine athletes who have had a concern raised based upon the history and exam.

Setting and Implementation

If the PPE is conducted in a location other than the office of the athlete's personal physician, the organizers should arrange a setting that ensures privacy, is comfortable for the athletes, and is conducive to maximizing the ability to perform the examination. For CV screening of groups of athletes from a school, program, or team, securing the use of patient examination areas in a medical facility is ideal. An individual exam room is preferred for reasons of privacy and the ability to have quiet space for auscultation. The use of gymnasiums, auditoriums, locker rooms, and other non-private areas is not recommended. Attempting to create a level of separation within a large room by using a "pipe and drape" setup is likewise not recommended.

In order to conduct a thorough exam, an appropriate amount of time should be allocated for each athlete being screened. The amount of time needed to conduct an exam for an individual athlete, the total number of athletes needing to be screened in a given time period, and the number of available examination rooms should be determined in advance. This will indicate the number of examiners needed and the total time required to perform a complete CV history and exam for a group of athletes.

Other factors to consider include whether an online questionnaire was completed in advance or a hard copy was completed on site. Online questionnaires must be completed on a secure website, and then viewed within an electronic medical record, or uploaded or printed and scanned to become part of the athlete's official medical record. If an online questionnaire or hard copy is to be completed on site, a private space should be provided for the athlete to complete the document. In either case, the athlete (or parent/guardian) must sign and date the questionnaire attesting to its accuracy.

Although uncommon, an athlete (or his parent/guardian) may withhold or misrepresent important medical information due to a concern that providing such information could jeopardize medical clearance for sport participation. Thus, it is important that the physician confirm that the acknowledgment is signed. In some cases, an athlete may view the history and exam as an unnecessary burden or "rubber stamp" process prior to the beginning of training. In these circumstances, an athlete may choose to select negative responses throughout the questionnaire in order to expedite the screening. This leads to substandard screening that could place the athlete at risk. In order to recognize if an athlete is not reading and responding to each question individually, and simply checking the "no column," it may be helpful to embed a question that requires a positive response. An example of such a question is "have you ever played a competitive sport?" Should the clinician feel that the athlete is providing inaccurate information, they should proceed to perform the history using a primary "interview" format, asking each question and clarifying each response verbally.

Personal and Family History

A detailed history and physical examination have been the cornerstones of the preparticipation evaluation of athletes in the United States for decades. However, given the high degree of variability and lack of standardization of cardiovascular assessment, the American Heart Association (AHA) convened an expert panel in 1996 to make recommendations for a standardized process for this component of the preparticipation evaluation [14] with an updated review of the recommendations in 2007 and 2014 [2, 11]. The result of this work was the development of a 14-point evaluation, which has now been widely embraced for the cardiovascular preparticipation screening of athletes (Table 1.1).

Perhaps the most important component of this 14-point evaluation is the personal and family history, since athletes with underlying yet undetected cardiovascular disease may present with warning signs (e.g., syncope or chest pain during exercise)

Table 1.1 The 14-element AHA recommendations for preparticipation cardiovascular screening of competitive athletes

Medical history[a]
Personal history
1. Chest pain/discomfort/tightness/pressure related to exertion
2. Unexplained syncope/near-syncope[b]
3. Excessive and unexplained dyspnea/fatigue or palpitations, associated with exercise
4. Prior recognition of a heart murmur
5. Elevated systemic blood pressure
6. Prior restriction from participation in sports
7. Prior testing for the heart, ordered by a physician
Family history
8. Premature death (sudden and unexpected, or otherwise) before 50 years of age attributable to heart disease in ≥ 1 relative
9. Disability from heart disease in dose relative < 50 years of age
10. Hypertrophic or dilated cardiomyopathy, long QT syndrome, or other ion channelopathies, Marfan syndrome, or clinically significant arrhythmias; specific knowledge of genetic cardiac conditions in family members
Physical examination
11. Heart murmur[c]
12. Femoral pulses to exclude aortic coarctation
13. Physical stigmata of Marfan syndrome
14. Brachial artery blood pressure (sitting position)[d]

AHA American Heart Association
[a]Parental verification is recommended for high school and middle school athletes
[b]Judged not to be of neurocardiogenic (vasovagal) origin; of particular concern when occurring during or after physical exertion
[c]Refers to heart murmurs judged likely to be organic and unlikely to be innocent; auscultation should be performed with the patient in both the supine and standing positions (or with Valsalva maneuver), specifically to identify murmurs of dynamic left ventricular outflow tract obstruction
[d]Preferably taken in both arms
Modified with permission form Maron et al. [3] Copyright © 2007, American Heart Association, Inc.

that may be revealed with a carefully obtained personal history. Furthermore, since most cardiovascular conditions leading to sudden death in athletes may be genetic or familial in nature, a revealing family history may be critical in raising suspicion for these disorders [15].

The AHA recommends that queries about the following elements be included in the personal history [2]:

1. Chest pain/discomfort/tightness/pressure related to exertion
2. Unexplained syncope/near-syncope
3. Excessive and unexplained dyspnea/fatigue or palpitations, associated with exercise
4. Prior recognition of a heart murmur
5. Elevated systemic blood pressure
6. Prior restriction from participation in sports

7. Prior testing for the heart, ordered by a physician

Positive or equivocal responses to these queries should be pursued with appropriate follow-up questions to probe and explore each response more deeply. An excellent list of follow-up questions for positive/equivocal responses to each of the above personal history elements has been included in the fifth edition of the *Preparticipation Physical Evaluation* monograph developed jointly by the American Academy of Family Physicians (AAFP), American Academy of Pediatrics (AAP), American College of Sports Medicine (ACSM), American Medical Society for Sports Medicine (AMSSM), American Orthopaedic Society for Sports Medicine (AOSSM), and American Osteopathic Academy for Sports Medicine (AOASM) and published by the AAP [1].

Similarly, the AHA recommends that questions about the following three elements be included in the family history [2]:

1. Premature death (sudden and unexpected or otherwise) before 50 years of age caused by heart disease in one or more relatives
2. Disability from heart disease in a close relative younger than 50 years of age
3. Hypertrophic or dilated cardiomyopathy, long QT syndrome, or other ion channelopathies, Marfan syndrome or clinically significant arrhythmias; specific knowledge of genetic cardiac conditions in family members

As with the personal history, positive or equivocal responses to questions for these elements should be probed further for more detailed information; suggested follow-up questions can be found in the PPE monograph cited above.

Finally, physicians, other providers, and organizations who conduct preparticipation screening should be aware of the Genetic Information Nondiscrimination Act of 2008 (GINA) [16]. This law prevents employers from using genetic information in employment decisions and prevents employers from requesting and requiring genetic information in employment decisions such as hiring, firing, promotions, pay, and job assignments (note that an important exception to Title II of GINA involves the US military). As such, when performing a PPE in a professional athlete, obtaining a personal or family history that includes questions regarding genetic disorders may be considered unlawful [17–19]. Because this information is essential to the cardiovascular history, the legal counsel of the team or organization and the relevant athlete union or player's association should determine if and how this key component of the PPE may be applied.

Physical Examination

The physical examination of the cardiovascular system should be comprehensive with particular attention to physical findings for conditions that may cause sudden death in athletes, such as physical stigmata suggestive of Marfan syndrome or the murmurs of aortic stenosis or obstructive hypertrophic cardiomyopathy. Documenting resting blood pressure is also a key component of the physical examination. The AHA recommends that the following elements be included in the physical examination [2]:

1. Auscultation for heart murmurs in both the supine and standing positions
2. Palpation of the femoral pulses to exclude aortic coarctation
3. Observation of physical stigmata of Marfan syndrome
4. Brachial artery blood pressure taken in the sitting position

It has been demonstrated that clinicians who conduct the PPE, regardless of experience or level of training, may be unable to distinguish pathological murmurs from physiological murmurs by auscultation [1, 20]. Simplifying the cardiac examination allows for better differentiation between benign and pathological murmurs. The following murmurs deserve further evaluation and referral [1]:

1. Loud (>grade 2/6) or harsh murmurs
2. Radiation of a murmur laterally rather than upward
3. A mid- or late systolic murmur accompanied by a click
4. Any murmur that becomes louder with dynamic maneuvers (standing, squatting) or Valsalva
5. Any holosystolic or diastolic murmur

The examining clinician should carefully look for any physical stigmata of Marfan syndrome which can predispose to aortic dissection and sudden death during exercise. These features include, but are not limited to, wrist and thumb signs, chest wall deformity, hind-foot deformity, diminished upper body to lower body segment ratio, increased arm span to height ratio, skin striae, scoliosis, or the murmur of mitral valve prolapse. A high index of suspicion for this syndrome based upon the presence of significant physical findings should prompt referral for further evaluation and diagnosis.

Blood pressure should be preferably measured in both arms. It should be measured with the athlete in the seated position with an appropriately sized cuff on the bare arm at the heart level after he or she has been sitting at rest in a quiet room for several minutes. Each of these conditions is critically important in obtaining an accurate measurement [21]. Cuff size is especially important in larger athletes as inadequate cuff size may result in a spuriously elevated blood pressure. Large adult size cuffs and thigh cuffs should be available to avoid this potential problem. If the blood pressure is measured appropriately and is elevated, re-measurement should be undertaken only after the athlete has sat or lied quietly for 5–10 minutes. Persistently elevated measurements should prompt further workup and evaluation.

Limitations of the History and Physical Examination

No studies have demonstrated the ability of the cardiovascular preparticipation examination to prevent cardiac sudden death. A single Italian study, performed to assess nationally mandated cardiovascular screening in athletes, has shown a reduction in sudden death in screened athletes over the 30-year course of the program, specifically for arrhythmogenic right ventricular dysplasia and premature coronary artery disease [22]. A recent systematic review and meta-analysis [23] have documented the effectiveness of the cardiac PPE in detecting potentially lethal cardiovascular conditions. Specifically, the history was found to have a sensitivity and specificity of 20% and 94%, respectively, while the physical examination was found to have a sensitivity of 9% and a specificity of 97%. The positive likelihood ratios were 3.22 for the history and 2.93 for the physical exam, while the negative likelihood ratios were 0.85 for the history and 0.93 for the physical examination.

Determination of Clearance and Coordination of Follow-Up

For the active person diagnosed with a cardiac disorder, the determination of future athletic eligibility is a critical step in the care spectrum that begins with diagnosis, through decision-making and then possibly treatment. This process may be challenging for the patient, family, physician, and school/sporting organization. Until recently, the 2005 Bethesda Conference statement [24] served as the best clinical guide for these decisions. The Bethesda guidelines were largely binary yes/no statements about clearance for play based on diagnosis and were criticized for being overly paternalistic in nature and based, for the most part, on expert consensus or opinion. As our knowledge of specific diseases and their natural progressions has expanded in the last 10 years, the need for a new document emerged. In 2015, a competitive sport eligibility statement sponsored jointly by the American Heart Association, American College of Cardiology, and Heart Rhythm Society updated and replaced the Bethesda guidelines [25]. This new statement represented a paradigm shift in the approach to the athlete with established cardiovascular disease (CVD), even sudden cardiac death predisposing CVD, moving away from a doctor-driven model toward a patient-centered care model that supports shared decision-making for clinicians, patients, and families.

Rather than strict yes or no to participation, the 2015 document provides different classes which represent a new approach to the evidence, the risk level, and patient desires. For cases deemed Class I, participation is recommended; those deemed Class IIA and IIB, participation may be reasonable, and for those in Class III, participation is not recommended. The establishment of the Class II category creates a space between the strict yes (Class I) and no (Class III) binary model previously utilized. Within this Class II context, physicians are encouraged to present patients with scientific facts and the uncertainties relevant to their condition and to engage in a shared decision-making (SDM) process about subsequent management and clearance options. Acknowledging the incomplete evidence in some disease process allows individual clinicians to state "…participation is reasonable if…" or "participation in sports may be considered after…," which allows the decision, in those instances where the evidence and risk level is unclear, to be individualized by the physician and the patient. In these situations, it is very important for appropriate decision-making that the primary physician or team physician works with a consulting cardiologist who has experience with competitive athletes in providing recommendations on sport participation.

This new SDM framework often results in a more time-intensive process, which requires much discussion and education. In order to successfully implement this framework, there must be a confirmation of the diagnostic accuracy, as many of these disease processes may be difficult to adequately differentiate from normal adaptations of the athlete's heart and pathological manifestations. Next, risk stratification should be conducted to better understand the risks and possibly put in place measures to mitigate or reduce risk. Patient and family education are the most important steps in the SDM process to ensure that those involved in the decision have a thorough understanding of the disease, the risks, the possible further risks of continuing sport, and the benefits that derive from sport participation.

Following the ultimate participation recommendation, longitudinal care is essential for all athletes with established CVD, regardless of whether they choose to continue in sport. It is imperative that their disease progression be assessed, changes in the risk level noted, and appropriate timely management decisions provided. This may include highlighting important signs and symptoms for the athlete to recognize and to report immediately to their healthcare team if features of worsening or progression of their disease should manifest. During this longitudinal follow-up, changes in the disease process may require an upgrade or downgrade of their participation status [26].

As the model for clearance decisions has shifted, concern has arisen that physicians now must shoulder an increased legal liability, especially in cases where uncertainty still exists. It is imperative that decisions are based on reasonable medical practice with the athlete's best interest in mind [27, 28]. Further thorough documentation of the certainty of diagnosis; the known (and unknown risks) as well as the possible benefits of participation is needed. Despite the concern of additional risk borne by the physician, no legal precedent exists for holding a physician liable for refusing to clear a patient if the risks clearly exceed the benefits [29].

Conclusion

The cardiovascular history and physical exam remain essential to the preparticipation evaluation. Standardizing the use of the key elements of history and examination and the broad and consistent implementation of these components remain a challenge across the many levels of sport participation in the United States. Communication between the athlete, primary physician or team physician, and the consulting cardiologist is integral to sound interpretation and management of concerning findings.

References

1. American Academy of Family Physicians, American Academy of Pediatrics, American College of Sports Medicine, American Medical Society for Sports Medicine, American Orthopaedic Society for Sports Medicine, American Osteopathic Academy of Sports Medicine. Preparticipation physical evaluation. 5th ed. Itasca: American Academy of Pediatrics; 2019.
2. Maron BJ, Friedman RA, Kligfield P, et al. Assessment of the 12-lead electrocardiogram as a screening test for detection of cardiovascular disease in healthy general populations of young people (12–25 years of age): a scientific statement from the American Heart Association and the American College of Cardiology. J Am Coll Cardiol. 2014;64:1479–514.
3. Corrado D, Pelliccia A, Bjornstad HH, et al. Cardiovascular preparticipation screening of young competitive athletes for prevention of sudden death: proposal for a common European protocol. Consensus statement of the Study Group of Sport Cardiology of the Working Group of Cardiac Rehabilitation and Exercise Physiology and the Working Group of Myocardial and Pericardial Diseases of the European Society of Cardiology. Eur Heart J. 2005;26:516–24.
4. Dvorak J, Grimm K, Schmied C, et al. Development and implementation of a standardized precompetition medical assessment of international elite football players—2006 FIFA World Cup Germany. Clin J Sport Med. 2009;19:316–21.
5. Ljungqvist A, Jenoure P, Engebretsen L, et al. The International Olympic Committee (IOC) Consensus Statement on periodic health evaluation of elite athletes March 2009. Br J Sports Med. 2009;43:631–43.
6. Hainline B, Drezner JA, Baggish A, et al. Interassociation consensus statement on cardiovascular care of college student-athletes. J Am Coll Cardiol. 2016;67:2981–95.
7. Madsen NL, Drezner JA, Salerno JC. The preparticipation physical evaluation: an analysis of clinical practice. Clin J Sport Med. 2014;24:142–9.
8. Glover DW, Glover DW, Maron BJ. Evolution in the process of screening United States high school student-athletes for cardiovascular disease. Am J Cardiol. 2007;100(11):1709–12.
9. Charboneau ML, Mencias T, Hoch AZ. Cardiovascular screening practices in collegiate student-athletes. PM R. 2014;6(7):583–6.
10. Moulson N, Kuljic N, McKinney J, Taylor T, Hopman WM, Johri AM. Variation in preparticipation screening medical questionnaires and physical examinations across Canadian Universities. Can J Cardiol. 2018;34(7):933–6.
11. Maron BJ, Thompson PD, Ackerman MJ, et al. Recommendations and considerations related to preparticipation screening for cardiovascular abnormalities in competitive athletes: 2007 update a scientific statement from the American Heart Association Council on Nutrition, Physical Activity, and Metabolism. Circulation. 2007;115:1643–55.
12. Drezner JA, O'Conner FG, Harmon KG, et al. AMSSM Position statement on cardiovascular preparticipation screening in athletes: current evidence, knowledge gaps, recommendations, and future directions. Clin J Sport Med. 2016;26:347–61.
13. Corrado D, Pelliccia A, Bjørnstad HH, et al. Cardiovascular pre-participation screening of young competitive athletes for prevention of sudden death: proposal for a common European protocol. Consensus statement of the Study Group of Sport Cardiology of the Working Group of Cardiac Rehabilitation and Exercise Physiology and the Working Group of Myocardial and Pericardial Diseases of the European Society of Cardiology. Eur Heart J. 2005;26(5):516–24. https://doi.org/10.1093/eurheartj/ehi108.
14. Maron BJ, Thompson PD, Puffer JC, McGrew CA, Strong WB, Douglas PS, Clark LT, Mitten MJ, Crawford MH, Atkins DL, Driscoll DJ, Epstein AE. Cardiovascular preparticipation screening of competitive athletes: a statement for health professionals from the Sudden Death Committee (Clinical Cardiology) and Congenital Cardiac Defects Committee (Cardiovascular Disease in the Young), American Heart Association. Circulation. 1996;94:850–6.
15. Ranthe MF, Winkel BG, Andersen EW, et al. Cardiovascular disease in family members of young sudden cardiac death victims. Eur Heart J. 2013;34:503–11.

16. Genetic information nondiscrimination act of 2008. 42 USC 2000ff. https://www.eeoc.gov/statutes/genetic-information-nondiscrimination-act-2008.
17. Evans RB. 'Striking out': the genetic nondiscrimination act of 2008 and title II's impact on professional sports employers. N C J Law Technol. 2009;11(1):205–21.
18. Bland JA. There will be blood … testing: the intersection of professional sports and the genetic information nondiscrimination act of 2008. Vanderbilt J Entertain Technol Law. 2011;13(2):357–83.
19. Patel S, Varley I. Exploring the regulation of genetic testing in sport. Entertain Sports Law J. 2019;17:5, 1–13. https://doi.org/10.16997/eslj.223.
20. O'Connor FG, Johnson JD, Chapin M, Oriscello RG, Taylor DC. A pilot study of clinical agreement in cardiovascular preparticipation examinations: how good is the standard of care? Clin J Sports Med. 2005;15(3):177–9.
21. Whelton PK, Carey RM, Aronow WS, Casey DE Jr, Collins KJ, Dennison Himmelfarb C, DePalma SM, Gidding S, Jamerson KA, Jones DW, MacLaughlin EJ, Muntner P, Ovbiagele B, Smith SC Jr, Spencer CC, Stafford RS, Taler SJ, Thomas RJ, Williams KA Sr, Williamson JD, Wright JT Jr. 2017 ACC/AHA/AAPA/ABC/ACPM/AGS/APhA/ASH/ASPC/NMA/PCNA Guideline for the prevention, detection, evaluation, and management of high blood pressure in adults: executive summary: a report of the American College of Cardiology/American Heart Association Task Force on clinical practice guidelines. Hypertension. 2018;71:1269–324.
22. Corrado D, Basso C, Pavei A, Michieli P, Schiavon M, Thiene G. Trends in sudden cardiovascular death in young competitive athletes after implementation of a preparticipation screening program. JAMA. 2006;296:1593–601.
23. Harmon KG, Zigman M, Drezner JA. The effectiveness of screening history, physical exam, and ECG to detect potentially lethal cardiac disorders in athletes: a systematic review/meta-analysis. J Electrocardiol. 2015;48:329–38.
24. Maron BJ, Zipes DP. 36th Bethesda conference: introduction: eligibility recommendations for competitive athletes with cardiovascular abnormalities. J Am Coll Cardiol. 2005;45:1318–21.
25. Maron BJ, Zipes DP, Kovacs RJ, American Heart Association Electrocardiography and Arrhythmias Committee of Council of Council on Clinical Cardiology, Council on Cardiovascular Disease in Young, Council on Cardiovascular and Stroke Nursing, Council on Functional Genomics and Translational Biology, American College of Cardiology. Eligibility and disqualification recommendations for competitive athletes with cardiovascular abnormalities: preamble, principles, and general considerations: a scientific statement from the American Heart Association and American College of Cardiology. Circulation. 2015;132:e256–61. https://doi.org/10.1161/CIR.0000000000000236.
26. Baggish AL, Ackerman MJ, Putukian M, et al. Shared decision making for athletes with cardiovascular disease: practical considerations. Curr Sports Med Rep. 2019;18(3):76–81.
27. Baggish AL, Ackerman MJ, Lampert R. Competitive sport participation among athletes with heart disease: a call for a paradigm shift in decision making. Circulation. 2017;136:1569–71.
28. Mitten MJ. Emerging legal issues in sports medicine: a synthesis, summary and analysis. St John's Law Rev. 2002;76:5–86.
29. Di Luca TR. Medical malpractice and the modern athlete: a whole new ballgame…or is it? Westchester County Bar Assoc J. 2008;35:17–26.

Chapter 2
Using an Electrocardiogram as a Component of Athlete Screening

David J. Engel

Should Every Athlete Have an ECG Added to Their Pre-participation Screening Exam? Findings from Epidemiological Studies

The optimal pre-participation screening strategy to detect cardiac abnormalities that place athletes at risk for exercise-triggered sudden cardiac death (SCD) is unresolved. It has been customary in the USA and recommended by all major medical societies involved in the care of athletes that pre-participation screening of athletes should be performed and that this evaluation should include a history and physical exam (H&P) [1–4]. To assist with standardization and optimization of the H&P, the American Heart Association (AHA) has provided consensus recommendations for a 14-Element H&P to serve as a guideline for the performance of these exams [5]. While a careful H&P will uncover many previously undiagnosed cardiac disorders that can predispose to exercise-triggered SCD, the sensitivity and specificity of this exam are imperfect. To enhance screening, it has been advocated to incorporate a 12-lead electrocardiogram (ECG) universally into the pre-participation evaluation of athletes in order to improve the effectiveness of cardiac screening [2, 6, 7]. There remains significant discussion and debate, however, on this issue.

Controversies surrounding mass screening of asymptomatic athletes with ECGs relate to concerns regarding cost and resource allocation, the accuracy of the ECG to identify occult cardiovascular disease, and the consequences of false-positive ECGs. At the same time, there is a recognition that ECGs can increase the yield of screening to detect cardiac abnormalities that are associated with SCD in athletes [8, 9].

D. J. Engel (✉)
Division of Cardiology, Columbia University Irving Medical Center, New York, NY, USA
e-mail: de165@cumc.columbia.edu

© Springer Nature Switzerland AG 2021
D. J. Engel, D. M. Phelan (eds.), *Sports Cardiology*,
https://doi.org/10.1007/978-3-030-69384-8_2

A significant impetus for the promotion of universal ECG inclusion into athlete screening stems from data generated from the long-standing Italian national athlete screening program. In 1971 the Italian government instituted legislation requiring medical supervision of all competitive athletes, but in 1982, the law was signifi-cantly enhanced and formalized to require annual pre-participation medical screen-ing that included an H&P plus ECG [10, 11]. In a study of SCD rates in the Veneto region of Italy between 1979 and 2004, the introduction of ECG-inclusive athlete screening resulted in an 89% reduction (3.6 deaths per 100,000 person-years to 0.4 deaths per 100,000 person-years) in the SCD rate of athletes, most of which was attributable to the detection of cardiomyopathies uncovered by screening, while no such trend during this time period was observed in unscreened age-matched nonath-letes [12] (Fig. 2.1).

Other large-scale initiatives to universally incorporate ECGs into pre-participation evaluations, however, have not replicated the Italian findings. In 1997, Israel enacted the Israeli Sport Law which mandated pre-participation medical screening of com-petitive athletes including an annual H&P and ECG, plus a treadmill ECG stress test every 4 years (yearly stress tests for athletes $\geq$35 years of age) [13, 14]. In a study of athlete SCD rates in Israel between 1985 and 2009 (12 years before and 12 years after the initiation of this legislation), no measurable differences in athlete SCD rates were observed (2.66 events per 100,000 person-years prior to legislation vs 2.54 events per 100,000 person-years after legislation, $P = 0.88$) [14]. Additionally, in a study comparing athlete SCD rates over an 11-year period (1993–2004) in Veneto, where athlete screening included an ECG, and Minnesota, a

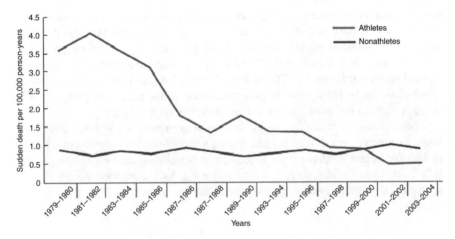

Fig. 2.1 Annual sudden cardiac death rates among screened competitive athletes and unscreened nonathletes in the Veneto region of Italy from 1979 to 2004. (Reprinted with permission from Corrodo et al. [10], Elsevier)

demographically similar area to Veneto and where athlete pre-participation screening was limited to H&P only, no differences in SCD rates were observed [15]. These studies that formed different conclusions from the Italian study regarding the utility of the ECG for SCD prevention have raised questions regarding the appropriateness of the universal incorporation of ECGs into screening.

Strengths and Pitfalls of the ECG in Athlete Screening

The determination of policies and practice regarding the optimal use of the ECG in athlete screening cannot be based solely on data generated from large-scale epidemiological studies. Analyses of the strengths and pitfalls of the ECG itself are also essential to assist with the formulation of a strategy. Assessments of the intrinsic characteristics of the ECG are integral components of the guideline recommendations and position statements regarding athlete screening currently put forth by leading medical organizations. Important strengths and pitfalls of the ECG as related to athlete screening are summarized in Table 2.1.

Table 2.1   Strengths and pitfalls of the ECG for athlete screening

Strengths of the ECG	Pitfalls of the ECG
The ECG is abnormal in a high proportion of athletes with cardiomyopathies	False-positive ECGs occur despite the use of athlete-specific ECG interpretation criteria
The ECG is the best initial screening tool to detect intrinsic conduction abnormalities that are associated with SCD in athletes including ventricular pre-excitation, ion channelopathies, and long QT syndrome	Several cardiovascular disorders associated with SCD in athletes will not be detected by an ECG including atherosclerotic coronary artery disease, anomalous coronary arteries, bicuspid aortic valves, and Marfan Syndrome
The ECG increases the sensitivity above H&P alone to detect cardiovascular disorders that can predispose to exercise-triggered SCD	Downstream testing required to evaluate a large number of athletes with ECGs classified as abnormal can adversely affect an athlete's participation status and place a significant strain on healthcare systems to provide streamlined and affordable testing
The ECG is non-expensive and fast	Technical factors including lead placement variability, inaccuracies in interval (esp. QT interval) measurements, and interobserver variability in ECG interpretation adversely affect the reliability of the test
There are low false-positive rates with the newest sets of athlete-specific ECG interpretation criteria	The incidence of SCD in athletes is low, and false-positive ECGs vastly outnumber true positives. Risk/benefit of an ECG for an asymptomatic athlete not entirely clear

Strengths of the ECG

The ECG is an effective diagnostic tool for the detection of underlying structural heart disease as an ECG will be abnormal in a high proportion of individuals with cardiomyopathies. Additionally, the cost of an ECG is low and the test requires only a few minutes to perform. Numerous studies have shown that ECG abnormalities are present in approximately 75–95% of individuals with hypertrophic cardiomyopathy (HCM), a prominent cause of exercise-triggered SCD [16–19]. ECG abnormalities are similarly seen in a high proportion of patients with arrhythmogenic right ventricular cardiomyopathy (ARVC) [20–22]. The value of an ECG for diagnosing arrhythmic disorders is even greater than that for detecting underlying structural heart disease. The ECG is the initial diagnostic modality of choice for identifying conduction abnormalities that are associated with SCD in athletes including ventricular pre-excitation and ion channelopathies such as long QT syndrome.

Owing to these intrinsic capabilities to detect important cardiac disorders associated with SCD in athletes, the ECG has been shown to increase the power and sensitivity of athlete screening when added to the H&P. The use of the ECG as part of the Italian national athlete screening program in the Veneto region over a 17-year period (1979–1996) was shown to significantly increase the yield for the detection of HCM over the H&P alone [8]. Similarly, within the USA, prospective studies of ECG-inclusive screening programs in high school [23, 24] and collegiate [9, 25, 26] athletes demonstrated that the ECG increased the detection and had increased sensitivity and specificity for identifying potentially lethal cardiac conditions than the H&P alone. A National Collegiate Athletic Association (NCAA) sponsored prospective study across 35 universities that included over 5000 athletes reported that the sensitivity for the ECG in detecting serious underlying cardiac disorders was 100% in comparison with 15.4% for the H&P [27]. These analyses and review of the strengths of the ECG to enhance screening are fundamental components of the arguments favoring the universal inclusion of an ECG in the pre-participation examination of athletes.

Pitfalls of the ECG

Notwithstanding these arguments favoring the standard inclusion of an ECG in athlete screening, several properties of the ECG, plus realities that healthcare providers and athletes encounter when ECGs are utilized in this capacity, need also be considered. False-positive ECGs continue to exist despite the formulation and use of expert consensus athlete-specific ECG interpretation criteria [28]. Even with the most current and specific athlete ECG criteria published to date (International Recommendations [29]), false-positive rates can reach as high as 6.8–15.6% when these ECG criteria are applied and studied prospectively in athlete groups [30–32]. In addition to false-positives, an ECG may not always demonstrate typical patterns or alert to the presence of underlying structural heart disease. False-negative ECGs can be present in up to 10% of cases of HCM and up to 1/3 of cases of ARVC [33, 34]. With respect to HCM in particular, it is known that the phenotype and ECG expression of this disorder can develop during adolescence or early adulthood, a time period that coincides with the majority of competitive athlete careers, thus requiring repetitive screening to optimally employ ECGs in this setting [35, 36]. In addition to issues surrounding false-positives and false-negatives, ECGs will not detect several important cardiovascular disorders that are known to be associated with SCD in athletes including atherosclerotic coronary artery disease, anomalous coronary artery origins, bicuspid aortic valves, and Marfan syndrome.

Technical factors inherent in ECG acquisition also provide a basis to advise caution with respect to mass screening of athletes with ECGs. The appearance of the waveforms on the ECG tracing is highly dependent on limb and precordial lead placement, and variability in lead placements that inevitably occur in the widespread performance of ECGs leads to significant inconsistencies in the accuracy and interpretation of the test [37–39]. Similarly, variabilities and difficulties in obtaining accurate interval measurements, especially as they relate to precise QT interval measurement, are another important source of inconsistency that affect the reliability and interpretation of the ECG [40, 41]. These technical factors contribute to significant interobserver variability in the interpretation of ECG tracings and are principal elements impacting quality control that have important implications for athlete screening both on an individual and population bases [42, 43].

The classification of an athlete's screening ECG as abnormal will necessitate further evaluation and downstream testing to ensure athlete health and safety. These evaluations often have immediate and potentially long-term adverse effects on an individual athlete's participation status as well as significant impacts on health resource utilization. Typical next steps to evaluate athletes with abnormal ECGs include subspecialist consultations, echocardiograms, stress tests, extended rhythm monitoring, cardiac MRI (CMR), or potentially invasive cardiac testing. With many millions of athletes worldwide competing at high school, collegiate, adult amateur, and professional levels, even an exceptionally small percentage of asymptomatic athletes required to undergo further evaluation because of abnormal ECG classification would place a tremendous strain on healthcare systems to provide streamlined and affordable downstream testing. The debate and discussion remain, given low published estimated incidences of SCD in athletes ranging from 0.6 to 1.2 per 100K athlete-years [15, 44, 45] without universal ECG screening, on the ultimate risks and benefits of ECG use in screening.

Medical Society Guidelines and Position Statements

At the present time, there is no universal agreement among leading medical organizations on recommendations for the use of ECGs in athlete pre-participation screening examinations. Table 2.2 summarizes the current position statements of these medical organizations regarding the standard inclusion of ECGs into pre-participation

Table 2.2 Position statements of leading medical organizations regarding the standard inclusion of ECGs into pre-participation screening programs

Medical organization/society	Routine use of ECG in athlete pre-participation screening	Position statement source
American Heart Association/ American College of Cardiology (AHA/ACC)	Not recommended	Eligibility and disqualification recommendations for competitive athletes with cardiovascular abnormalities: task force 2: pre-participation screening for cardiovascular disease in competitive athletes – a scientific statement from the American Heart Association and American College of Cardiology Circulation 2015; 132: e267–e272
National Collegiate Athletic Association (NCAA)	No formal recommendation for or against universal incorporation of ECGs – guidelines for optimal processes provided for member institutions who choose to implement	Interassociation consensus statement on cardiovascular care of college student-athletes J Am Coll Cardiol 2016; 67: 2981–95
European Society of Cardiology (ESC)	Recommended	Pre-participation cardiovascular evaluation for athletic participants to prevent sudden death: position paper from the EHRA and the EACPR, branches of the ESC. Endorsed by APHRS, HRS, and SOLAECE Eur J Prev Cardiol 2017; 24: 41–69
International Olympic Committee (IOC)	Recommended	The International Olympic Committee (IOC) consensus statement on periodic health evaluation of elite athletes, March 2009 Clin J Sport Med 2009; 19: 347–60
Canadian Cardiovascular Society/Canadian Heart Rhythm Society (CCS)	Not recommended	Canadian Cardiovascular Society/ Canadian Heart Rhythm Society Joint Position Statement on the cardiovascular screening of competitive athletes Can J Cardiol. 2019; 35: 1–11
American Medical Society of Sports Medicine (AMSSM)	No formal recommendation for or against universal incorporation of ECGs	AMSSM position statement on cardiovascular pre-participation screening in athletes: current evidence, knowledge gaps, recommendations, and future directions Clin J Sport Med 2016; 26: 347–361

screening programs. While recommendations differ, a key concept emphasized by all guidelines and position statements is that any institution or organization that chooses to include ECGs into the pre-participation screening process must have a thorough understanding of both the strengths and pitfalls of the ECG, as well as the potential benefits and risk to the athlete. Safeguards and essential elements for this process include that ECG interpretation must be performed by healthcare professionals familiar with the spectrum of ECG findings in athletes and that experts in the cardiovascular care of athletes are closely aligned to provide oversight and to efficiently and expeditiously manage downstream testing [2–4, 46–48].

How Do We Interpret Athlete ECGs?

Development of Athlete-Specific ECG Interpretation Criteria

When the decision has been made to perform an ECG on an athlete, whether it is for the purpose of screening or to evaluate a clinical concern, healthcare providers must next try and determine whether the observed ECG findings are normal or abnormal requiring further evaluation. It is appreciated that long-term and intensive athletic training results in physiologic, adaptive cardiac remodeling [49–51]. As such, surface ECGs that reflect underlying cardiac structure can frequently be different in well-trained athletes than in age-matched nonathletes [52, 53]. The challenge for healthcare providers in this setting is to distinguish physiologic, training-related ECG changes from findings that may suggest an underlying cardiac disorder. To assist in this process, with the goal to increase specificity and minimize false-positive rates in ECG interpretation, expert consensus athlete-specific ECG interpretation criteria have been developed. The first formalized set of athlete-specific ECG interpretation criteria was compiled by the European Society of Cardiology (ESC) in 2005 [54]. These criteria provided a table of abnormal ECG findings that, if present, suggested a need for further evaluation. When these criteria were applied prospectively in athlete groups, however, false-positive ECG rates were found to be unacceptably high, with a comprehensive study of 1005 elite mixed-sports athletes showing a false-positive rate of 40% using these criteria [52]. The ESC subsequently developed and published a modernized set of criteria in 2010 that separated ECG findings into common and physiologic "training-related ECG findings" and findings that were not to be expected as a result of athletic training and classified as "abnormal" [55]. These newer criteria did improve specificity and lower false-positive rates in comparison with the 2005 criteria, but abnormal ECG classification rates of approximately 10% were still observed in cohorts of athletes engaged in a cross section of sports [56]. An important additional limitation of the 2010 ESC criteria stemmed from the fact that these criteria were derived from analyses of ECGs in primarily white athletes and they did not incorporate emerging data highlighting different repolarization and T wave patterns between white and black athletes [57–59].

Based on these observed ethnic differences in repolarization, and in the effort to further improve ECG specificity, an international summit of sports cardiologists and sports medicine physicians convened in Seattle in 2012 to derive an improved set of criteria, and these "Seattle Criteria" were published in 2013 [60]. The Seattle criteria classified a pattern of convex ST elevation combined with T wave inversion

(TWI) in leads V1–V4 as a normal ECG variant in black athletes based on data demonstrating that this T wave pattern was not associated with underlying cardiac pathology in black athletes [59, 60]. In addition, the Seattle criteria shortened cut-offs to define QT prolongation and lengthened cutoffs to define abnormal QRS widening [60].

Subsequent to the publication of the Seattle criteria, a large-scale analysis that included over 2500 mixed-sports athletes and nearly 10,000 controls demonstrated that the ECG findings of atrial enlargement and axis deviation in isolation, findings classified as abnormal by Seattle criteria, were not associated with cardiac pathology when matched ECG and echocardiographic data were compared. Removal of these ECG findings from abnormal ECG classification reduced false-positive ECG rates from 13% to 7.5% [61]. The incorporation of this data led to the creation of the "Revised Criteria" published in 2014 which added a category of borderline ECG findings in addition to training-related and abnormal ECG findings [62]. Borderline variants, when present in isolation, were no longer classified as abnormal ECG findings, but if two or more borderline variants were present, then the ECG would be classified as abnormal.

A summary of the evolution of these athlete-specific ECG interpretation criteria, as well as the designation of ECG findings within each set of these criteria, is shown in Fig. 2.2. While specificity has improved with each updated set of criteria, it is important to recognize inherent limitations of these criteria. The designation of individual ECG findings as normal or abnormal was based primarily on expert consensus opinion. In addition, the criteria were not sport-specific, and they did not

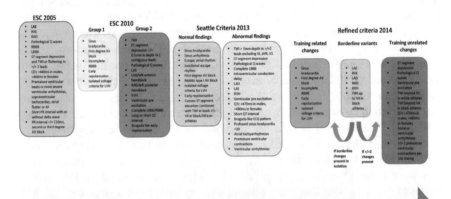

Fig. 2.2 Evolution of athlete-specific ECG interpretation criteria. (Reprinted without modification from Basu and Malhotra [70]. Springer Nature (http://creativecommons.org/licenses/by/4.0/)). *LAE* left atrial enlargement, *RAE* right atrial enlargement, *LVH* left ventricular hypertrophy, *RVH* right ventricular hypertrophy, *LAD* left axis deviation, *RAD* right axis deviation, *RBBB* right bundle branch block, *LBBB* left bundle branch block, *TWI* T wave inversion, *QTc* corrected QT interval, *AF* atrial fibrillation, *AV* atrioventricular

incorporate how varied hemodynamic demands of different sports, or the level or years of intensive training, may alter adaptive cardiac remodeling and ECG manifestations of these cardiac structural and electrical changes. Rather, the criteria were designed to be used in a "one size fits all" approach. A further limitation was the fact that the criteria sets were not studied prospectively to test or assess their accuracy in athlete groups prior to publication. Nonetheless, these expert consensus criteria have provided a vitally important frame of reference for healthcare providers to evaluate athlete ECGs. All practitioners who perform and interpret ECGs in athletes should be intimately familiar with the newest and most up-to-date versions of these criteria.

2017 International Recommendations

The most recent set of athlete-specific ECG interpretation criteria was published in 2017 by an international group of experts in sports cardiology, inherited cardiac disease, and sports medicine [29]. The International Recommendations put forth by this group represent the most current and specific guideline recommendations for the interpretation of ECGs in athletes. The International Recommendations further increase specificity from prior ECG criteria sets by re-classifying right bundle branch block (RBBB) from an abnormal ECG finding to a borderline variant, based on data demonstrating that RBBB was more prevalent in athletes than nonathletes but that this ECG pattern was not inherently reflective of underlying structural heart disease in athletes [63]. In addition, the definition of an abnormal Q wave was made more stringent. Since their publication, while false-positive rates are still shown to exist, the International Recommendations have outperformed the previous ESC, Seattle, and refined criteria and reduce false-positive ECG rates in studies of pediatric athletes, professional cyclists, and professional basketball players in the National Basketball Association (NBA) [30–32].

The flowchart to evaluate an athlete's ECG using the International Recommendations is shown in Fig. 2.3. ECG findings in green are classified as physiologic, training-related findings that do not warrant further evaluation without other clinical indications. Sample ECG tracings of common training-related ECG patterns are shown in Fig. 2.4. ECG findings in yellow are classified as borderline ECG changes – included in this category are axis deviation, atrial enlargement, and complete RBBB. These findings in isolation do not warrant further evaluation, but two or more borderline findings would change the ECG classification to abnormal. ECG findings in red are classified as abnormal and are findings not known to be connected to athletic remodeling. Further evaluation is recommended for ECG findings in this category. The precise definitions used for each abnormal ECG finding are shown in Table 2.3. Sample tracings representing ECG patterns in this category are shown in Fig. 2.5.

An additional component of the International Recommendations that helped to further distinguish it from prior athlete ECG criteria sets was the placement of

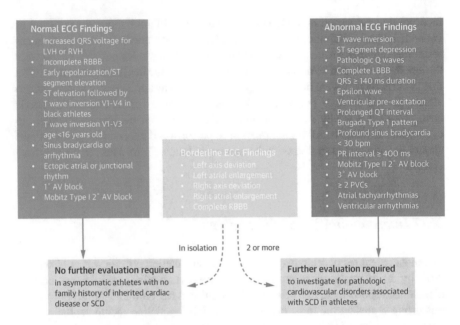

Fig. 2.3 Flowchart for ECG interpretation using the International Recommendations. (Reprinted with permission from Sharma et al. [27], Elsevier)

greater emphasis on the recognition of abnormal TWI. While there are patterns of TWI that have been demonstrated to be relatively common in athletes and not associated with underlying cardiac pathology, including TWI confined to V1 and V2 in white athletes [64], TWI in leads V1–V3 in pediatric athletes <16 years old (juvenile TWI) [65], and TWI in V1–V4 preceded by convex ST elevation in black athletes (Fig. 2.4d) [59, 60], other patterns of TWI are not prevalent findings in athletes. TWI that involves the inferolateral leads are highly uncommon in athletes regardless of ethnicity [35, 59, 66]. Given also the fact that TWI involving the inferior and lateral leads is frequently present in HCM [33, 67, 68], the presence of inferolateral TWI in an athlete warrants further investigation. Sample tracings demonstrating abnormal inferolateral TWI are shown in Fig. 2.6.

Data generated by large-scale and longitudinal studies of athletes with inferolateral TWI helped to further shape the guideline recommendations that are included in the International Recommendations for athletes with this ECG pattern. In a database of over 12,000 Italian mixed-sports asymptomatic athletes, 0.6% had baseline abnormal TWI (the majority in the inferolateral leads) but otherwise normal cardiovascular screening exams. When these athletes were followed over a mean period of 9 years, 6% of these athletes were subsequently observed to develop a cardiomyopathy, and 7% were observed to develop other cardiac disorders [35]. In a separate study of over 6000 mixed-sports athletes in which 2.4% were detected to have abnormal TWI (83.9% involving inferior or lateral leads), 44.5% of these athletes were ultimately found to have cardiac disease [66]. In these cases of established

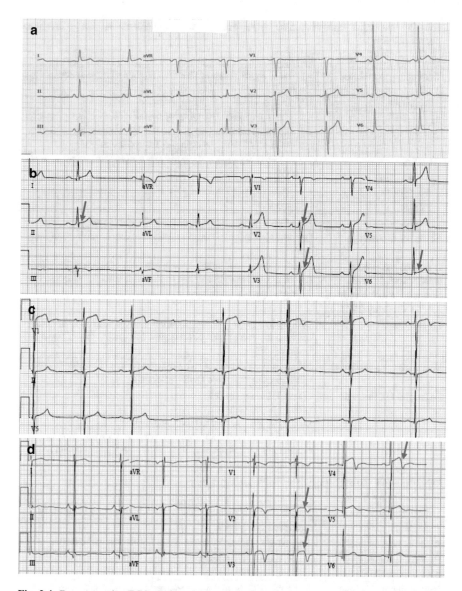

Fig. 2.4 Representative ECG tracings for common "training-related" ECG patterns. (**a**) Voltage criteria for left ventricular hypertrophy (Sokolow-Lyon criteria). (**b**) Early repolarization seen by diffuse elevation of the QRS-ST junction (J point) (blue arrows). (**c**) Sinus rhythm with type I atrioventricular block (Wenckebach). (**d**) Convex ST elevation with T wave inversion V1–V4 in a black athlete (blue arrows)

Table 2.3 Abnormal and borderline ECG findings with definitions as per international recommendations

Abnormal ECG findings	Definition
Abnormal T wave inversion (TWI)	≥1 mm in depth in two or more contiguous leads; excludes aVR, III, and V1
Anterior	V2–V4
	Excludes black athletes with J-point elevation and convex ST elevation followed by TWI in V2–V4; athletes age <16 with TWI in V1–V3; and biphasic T waves in only V3
Lateral	I and aVL, V5 *and/or* V6 (only one lead of TWI required in V5 or V6)
Inferolateral	II and aVF, V5–V6, I and aVL
Inferior	II and aVF
ST depression	≥0.5 mm in depth in two or more contiguous leads
Abnormal Q waves	Q/R ratio ≥0.25 or ≥40 ms in duration in two or more contiguous leads
Complete left bundle branch block (LBBB)	QRS ≥120 ms, predominately negative QRS complex in lead V1 (QS or rS), and upright notched or slurred R wave in leads I and V6
Nonspecific intraventricular conduction delay (IVCD)	Any QRS duration ≥140 ms
Epsilon wave	Distinct low amplitude signal (small positive deflection or notch) between the end of the QRS complex and onset of the T wave in leads V1–V3
Ventricular pre-excitation	PR interval <120 ms with a delta wave (slurred upstroke in the QRS complex and wide QRS (≥120 ms)
Prolonged QT interval	QTc ≥470 ms (female) QTc ≥480 ms (male) QTc ≥500 ms (marked QT prolongation)
Brugada type 1 pattern	Coved pattern: initial ST elevation ≥2 mm (high take-off) with downsloping ST elevation followed by a negative symmetric T wave in >1 leads in V1–V3
Profound sinus bradycardia	<30 beats/min or sinus pauses ≥3 s
Profound 1° AV block	≥400 ms
Mobitz type II 2° AV block	Intermittently non-conducted P waves with a fixed PR interval
3° AV block	Complete heart block
Atrial tachyarrhythmias	Supraventricular tachycardia, atrial fibrillation, atrial flutter
Premature ventricular contractions (PVC)	≥2 PVCs per 10 s tracing
Ventricular arrhythmias	Couplets, triplets, and non-sustained ventricular tachycardia
Borderline ECG findings	*These ECG findings in isolation do not represent pathologic cardiovascular disease in athletes, but the presence of two or more borderline findings may warrant further investigation*
Left axis deviation	−30° to −90°
Left atrial enlargement (LAE)	Prolonged P wave duration of >120 ms in leads I or II with negative portion of the P wave ≥1 mm in depth and ≥40 ms in duration in lead V1
Right axis deviation	> 120°
Right atrial enlargement	P wave ≥2.5 mm in II, III, or aVF
Complete right bundle branch block (RBBB)	rSR' pattern in lead V1 and an S wave wider than R wave in lead V6 with QRS duration >120 ms

Adapted from Sharma et al. [27]

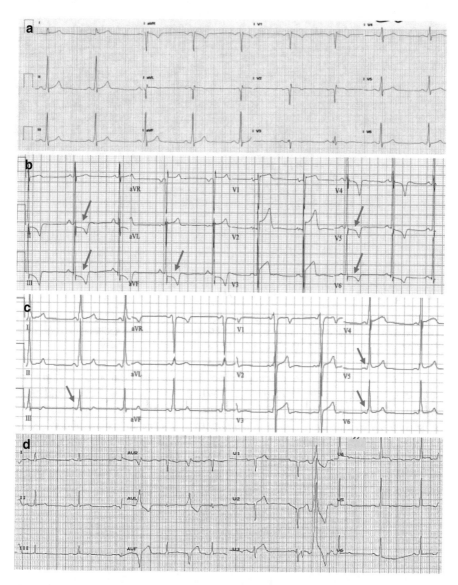

Fig. 2.5 Representative ECG tracings for abnormal ECG patterns in athletes. (**a**) Abnormal Q waves (V1–V2). (**b**) ST depressions with inferolateral T wave inversions (V5, V6, II, III, aVF) (blue arrows). (**c**) Ventricular pre-excitation (delta waves) (blue arrows). (**d**) Frequent PVCs

disease, echocardiography detected underlying cardiac pathology in 53.6% of cases. CMR, however, led to a diagnosis of cardiomyopathy in an additional 16.5% of cases in athletes where the echocardiogram interpretation was normal and an additional 30% of cases in athletes where the echocardiogram findings were suspicious [66]. In a 1-year follow-up of the athletes with abnormal TWI but normal echo and CMR, 7.2% were subsequently found to develop signs of a cardiomyopathy [66].

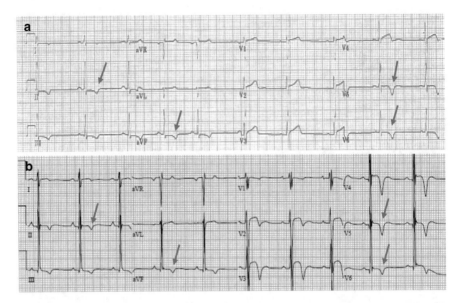

Fig. 2.6 Blue arrows demonstrate T wave inversions in the inferolateral leads. These T wave inversions are not considered training-related ECG findings and warrant additional investigation, including use of cardiac MRI with gadolineum, to exclude structural heart disease

The International Recommendations incorporated this data and highlight the importance of recognizing inferolateral TWI in athletes. The recommendations state that if echocardiography is not diagnostic, then CMR with gadolinium should be performed to further evaluate athletes with lateral or inferolateral TWI [29]. Cited advantages of CMR in this setting are that CMR can provide better delineation of myocardial hypertrophy of the LV apex if echocardiographic images are technically suboptimal and that late gadolinium enhancement, if present, could suggest myocardial fibrosis [29]. In addition, serial follow-up examinations are recommended for athletes with this ECG pattern [29].

Conclusions

Debate and discussion continue to surround the issue as to whether an ECG should universally be included in pre-participation screening examinations of asymptomatic athletes. Powerful arguments for and against the standard inclusion of an ECG are currently advanced by leading medical organizations throughout the world. At the present time, most organizations, including those in the USA, do not recommend adding an ECG to the screening process of asymptomatic athletes. While there is not universal agreement regarding policy, a consistent guideline recommendation is that if healthcare systems are to include an ECG as part of the standard pre-participation exam, then detailed protocols should be in place to efficiently manage the downstream testing that will inevitably occur. Additionally, ECG interpretation should be performed by sports cardiologists or other healthcare providers with expertise in the cardiac evaluation and interpretation of ECGs in athletes.

It can be challenging and remains a clinical conundrum for healthcare providers to distinguish training-related ECG changes that occur as a consequence of athletic cardiac remodeling from ECG changes that could represent underlying cardiac pathology. Significant achievements have been made to develop athlete-specific ECG interpretation criteria that improve the accuracy of ECG interpretation and lower false-positive rates. The newest International Recommendations additionally highlight important ECG patterns that have a higher probability of portending cardiac disease. Further refinements of these ECG criteria, however, are needed. Given that varied hemodynamic demands of different sports variably affect training-related cardiac structural adaptation and ECG change, more sports-specific ECG standards are required. A "one size fits all" approach to ECG interpretation may not be the best approach. As highlighted by the American College of Cardiology Sports and Exercise Physiology Think Tank [69], the generation of more sport-specific normative cardiac data is needed to allow for more accurate interpretation of test results in athletes and to help further refine best practices to promote athlete health and safety. Similarly, the optimal strategy for the use of the ECG in athlete screening may not be to apply a uniform approach across all athlete groups, but to integrate athlete-specific and sport-specific data to serve the best interests of the athlete.

References

1. Maron BJ, Thompson PD, Ackerman MJ, et al. Recommendations and considerations related to preparticipation screening for cardiovascular disorders in competitive athletes: 2007 update: a scientific statement from the American Heart Association Council on Nutrition, Physical Activity, and Metabolism. Circulation. 2007;115:1643–55.
2. Mont L, Pellicia A, Sharma S, et al. Preparticipation cardiovascular evaluation for athletic participants to prevent sudden death: position paper from the EHRA and the EACPR, branches of the ESC. Endorsed by APHRS, HRS, and SOLACE. Europace. 2017;19:139–63.
3. Hainline B, Drezner JA, Baggish A, et al. Interassociation consensus statement on cardiovascular care of college student-athletes. J Am Coll Cardiol. 2016;67:2981–95.
4. Johri AM, Poirier P, Dorian P, et al. Canadian Cardiovascular Society/Canadian Heart Rhythm Society Joint Position Statement on the cardiovascular screening of competitive athletes. Can J Cardiol. 2019;35:1–11.
5. Maron BJ, Friedman RA, Kligfield P, et al. Assessment of the 12-lead ECG as a screening test for detection of cardiovascular disease in healthy general populations of young people (12–25 years of age): a scientific statement from the American Heart Association and the American College of Cardiology. Circulation. 2014;130:1303–34.
6. Asif IM, Drezner JA. Cardiovascular screening in young athletes: evidence for the electrocardiogram. Curr Sports Med Rep. 2016;15:76–80.
7. Myerburg RJ, Vetter VL. Electrocardiograms should be included in preparticipation screening of athletes. Circulation. 2007;116:2616–26.
8. Corrado D, Basso C, Schiavon M, Thiene G. Screening for hypertrophic cardiomyopathy in young athletes. N Engl J Med. 1998;339(6):364–9.

9. Baggish AL, Hutter AM, Wang F, et al. Cardiovascular screening in college athletes with and without electrocardiography: a cross-sectional study. Ann Intern Med. 2010;152:269–75.
10. Corrado D, Basso C, Schiavon M, et al. Pre-participation screening of young competitive athletes for prevention of sudden cardiac death. J Am Coll Cardiol. 2008;52:1981–9.
11. Decree of the Italian Ministry of Health, February 18, 1982. Norme per la tutela sanitaria dell'attività sportiva agonistica [rules concerning the medical protection of athletic activity]. Gazzetta Ufficiale della Repubblica Italiana. March 5, 1982:63. Accessed 8 Feb 2019.
12. Corrodo D, Basso C, Pavel A, et al. Trends in cardiovascular death in young competitive athletes after implementation of a preparticipation screening program. JAMA. 2006;296:1593–601.
13. Israel Ministry of Health Athlete pre-participation medical screening guidelines. Ministry of Health website. Available at: http://www.health.gov.il. Accessed 15 Feb 2019.
14. Steinvil A, Chundadze T, Zeltser D, et al. Mandatory electrocardiographic screening of athletes to reduce their risk for sudden death. Proven fact or wishful thinking? J Am Coll Cardiol. 2011;57:1291–6.
15. Maron BJ, Haas TS, Doerer JJ, et al. Comparison of U.S. and Italian experiences with sudden cardiac deaths in young competitive athletes and implications for preparticipation screening strategies. Am J Cardiol. 2009;104:276–80.
16. Ryan MP, Cleland JG, French JA, et al. The standard electrocardiogram as a screening test for hypertrophic cardiomyopathy. Am J Cardiol. 1995;76:689–94.
17. Maron BJ, Mathenge R, Casey SA, Poliac LC, Longe TF. Clinical profile of hypertrophic cardiomyopathy identified de novo in rural communities. J Am Coll Cardiol. 1999;33:1590–5.
18. Pellicia A, DiPaolo FM, Corrado D, Buccolieri C, et al. Evidence for efficacy of the Italian national pre-participation screening programme for identification of hypertrophic cardiomyopathy in competitive athletes. Eur Heart J. 2006;27:2196–200.
19. Maron BJ. Hypertrophic cardiomyopathy: a systematic review. JAMA. 2002;287:1308–20.
20. Marcus FI. Prevalence of T-wave inversion beyond V1 in young normal individuals and usefulness for the diagnosis of arrhythmogenic right ventricular cardiomyopathy/dysplasia. Am J Cardiol. 2005;95:1070–1.
21. Marcus FI. Electrocardiographic features of inherited diseases that predispose to the development of cardiac arrhythmias, long QT syndrome, arrhythmogenic right ventricular cardiomyopathy/dysplasia, and Brugada syndrome. J Electrocardiol. 2000;33(Suppl):1–10.
22. Gemavel C, Pellicia A, Thompson PD. Arrhythmogenic right ventricular cardiomyopathy. J Am Coll Cardiol. 2001;38:1773–81.
23. Price DE, McWilliams A, Asif IM, et al. Electrocardiography-inclusive screening strategies for detection of cardiovascular abnormalities in high school athletes. Heart Rhythm. 2014;11:442–9.
24. Williams EA, Pelto HF, Toresdahl BG, et al. Performance of the American Heart Association (AHA) 14-point evaluation versus electrocardiography for the cardiovascular screening of high school athletes: a prospective study. J Am Heart Assoc. 2019;8:e012235.
25. Le VV, Wheeler MT, Mandic S, et al. Addition of the electrocardiogram to the preparticipation examination of college athletes. Clin J Sport Med. 2010;20:98–105.
26. Harmon KG, Suchsland MZ, Prutkin JM, Petek BJ, Malik A, Drezner JA. Comparison of cardiovascular screening in college athletes by history and physical examination with and without an electrocardiogram: efficacy and cost. Heart Rhythm. 2020;S1547–5271(20):30406–9.
27. Drezner JA, Owens DS, Prutkin JM, et al. Electrocardiographic screening in National Collegiate Athletic Association athletes. Am J Cardiol. 2016;118:754–9.
28. Harmon KG, Zigman M, Drezner JA. The effectiveness of screening history, physical exam and ECG to detect potentially lethal cardiac disorders in athletes: a systematic review/meta-analysis. J Electrocardiol. 2015;48:329–38.
29. Sharma S, Drezner JA, Baggish A, et al. International recommendations for electrocardiographic interpretation in athletes. J Am Coll Cardiol. 2017;69:1057–75.
30. McClean G, Riding NR, Pieles G, et al. Diagnostic accuracy and Bayesian analysis of new international ECG recommendations in paediatric athletes. Heart. 2019;105:152–9.

31. Beale AL, Julliard MV, Maziarski P, Zittener JL, Burri H, Meyer P. Electrocardiographic findings in elite professional cyclists: the 2017 international recommendations in practice. J Sci Med Sport. 2019;22:380–4.
32. Waase MP, Mutharasan RK, Whang W, et al. Electrocardiographic findings in National Baskebtall Association athletes. JAMA Cardiol. 2018;3:69–74.
33. Rowin EJ, Baron BJ, Appelbaum E, et al. Significance of false negative electrocardiograms in preparticipation screening of athletes for hypertrophic cardiomyopathy. Am J Cardiol. 2012;110:1027–32.
34. Zaidi A, Sheikh N, Jongman JK, et al. Clinical differentiation between physiological remodeling and arrhythmogenic right ventricular cardiomyopathy in athletes with marked repolarization abnormalities. J Am Coll Cardiol. 2015;65:2702–11.
35. Pellicia A, Di Paolo FM, Quattrini FM, et al. Outcomes in athletes with marked ECG repolarization abnormalities. N Engl J Med. 2008;358:152–61.
36. Maron BJ. Clinical course and management of hypertrophic cardiomyopathy. N Engl J Med. 2018;379:655–68.
37. Herman MV, Ingram DA, Levy JA, et al. Variability of electrocardiographic precordial lead placement: a method to improve accuracy and reliability. Clin Cardiol. 1991;14:469–76.
38. Wenger W, Kligfield P. Variability of precordial electrode placement during routine electrocardiography. J Electrocardiol. 1996;29:179–84.
39. Angeli F, Verdecchia P, Angeli E, et al. Day-to-day variability of electrocardiographic diagnosis of left ventricular hypertrophy in hypertensive patients: influence of electrode placement. J Cardiovasc Med. 2006;7:812–6.
40. Hill AC, Miyake CY, Grady S, Dubin AM. Accuracy of interpretation of preparticipation screening electrocardiograms. J Pediatr. 2011;159:783–8.
41. Viskin S, Rosovski U, Sands AJ, et al. Inaccurate electrocardiographic interpretation of long QT: the majority of physicians cannot recognize a long QT when they see one. Heart Rhythm. 2005;2:569–74.
42. Berte B, Duytschaever M, Elices J, et al. Variability in interpretation of the electrocardiogram in young athletes: an unrecognized obstacle for electrocardiogram-based screening protocols. Europace. 2015;17:1435–40.
43. Lampert R. ECG screening in athletes: differing views from two sides of the Atlantic. Heart. 2018;104:1037–43.
44. Maron BJ, Doerer JJ, Tierney DM, Mueller FO. Sudden deaths in young competitive athletes: analysis of 1866 deaths in the United States, 1980–2006. Circulation. 2009;119:1085–92.
45. Maron BJ, Haas TS, Murphy CJ, Ahluwalia A, Rutten-Ramos S. Incidence and causes of sudden death in U.S. college athletes. J Am Coll Cardiol. 2014;63:1636–43.
46. Maron BJ, Levine BD, Washington RL, Baggish AL, Kovacs RJ, Marson MS. Eligibility and disqualification recommendations for competitive athletes with cardiovascular abnormalities: task force 2: preparticipation screening for cardiovascular disease in competitive athletes. A scientific statement from the American Heart Association and American College of Cardiology. Circulation. 2015;132:e267–72.
47. Ljungqvist A, Jenoure P, Engebretsen L, et al. The International Olympic Committee (IOC) consensus statement on periodic health evaluation of elite athletes March 2009. Br J Sports Med. 2009;43:631–43.
48. Drezner JA, O'Connor FG, Harmon KG, et al. AMSSM Position statement on cardiovascular preparticipation screening in athletes: current evidence, knowledge gaps, recommendations, and future directions. Clin J Sport Med. 2016;26:347–61.
49. Pelliccia A, Maron BJ, Spataro A, Proschan MA, Spirito P. The upper limit of physiologic cardiac hypertrophy in highly trained elite athletes. N Engl J Med. 1991;324:295–301.
50. Bekaert I, Pannier JL, Van De Weghe C, Van Durme JP, Clement DL, Pannier R. Non-invasive evaluation of cardiac function in professional cyclists. Br Heart J. 1981;45:213–8.
51. Engel DJ, Schwartz A, Homma S. Athletic cardiac remodeling in US professional basketball players. JAMA Cardiol. 2016;1:80–7.

52. Pellicia A, Maron BJ, Culasso F, et al. Clinical significance of abnormal electrocardiographic patterns in trained athletes. Circulation. 2000;102:278–84.
53. Sharma S, Whyte G, Padula M, Kaushal R, Mahon N, McKenna W. Electrocardiographic changes in 1000 highly trained junior athletes. Br J Sports Med. 1999;33:319–24.
54. Corrodo D, Pellicia A, Bjornstad HH, et al. Cardiovascular preparticipation screening of young competitive athletes for prevention of sudden death: proposal for a common European protocol. Consensus statement of the study group of sport cardiology of the working group of cardiac rehabilitation and exercise physiology and the working group of myocardial and pericardial diseases of the European Society of Cardiology. Eur Heart J. 2005;26:516–24.
55. Corrodo D, Pellicia A, Heidbuchel H, et al. Recommendations for interpretation of 12-lead electrocardiogram in the athlete. Eur Heart J. 2010;31:243–59.
56. Weiner RB, Hutter AM, Wang F, et al. Performance of the 2010 European Society of Cardiology criteria for ECG interpretation in athletes. Heart. 2011;97:1573–7.
57. Sharma S, Ghani S, Papadakis M. ESC criteria for ECG interpretation: better but not perfect. Heart. 2011;97:1540–1.
58. Magalski A, Maron BJ, Main ML, et al. Relation of race to electrocardiographic patterns in elite American football players. J Am Coll Cardiol. 2008;51:2250–5.
59. Papadakis M, Carre F, Kervio G, et al. The prevalence, distribution, and clinical outcomes of electrocardiographic repolarization patterns in male athletes of African/Afro-Caribbean origin. Eur Heart J. 2011;32:2304–13.
60. Drezner JA, Ackerman MJ, Anderson J, et al. Electrocardiographic interpretation in athletes: the 'Seattle Criteria'. Br J Sports Med. 2013;47:122–4.
61. Gati S, Sheikh N, Ghani S, et al. Should axis deviation or atrial enlargement be categorized as abnormal in young athletes? The athlete's electrocardiogram: time for re-appraisal of markers of pathology. Eur Heart J. 2013;34:3641–8.
62. Sheikh N, Papadakis M, Ghani S, et al. Comparison of electrocardiographic criteria for the detection of cardiac abnormalities in elite black and white athletes. Circulation. 2014;129:1637–49.
63. Kim JH, Baggish AL. Electrocardiographic right and left bundle branch block patterns in athletes: prevalence, pathology, and clinical significance. J Electrocardiol. 2015;48:380–4.
64. Malhotra A, Dhutia H, Gati S, et al. Anterior T-wave inversion in young white athletes and nonathletes. Prevalence and significance. J Am Coll Cardiol. 2017;69:1–9.
65. Migliore F, Zorzi A, Michieli P, et al. Prevalence of cardiomyopathy in Italian asymptomatic children with electrocardiographic T-wave inversion at preparticipation screening. Circulation. 2012;125:529–38.
66. Schnell F, Riding N, O'Hanlon R, et al. Recognition and significance of pathological T-wave inversions in athletes. Circulation. 2015;131:165–73.
67. Sheikh N, Papadakis M, Schnell F, et al. Clinical profile of athletes with hypertrophic cardiomyopathy. Circ Cardiovasc Imaging. 2015;8:e003454.
68. Bent RE, Wheeler MT, Hadley D, et al. Systematic comparison of digital electrocardiograms from healthy athletes and patients with hypertrophic cardiomyopathy. J Am Coll Cardiol. 2015;65:2462–3.
69. Lawless CE, Asplund C, Asif IM, et al. Protecting the heart of the American athlete: proceedings of the American College of Cardiology Sports and Exercise Cardiology Think Tank October 18, 2012, Washington, DC. J Am Coll Cardiol. 2014;64:2146–71.
70. Basu J, Malhotra A. Interpreting the athlete's ECG: current state and future prospectives. Curr Treat Options Cardiovasc Med. 2018;20:104–14.

Chapter 3
Diagnostic Approach after Initial Abnormal Screening

Matthew W. Martinez

Introduction

Presentations of athletes with potential cardiac issues can vary considerably. Athletes can be asymptomatic but have concerning findings identified during routine or required pre-participation screening, or they may present with symptoms ranging from mild to severe. Rarely, an athlete may present to the health system with exercise-related cardiac arrest. Determining which athlete should undergo a targeted diagnostic assessment can be a clinical challenge when an athlete is asymptomatic or if signs or symptoms on an initial screening exam are nonspecific.

The cardiac evaluation of an athlete begins with a history and physical examination and sometimes includes a 12-lead electrocardiogram (ECG), depending upon local or organizational policies and practices. An understanding of symptoms and physical exam findings that warrant further evaluation, plus knowledge of expected and abnormal ECG findings in athletes, is essential to determine when, and if, further and more detailed downstream cardiac testing is required. When imaging beyond an ECG is indicated and requested, this downstream testing can encompass numerous cardiac tests and visits to subspecialists that have the potential to incur significant cost, time, anxiety, and continued uncertainty. Physicians who are responsible for ordering and interpreting these cardiac studies in athletes must first and foremost be familiar with the cardiac physiology of athletes to help optimize plans for downstream testing.

Adaptive changes in cardiac structure and function occur in response to regular physical training, and these manifestations of athletic remodeling are commonly encountered during the evaluation of athletes. A strong linear relationship exists

M. W. Martinez (✉)
Director of Sports Cardiology, Morristown Medical Center, Atlantic Health System, Morristown, NJ, USA
e-mail: matthew.martinez@atlantichealth.org

© Springer Nature Switzerland AG 2021
D. J. Engel, D. M. Phelan (eds.), *Sports Cardiology*,
https://doi.org/10.1007/978-3-030-69384-8_3

between the amount of training performed and resultant changes in cardiac dimensions [1]. Exercise-induced cardiac remodeling (EICR) is the term used to characterize the process by which the heart and vasculature change as a physiologic response to repetitive exercise [2]. Important determinants of the magnitude and geometry of EICR in an individual athlete include gender and ethnicity, genetics, duration of exercise exposure, as well as the hemodynamic attributes of the athlete's sport and training [3–5]. Not all athletes will develop EICR in the same way, and data as to what degree cardiac adaptations differ across the spectrum of sporting disciplines, gender and ethnicity, and individual training regimens is still emerging [6–10].

EICR commonly leads to imaging findings that overlap with similar appearing features of certain heart muscle diseases that are known to be associated with adverse cardiovascular risk. This observed overlap between EICR and pathology is referred to as the "gray zone." The most important task for providers who request, obtain, and interpret cardiac imaging studies in athletes is to try and differentiate EICR from potential underlying pathology [11, 12]. This process requires a comprehensive understanding of EICR fundamentals (a detailed discussion of EICR can be found in Chap. 8) as well as a recognition of cardiac findings that may be outside of the boundaries of EICR and suggestive of pathology.

Overview of Downstream Testing

Fundamental downstream tests commonly requested and used in the cardiac evaluation of highly active individuals and competitive athletes include transthoracic echocardiograms (TTE), cardiac magnetic resonance imaging (CMR), coronary computed tomography angiography (CCTA), and stress testing. An evaluation may include one or more imaging tests to evaluate valve disease, myocardial structure and function, or the aortic origins of coronary artery ostia. There is not a single imaging modality or algorithm for athlete assessment that will ever fit all scenarios. Most first-line evaluations will include a TTE. TTE can measure and characterize myocardial structure, systolic and diastolic function, valve morphology and function, and proximal coronary anatomy with sufficient accuracy to confirm or exclude the presence of clinically relevant disease in the majority of athletes. TTE has been the primary imaging method used in the study of EICR and in the establishment of normative EICR data in varied athlete groups. This growing reference TTE data helps for the distinction between EICR and pathology. Limitations of TTE imaging include occasional suboptimal visualization of the cardiac chambers due to thoracic rib acoustic shadowing, thereby preventing adequate determination of cardiac morphology and function. In addition, measurement errors due to difficulty in differentiating RV trabecular tissue from the left ventricular portion of the interventricular septum can result in inaccurate diagnoses.

In cases where TTE imaging is suboptimal, CMR has emerged as the reference standard for defining myocardial structure and myocardial tissue characterization and is increasingly utilized in the assessment of athletes [13]. CMR allows for definitive assessment of myocardial function, valve morphology and function, coronary artery origin, and anatomy of the great vessels. CMR examination can delineate the presence, severity, and symmetry of ventricular hypertrophy and/or dilation and assess ventricular tissue architecture using qualitative and quantitative assessments of myocardial fibrosis, tissue edema, and inflammation. Limitations of CMR include the cost, availability, and time required to obtain the test. In addition, CMR remains highly technical, and there is variability in the performance and interpretation of these studies across centers. At the present time, there is little reference CMR data for athletes.

The role of cardiac CT is less well established in the athlete but plays an important role in specific clinical situations. CT requires a very short image acquisition time to provide three-dimensional images with a high level of spatial resolution including cardiac motion if necessary. These features provide superb assessment of coronary artery anatomy and vessel course. In addition, CCTA can provide accurate assessment of the aortic origins of the coronary ostia, the presence of coronary artery atherosclerosis, and degree of stenosis, along with characterization of great vessel morphology.

Cardiovascular specialists familiar with EICR data and the strengths and weaknesses of the individual tests in the armamentarium of available downstream tests are well positioned to provide effective care for athletes as they can integrate and interpret multimodality diagnostic imaging as required on an individual case-by-case basis. Communication between the referring team and the imaging team to develop a plan prior to testing is vital. This collaboration will optimize testing protocols and reduce the need for unnecessary testing or a delay in determining risk.

This remainder of this chapter will focus on and outline how to best utilize multimodality imaging for the assessment of athletes who may present for an evaluation after a pre-participation screening exam, for athletes with new or evolving symptoms, for asymptomatic older athletes, and for younger athletes with congenital heart disease. A summary of these recommendations can be found in the accompanying Table 3.1.

Use of Downstream Testing Following an ECG

When to Avoid Downstream Testing

Athletes without symptoms and that have expected ECG features associated with athletic training do not generally require any additional investigations. Examples include sinus bradycardia, first-degree atrioventricular (AV) block, Mobitz type I second-degree AV block (Wenckebach), ectopic atrial arrhythmia, and sinus arrhythmia [14]. These commonly encountered findings are classified as training-related ECG findings and result from physiologic adaptations that typically do not warrant

Table 3.1 Important cardiac conditions and presenting signs/symptoms in athletes with recommended downstream testing approach

Suspected disease or clinical finding	First-line imaging	Additional imaging as needed
Hypertrophic cardiomyopathy	TTE and CMR	Ambulatory ECG, stress imaging
Arrhythmogenic ventricular cardiomyopathy	TTE and CMR	Ambulatory ECG
Familial/idiopathic dilated cardiomyopathy	TTE and CMR	
Left ventricular non-compaction cardiomyopathy	TTE and CMR	Stress imaging
Toxic cardiomyopathy (alcohol, illicit anabolic steroids, etc.)	TTE and CMR	
Myocarditis	TTE and CMR	Stress imaging, Ambulatory ECG
Complex congenital heart disease	TTE	CMR and CT, Stress imaging
Disorders of cardiac conduction		
Ventricular pre-excitation/Wolff-Parkinson-White syndrome	TTE and stress imaging	Ambulatory ECG, CMR or CTA
Congenital long-QT syndrome	Stress imaging	Ambulatory ECG
Catecholaminergic polymorphic ventricular tachycardia	Stress imaging	Ambulatory ECG
Idiopathic ventricular tachycardia	Stress imaging	Ambulatory ECG
Disorders of coronary circulation		
Congenital anomalies of coronary arterial origin and course	CTA or CMR or TTE	Exercise stress testing
Acquired atherosclerotic disease	TTE	Stress imaging or CMR
Disorders of the heart valves		
Bicuspid aortic valve (with stenosis +/− aortopathy)	TTE	CMR or CTA
Pulmonic stenosis (with ≥ moderate stenosis)	TTE	
Mitral valve prolapse (with corollary arrhythmogenicity)	TTE	Ambulatory ECG
Disorders of the aorta		
Bicuspid aortic valve aortopathy	CTA or CMR or TTE	
Familial aortopathy/TAA/Idiopathic aortopathy	CTA or CMR or TTE	
Marfan syndrome/Loeys-Dietz syndrome/ Ehlers-Danlos vascular type (IV)	CTA or CMR or TTE	
Symptoms or signs		
Murmur	TTE	CMR
Exertional chest pain/pressure or breathlessness	TTE and stress imaging	
Syncope	TTE	CMR
Loss of power	TTE and stress imaging	
Bradycardia	ECG	TTE

CMR cardiac magnetic resonance imaging, *CTA* computed tomographic angiography, *ECG* electrocardiogram, *TAA* thoracic aortic aneurysm, *TTE* transthoracic echocardiography additional testing. In my experience, in the absence of symptoms, a formal exercise test is not needed for the above-described findings, but rather physical activity can be performed on the spot (i.e., walking stairs or in the hallway), even while in the office setting, for reassurance and to ensure an appropriate rate and rhythm response to exertion. After the limited exertion, a repeat "resting" ECG can be performed to confirm and document the return of normal sinus node activity. In rare instances, such as in those athletes with potential symptoms that could be correlated with the ECG findings, a standard treadmill ECG stress test can be performed to document appropriate sinus and AV node function.

When Downstream Testing Is Optional

Electrocardiographic changes may fall in the "gray zone" and be considered border-line abnormal in the context of surrounding clinical circumstances. Currently classified borderline ECG abnormalities, as described by the international ECG criteria for athletes [15], include left or right axis deviation, left or right atrial enlargement, and complete RBBB. These findings are considered probable normal variants in athletes in most cases. In this regard, an isolated borderline athletic ECG finding, with or without other expected training-related ECG patterns, does not typically warrant additional testing in an asymptomatic athlete. In contrast, identification of two or more borderline ECG findings on an ECG tracing would move the athlete into the abnormal category, prompting imaging with a TTE for myocardial structure and function assessment. If the TTE is inconclusive for exclusion of underlying cardiac pathology, then CMR would be the next best subsequent study to assess for underlying structural heart disease.

Left Ventricular Hypertrophy Voltage Criteria

Athletes often meet criteria for left ventricular hypertrophy (LVH) using accepted QRS voltage criteria [16–21]. Isolated increased QRS voltage that fulfils voltage criteria for LVH in the absence of other ECG or clinical markers suggestive of pathology is expected physiologic ECG changes and usually do not require further evaluation. Pathological LVH should be suspected when QRS voltage criteria are associated with ECG features such as T wave inversions (TWI) involving the inferior and/or lateral leads, ST segment depression, or abnormal Q waves [22, 23]. LVH in conjunction with these findings should raise suspicion for an underlying cardiomyopathy and warrants downstream imaging with TTE for myocardial structure and function assessment. If the TTE is abnormal or inconclusive for exclusion of LV and/or RV pathology, CMR should be performed as a subsequent study.

When Downstream Testing Is Required

Electrocardiographic changes may fall in the abnormal category as classified by the international ECG criteria for athletes [15]. Abnormal ECG findings such as TWI (anterior, inferior, or lateral), ST segment depression, pathologic Q waves, and left bundle branch block (LBBB) are all recognized ECG findings that can be present in hereditary cardiomyopathic disorders and ischemic heart disease. The ECG patterns of primary electrical diseases such as ventricular pre-excitation, long QT syndrome (LQTS), and Brugada syndrome are also classified as abnormal ECG findings per the international criteria [15]. None of these abovementioned abnormal ECG findings are considered to represent physiologic athletic adaptation or features of athletic training and, in general, always require downstream testing to exclude the presence of intrinsic cardiac disease.

T Wave Inversions (TWI)

Negatively deflected T waves are referred to as TWI and are commonly encountered in patients with cardiomyopathy and may be found in athletes without overt pathology [24]. TWI ≥ 1 mm in depth in two or more contiguous leads (excluding leads aVR, III, and V1) in the anterior, lateral, inferolateral, or inferior leads should alert for the possible presence of an underlying cardiac disorder and warrants further assessment in most cases.

Anterior TWI is a normal variant in asymptomatic adolescent athletes aged <16 years (V1–V3) and in black athletes (V1–V4) when preceded by J-point elevation and convex ST segment elevation [25]. In a study of 80 athletes of mixed ethnicity, TWI up to lead V4 with J-point elevation ≥ 1 mm excluded LV/RV cardiomyopathy with 100% negative predictive value, regardless of ethnicity [25]. Anterior TWI extending to lead V3 has also been reported in a proportion (14.3%) of healthy white adult endurance athletes [14]. Malhotra et al., however, examined 14,646 young white individuals, 20% of which were athletes, and found that anterior TWI beyond V2 was present in only 1.2% of women and 0.2% of men [26]. Based on available data regarding anterior TWI, it appears justifiable to consider investigation of asymptomatic athletes with anterior TWI beyond V2 (without preceding J-point elevation) with downstream testing [26].

Lateral or inferolateral lead TWI, in any athlete, may be associated with the presence of quiescent cardiomyopathy [18, 27–29]. TWI in this distribution has been associated with both LV and RV forms of structural heart disease including hypertrophic cardiomyopathy (HCM), arrhythmogenic right ventricular cardiomyopathy (ARVC), dilated cardiomyopathy (DCM), isolated left ventricular non-compaction, and acute or resolving myocarditis. For example, in a study comparing 1124 athletes with 255 patients with HCM, TWI in V4–V6 was present in <1% of athletes compared with 38% in patients with HCM [30]. For those athletes with lateral or inferolateral TWI where there could be suspicion for HCM or ARVC, TTE is the first-line imaging test for evaluation. TTE quality, however, is variable and may not provide adequate assessment of the LV apex, inferior septum, anterior lateral wall, or the right ventricle [31]. Thus, a multimodality approach is suggested utilizing both TTE and CMR [17, 25, 32–38]. Contrast-enhanced CMR provides superior assessment of LV regional and global myocardial hypertrophy, as well as RV structure, while also evaluating for edema and fibrosis/scarring. CMR should be a standard component of the assessment for abnormal TWI involving the lateral and inferior leads [30, 39]. If CMR is not available, echocardiography with contrast should be considered as an alternative investigation for apical HCM [33].

Further assessment beyond CMR for lateral and inferolateral TWI is often indicated due to the complex relationship between underlying disease and athletics. An exercise treadmill test, ambulatory rhythm monitoring, and signal-averaged ECG should be considered. In those cases where a diagnosis is unclear despite imaging, such as with mild hypertrophy (LV wall thickness 13–15 mm) without fibrosis or a dilated RV in which a pathologic diagnosis remains uncertain, these additional evaluations can be especially helpful. In such cases, the presence of ventricular tachycardia during exercise or ambulatory ECG monitoring may support a pathological diagnosis and is useful in risk stratification [40].

Isolated inferior lead TWI without ST segment depression (II, III, and aVF) has not been studied in detail. To date, TWI confined to the inferior leads without ST segment depression has not been found to be a strong predictor of pathologic myocardial disease in the absence of clinical concerns or other abnormal ECG features. In my experience, abnormal results in downstream testing are rare in the presence of isolated inferior TWI without ST depression. However, isolated inferior TWI cannot be definitively attributed to athletic physiological changes at this time and thus warrants further investigation until studies prove otherwise. CMR should be considered based on the echocardiographic findings or clinical suspicion but is often not required.

Continued surveillance is required for those with TWI. Regular follow-up with serial cardiac imaging is necessary even when the initial evaluation does not yield pathology, in order to monitor for the potential development of a cardiomyopathic phenotypic expression.

ST Segment Depression

ST segment depression is common in cardiomyopathy and is not an ECG feature of athletic training. ST segment depression of ≥ 0.5 mm in depth in two or more leads has a prevalence of approximately 67% in patients with HCM, has been associated with the risk of sudden cardiac arrest, and should be considered an abnormal finding on an athlete's ECG [18, 23, 30, 41–44]. Given the strong association with cardiomyopathy, TTE is the minimum downstream evaluation required for athletes with ST segment depression. CMR should be considered based on the echocardiographic findings or if there is a high clinical suspicion for pathology.

Pathologic Q Waves

Pathologic Q waves (Q/R ratio $\geq$ 0.25 or 40 ms in duration in two or more leads excluding III and aVR) [15] are not a physiologic adaptation expected in athletes and require investigation by TTE. If pathologic Q waves are present along with other ECG abnormalities, such as ST segment depression or TWI, or if concerning clinical findings are present, CMR should be considered. In athletes $\geq$30 years old, especially in the presence of risk factors for coronary artery disease (CAD), assessment for CAD with stress testing or CCTA is suggested. If the TTE is normal and there are no other concerning clinical findings or additional ECG abnormalities, no additional testing may be necessary. Additionally, any ECG with abnormal Q waves should be carefully examined for the possibility of a bypass tract, looking for a short PR interval or evidence of a delta wave.

Wolff-Parkinson-White (WPW) ECG Pattern

A short PR interval associated with a delta wave without a history of arrhythmia is consistent with the WPW pattern [45]. The finding of the WPW, or pre-excitation, and ECG pattern is relatively common, and not all those with a WPW pattern will be symptomatic or need intervention. WPW pattern often occurs in structurally normal hearts but may be associated with Ebstein's anomaly or other forms of cardiomyopathy; therefore TTE is indicated. A short PR interval may be identified in isolation without a widened QRS or delta wave in an asymptomatic athlete. This scenario does not represent WPW pattern or require further assessment. WPW syndrome is when the ECG pattern is accompanied by symptoms associated with tachyarrhythmias.

   With or without symptoms, further assessment of the refractory period of the accessory pathway is warranted in athletes. Non-invasive risk stratification for WPW begins with an exercise stress test in which abrupt, complete loss of pre-excitation at higher heart rates suggests a low-risk accessory pathway [46, 47]. If non-invasive testing cannot confirm a low-risk pathway, or is inconclusive, then electrophysiology testing should be considered to determine the shortest pre-excited RR interval [46]. The finding of a pre-excited RR interval that is $\leq$250 ms (240 bpm) classifies the accessory pathway as high-risk and shared decision-making should occur regarding pursuit of pathway ablation [45, 46]. Some have advocated that all competitive athletes with a WPW ECG pattern should be evaluated by an electrophysiological study. Ambulatory monitors may provide more data to determine whether an athlete has occult arrhythmias. Clinicians should be mindful of the risks of an invasive procedure with or without ablation [48]. In my practice, I do not routinely perform electrophysiological evaluation or ablation for the incidental findings of a WPW ECG pattern.

Complete Left Bundle Branch Block (LBBB)

LBBB is common in patients with cardiomyopathy and ischemic heart disease but a rare finding in athletes without structural disease [23, 30, 49–51]. LBBB should always be considered abnormal until proven otherwise and requires a comprehensive evaluation. A complete investigation should include both TTE and CMR to exclude pathology. In patients older than 30 years old, an ischemic workup to exclude CAD is appropriate. Specific patient characteristics, clinical suspicion, and institutional expertise are factors to determine whether a nuclear perfusion scan, stress echocardiogram, or coronary artery assessment (invasive angiography or CCTA) should be employed.

Epsilon Waves

Epsilon waves are associated with ARVC [52]. An epsilon wave is unlikely to be present in isolation without other ECG abnormalities and may be found in combination with right precordial TWI or delayed S wave upstroke. All those with an epsilon wave require downstream imaging with TTE and CMR [39]. A diagnosis of ARVC can be challenging, and the continuum of disease findings can vary from mild to severe. Disease progression is common and may require serial imaging for surveillance of the disease and/or disease exclusion [39, 53, 54]. If initial imaging is normal, equivocal, or only mildly abnormal, then continued surveillance is suggested, and early involvement of an expert in ARVC to facilitate evaluation and management is suggested. Additional assessment with an ambulatory ECG, exercise test, and signal-averaged ECG should be considered in an individualized basis [55].

When Continued Surveillance Is Required

ECG abnormalities often precede the development of overt structural heart disease identified by imaging in those with a genetic predisposition to cardiomyopathy [23, 28, 29]. Athletes who demonstrate one or more overtly abnormal ECG findings may therefore undergo comprehensive clinical evaluations that reveal no definitive evidence of true pathology. Athletes with markedly abnormal ECG findings, such as inferolateral TWI or ST depressions, and structurally normal hearts remain at risk for future manifestation of disease. Limited data suggests that progression to overt cardiomyopathy occurs in ~5–6% of abnormal ECGs without concurrent initial pathologic imaging findings [28, 29]. Continued longitudinal surveillance on an annual basis or more frequently based on clinician discretion is advised. Athletes with abnormal ECGs suggestive of cardiomyopathy without pathologic findings after a complete clinical evaluation, in my opinion, may participate in competitive activities without restriction. Athletes should be educated about the importance of regular follow-up and the risks of non-adherence. To that end, subsequent serial evaluations should be ongoing both during and after their competitive athletic career is completed.

Symptoms That May Warrant Downstream Testing

Many athletes present for an evaluation after a presumed cardiac "event" or newly recognized symptom. Common symptoms that warrant downstream testing include unexplained syncope and exertional symptoms such as chest discomfort/tightness or progressive, inappropriately labored breathing. Additionally, the presence of a family history of sudden cardiac death in a first-degree relative and an abnormality on physical examination such as a non-physiologic murmur, hypertension, or physical features suggestive of a genetic aortopathy necessitates downstream testing to exclude pathology [56]. Recommendations for downstream testing for specific symptoms are provided below.

Exertional Chest Discomfort

Chest discomfort is a common presenting complaint among athletes. Cardiac and non-cardiac etiologies can result in chest discomfort complaints with true cardiac etiologies accounting for only ~5% of diagnoses, but these cases can be associated with adverse outcomes [57]. Assessment begins with a detailed medical history, complete physical examination, and ECG which is often enough to identify a non-cardiac etiology without further diagnostics. In those with a suspected cardiac etiology, non-invasive imaging with TTE and stress testing is the first-line assessment with additional testing pursued in selected cases. In those athletes where there is a high suspicion of, or confirmed, LV or RV myocardial pathology, CMR is indicated after TTE due to its superior diagnostic and prognostic accuracy especially for RV assessment [39].

High fitness levels in athletes lessen the usefulness of a standardized and graded exercise test. An individualized protocol that reflects the scenario responsible for the presenting symptoms, with appropriate supplementation of imaging, is the optimal means for conducting a stress test [58]. To that end, assessments should utilize symptom-driven protocols rather than typical protocols where the test is terminated at a predetermined heart rate (i.e., 85% maximal age-gender predicted). Reproduction of symptoms may not manifest without achieving high workloads; therefore termination should be based on athlete fatigue, reproduction of athlete symptoms, or the development of high-risk findings. If utilizing stress echocardiography for ischemia assessment, the sonographer and interpreting physician should be cognizant of the rapid recovery of ischemic changes in athletes. Resolution can be brisk necessitating immediate post-exercise imaging to avoid false-negative findings. As such, stress echocardiography should be limited to centers with extensive experience and expertise performing stress echocardiography given the potential limitations of the modality. If institutional expertise affords the opportunity, CCTA may be the best first-line assessment for chest pain suspected to be related to obstructive CAD. CCTA provides an assessment of the coronary anatomy with high sensitivity for detecting CAD and excluding flow-limiting coronary artery stenosis [13].

If an anomalous coronary artery cannot be excluded using TTE, tomographic imaging either by CCTA or CMR is recommended, depending on patient characteristics and institutional expertise. CCTA is most often the imaging modality of choice to delineate coronary artery origin, vessel course (between the great vessels), and assessment of high-risk features [13].

Syncope or Near Syncope

Syncope, or transient loss of consciousness, followed by spontaneous and complete recovery is a common presenting complaint among athletes representing both pathologic and benign conditions [59, 60]. The etiology is best determined by a detailed history describing the event. Most often, syncope in athletes is attributed to neural mechanisms. Neurally mediated syncope manifests as classic "vasovagal" episodes that are unrelated to exercise or as post-exertional syncope which typically occurs within minutes of abrupt exercise termination and carries, in general, a benign prognosis [61]. A complete medical history, physical examination, and ECG should be performed in all athletes who present with syncope. This assessment is often enough to confirm a neurally mediated etiology and obviate the need for additional evaluation.

In contrast, symptoms of abrupt loss of consciousness during exercise, especially when the event is severe enough to cause musculoskeletal injury, should be attributed to underlying cardiovascular etiology necessitating additional evaluation. In these scenarios, cardiac etiologies may include obstructive valve disease, inducible myocardial ischemia, or electrical conduction disease related to acquired or congenital pathologies. Initial imaging should include TTE to investigate for the presence of obstructive valvular disease including LV/RV outflow pathology or cardiomyopathies with arrhythmic and/or ischemic predisposition and high-risk anomalous coronary anatomy. This evaluation may be enough to exclude or identify an etiology, with inconclusive findings prompting further evaluation including exercise testing and/or tomographic imaging using CT or MRI.

Palpitations and Arrhythmias

Benign ectopic arrhythmias are a common presenting symptom in athletes, and many will not require downstream testing. The assessment may be prompted by a diagnosis of "low heart rate" or after recognition of skipped beats with or without symptoms of palpitations. The evaluation of palpitations and/or arrhythmias begins with a comprehensive medical history, physical examination, and ECG. The objective is to differentiate ventricular arrhythmias from arrhythmias arising from the atria and to identify whether exercise precipitates or intensifies the symptoms. Documentation of the arrhythmia by ECG, ambulatory rhythm monitoring, or an exercise test to provoke the arrhythmia may be required. Occasionally, an implantable recorder will be necessary.

Imaging to identify or exclude myocardial abnormalities via TTE is usually employed, especially in the presence of ventricular arrhythmias. Abnormal myocardial substrate (hereditary or acquired), such as seen with ischemic disease, clinical myocarditis, congenital coronary anomalies, or pressure/volume overload changes related to valvular disease, would change the importance of any identified arrhythmia. In the absence of abnormal myocardial structure, arrhythmias may be attributable to conduction abnormalities from ventricular pre-excitation or hereditary channelopathies. The presence of ventricular pre-excitation should prompt imaging to exclude associated cardiac conditions including Ebstein's anomaly, PRKAG2 gene-mediated hypertrophic cardiomyopathy, or other congenital heart diseases [62, 63]. Primary channelopathies, such as LQTS, catecholaminergic polymorphic ventricular tachycardia (CPVT), Brugada pattern/syndrome, and idiopathic ventricular tachycardia, are typically detected without underlying structural abnormalities [64, 65]. CCTA or CMR should be the second-line assessment with use determined by clinical suspicion or to confirm pathology.

Atrial fibrillation is the most common arrhythmia encountered in elite athletes, particularly in middle-aged men [66]. The prevalence has been reported to be as high as 9% depending on the population studied [67, 68]. The pathophysiology remains unclear but is clearly multifactorial in origin and associated with sustained endurance training and increased vagal tone. Atrial ectopy and shortened atrial effective refractory period from enhanced parasympathetic activity serve as triggers [69]. Routine evaluation of atrial fibrillation in athletes should include a comprehensive history to identify medical etiologies such as thyroid dysfunction or a sleep disturbance and to assess for the use of performance-enhancing or illicit drugs, as well as alcohol. Imaging should include TTE to identify or exclude myocardial abnormalities [70]. Atrial fibrillation in an adolescent athlete should also raise the suspicion for an accessory pathway and consideration of an ambulatory monitor or serial ECGs to look for intermittent pre-excitation is appropriate.

Inappropriate Exertional Dyspnea

Breathlessness during recreational activity, athletic training, and athletic competition is common but when persistent or even progressive may represent an underlying cardiovascular disorder [71, 72]. A careful history focused on the duration and intensity of exercise is often sufficient to determine whether the perceived breathlessness is expected or disproportionate. Subjective breathlessness is typically appropriate for those at their upper limits of exercise capacity, when escalating a training regimen, with changing an exercise routine, or after prolonged deconditioning related to injury or illness. New dyspnea at a previously tolerated intensity, dyspnea that requires a reduction in exercise intensity, or dyspnea without a change in training regimen should be considered inappropriate. Attention to associated symptoms such as stridor, wheezing, chest tightness/pain syndromes, palpitations, or near syncope/syncope is helpful to determine specific downstream testing plans [73].

After a careful history and physical examination, in many young athletes, a noncardiac etiology related to reactive airway disease, exercise-induced bronchospasm, paradoxical vocal fold dysfunction, upper respiratory infection, allergic and non-allergic rhinitis, or dysfunctional breathing may be found to be the causative etiology [74]. If these diagnoses are suspected, then no cardiac imaging is required. If no subsequent diagnosis is identified or there is failure to respond to therapy, a cardiac etiology should be pursued.

Initial cardiac testing for all athletes with inappropriate or unexplained exertional dyspnea should include an ECG and TTE. Exercise testing, with or without concomitant imaging, should be performed with an aim to reproduce symptoms and exclude cardiac pathology. Gas exchange assessment, via pulmonary function testing and cardiopulmonary exercise testing, is often valuable in this scenario and is the suggested stress modality when institutional expertise allows [75]. CCTA or CMR should be reserved as second-line assessment for as dictated by suspected or confirmed pathology or if based on a high clinical suspicion.

Athletic Performance Decrement or Loss of Power

Clinical evaluation for a perceived or objective performance decrement poses a difficult diagnostic dilemma. A comprehensive history and physical should include a review of dietary intake to ensure adequate energy balance, an assessment for suboptimal sleep patterns or mood disturbance, and assessment for signs and symptoms of common organic pathologies such as endocrine disorders (i.e., thyroid, adrenal disorders, diabetes), infectious etiologies, inflammatory diseases, electrolyte deficiencies, and anemia [76]. Training in unfamiliar conditions (altitude, heat, or cold) or a significant increase in training load or change in training pattern should be determined and considered. Overtraining syndrome is common, occurring in both elite and non-elite runners, but should be considered as a diagnosis of exclusion [77]. The evaluation of this broad differential is best performed by experienced sports cardiologists and often requires multiple other specialist visits that include a sports medicine physician. A thorough medical history and physical examination can help avoid broad testing and subsequent irrelevant diagnoses. An ECG is appropriate but very low yield. The use of TTE for those with historical and physical examination or ECG findings suggestive of myocardial, coronary, or valvular pathology is typically first line. Documentation of exercise capacity and effort-utilizing cardiopulmonary exercise testing along with isch-emia assessment is often valuable and the recommended stress modality when institutional expertise allows. Stress perfusion imaging and stress echocardiogra-phy are appropriate with the caveats previously discussed in the chapter. CT and MRI should be reserved for individual situations as dictated by suspected or con-firmed pathology.

Special Populations

Athletes 40 Years and Older

Athletes 40 years and older are at a higher risk of atherosclerotic coronary disease, atrial tachyarrhythmias particularly atrial fibrillation, degenerative aortic and mitral valve disease, and hypertensive heart disease [56, 78]. Symptoms of athletes in this age group are often attributable to these conditions rather than hereditary forms of heart disease and should be thought of and sought out initially.

Athletes often have a predicted low-risk CAD profile given a relative infrequency of traditional atherosclerotic risk factors (hypertension, dyslipidemia, family his-tory of CAD, and prior/on-going tobacco use), and as a result, the use of the Framingham risk score has been shown to underestimate CAD risk in athletes [79]. Therefore, exercise stress testing and coronary artery imaging are key components to a diagnostic evaluation. In general, I recommend symptom-limited exercise test-ing in older athletes with suspected or elevated risk of CAD. As previously men-tioned, when using stress echocardiography, careful attention to immediate imaging after stress is critical due to the rapid recovery of athletes and a higher potential for false-negative results.

Non-invasive coronary artery imaging with either coronary artery calcium (CAC) scoring or CCTA may be helpful for athletes with a high suspicion or persistent symptoms after unrevealing stress testing. The utility of CAC scoring among ath-letes is controversial, with some studies showing increased CAC scores in older endurance athletes in comparison with age-matched non-athletes and athletes with less exercise exposure [80, 81]. The mechanism of this seeming paradox is not clear and has led to speculation that long-term and intensive exercise training could potentially be detrimental, as data among athletes and non-athletes has shown that a zero-calcium score carries the best prognostic risk for future events [82–84]. However, more recent and large-scale data has shown that while there is more CAC in athletes with the most exercise exposure, these athletes still had better cardiovas-cular outcomes than those athletes with less exercise exposure and lower CAC scores [81]. Additional investigation regarding the full prognostic implications of CAC and its relationship to risk in highly active individuals is ongoing. For those athletes with a higher suspicion of obstructive CAD based on symptoms or tradi-tional CAD risk factors, where assessment of coronary luminal anatomy is required, invasive coronary angiography may be an appropriate approach instead of CCTA, based on patient and provider preference.

Atrial fibrillation and atrial flutter are often encountered in competitive athletes and are the most common arrhythmias encountered in elite athletes, particularly in middle-aged men [66]. Specific mechanisms underlying these arrhythmias in athletes are emerging, with appreciated associated factors of longer duration and intensity of athletic activity and increased vagal tone [85, 86]. Symptoms plus resting or ambulatory ECG are the usual means to make a diagnosis. Routine evaluation should include a comprehensive history to identify etiologies such as performance-enhancing or illicit drugs, excessive alcohol use, thyroid dysfunction, family history of cardiomyopathy, or the presence of a sleep apnea. Initial downstream testing should include TTE to identify or exclude structural heart disease (myocardial or valvular) and to exclude tachycardia-mediated cardiomyopathy [70]. Exercise may be the trigger that the arrhythmia and stress testing or prolonged ambulatory ECG monitoring may be required to document the arrhythmia. CMR and CCTA may be helpful as second-line imaging for a cardiomyopathy or clarification of the presence/extent of CAD. In addition, CCTA or CMR as tomographic imaging may also be utilized for anatomic mapping in those scenarios where an invasive catheter-based ablation strategy will be employed.

Pediatric Athletes and Congenital Heart Disease (CHD)

Children and adolescents represent a significant population of athletes [46, 87]. Many inherited cardiac conditions associated with an increased risk of sudden death become clinically apparent in this age group. There is rapid growth and variation in cardiac dimensions within this group, thereby making the distinction between normal growth-related changes, athletic adaptive physiology, and potential emerging pathology difficult. Challenges in differentiating normal physiology from pathology are further compounded by the relative dearth of age-specific normative cardiac data in pediatric athletes.

Many patients with repaired and unrepaired congenital heart defects participate as athletes in a variety of sporting activities [87]. There is a broad range of congenital cardiac malformations with varied severity and varied needs for therapeutic interventions. A clear understanding of the individual patient's anatomy is necessary to determine a risk assessment. The safety of competitive sport participation among patients with CHD has not been rigorously studied [87, 88], with competitive sport eligibility recommendations based predominantly on expert opinion [89, 90]. Although the guideline recommendations provide a useful initial template, the wide variety of patients included in this category, as well as variations in clinical practice, makes an individualized approach to physical activity recommendations the most often employed strategy [91]. With these factors in mind, a collaborative approach is strongly encouraged with inclusion of pediatric cardiologists and CHD trained physicians, respectively [88].

Recommendations for pediatric and CHD patients are often consistent with adult recommendations, but consultation with specialists is required to help determine the optimal imaging plan for these patients [92]. Initial imaging with TTE is the predominant first-line downstream test followed by CMR or CCTA as directed by the CHD expert and dictated by disease type and severity. Symptom-limited functional exercise testing may be employed in a similar collaborative approach for assessment of exercise capacity or when eliciting for exercise-triggered symptoms or arrhythmias.

Conclusions

Differentiating EICR from mild forms of cardiac pathology remains challenging in clinical practice. The sports cardiologist should be prepared to evaluate historical and physical examination findings along with ECG and imaging features that are both expected and suspicious among athletes. Individual patient characteristics and symptoms should dictate the downstream imaging strategy to identify or exclude abnormalities and to provide risk stratification in the presence of disease. Optimal use of multimodality imaging requires an understanding of EICR and the strengths and weaknesses of the available imaging techniques. A well-constructed plan for downstream testing can diagnose and risk stratify athletes in a streamlined fashion. Utilizing sports cardiologists as experts in this process will provide accurate diagnoses and limit unnecessary testing and expense while avoiding a prolonged return-to-play timeline.

References

1. Prior DL, La Gerche A. The athlete's heart. Heart. 2012;98:947–55.
2. Astrand PO, Cuddy TE, Saltin B, Stenberg J. Cardiac output during submaximal and maximal work. J Appl Physiol. 1964;19:268–74.
3. Weiner RB, Wang F, Isaacs SK, Malhotra R, Berkstresser B, Kim JH, Hutter AM Jr, Picard MH, Wang TJ, Baggish AL. Blood pressure and left ventricular hypertrophy during American-style football participation. Circulation. 2013;128:524–31.
4. Baggish AL, Weiner RB, Kanayama G, Hudson JI, Lu MT, Hoffmann U, Pope HG Jr. Cardiovascular toxicity of illicit anabolic-androgenic steroid use. Circulation. 2017;135:1991–2002.
5. Sharma S, Merghani A, Mont L. Exercise and the heart: the good, the bad, and the ugly. Eur Heart J. 2015;36:1445–53.
6. Whyte GP, George K, Nevill A, Shave R, Sharma S, McKenna WJ. Left ventricular morphology and function in female athletes: a meta-analysis. Int J Sports Med. 2004;25:380–3.
7. Sun B, Ma JZ, Yong YH, Lv YY. The upper limit of physiological cardiac hypertrophy in elite male and female athletes in China. Eur J Appl Physiol. 2007;101:457–63.
8. Whyte GP, George K, Sharma S, Firoozi S, Stephens N, Senior R, McKenna WJ. The upper limit of physiological cardiac hypertrophy in elite male and female athletes: the British experience. Eur J Appl Physiol. 2004;92:592–7.

9. Howden EJ, Perhonen M, Peshock RM, Zhang R, Arbab-Zadeh A, Adams-Huet B, Levine BD. Females have a blunted cardiovascular response to one year of intensive supervised endurance training. J Appl Physiol (1985). 2015;119:37–46.

10. Weiner RB, DeLuca JR, Wang F, Lin J, Wasfy MM, Berkstresser B, Stöhr E, Shave R, Lewis GD, Hutter AM Jr, Picard MH, Baggish AL. Exercise-induced left ventricular remodeling among competitive athletes: a phasic phenomenon. Circ Cardiovasc Imaging. 2015;8:e003651.

11. Caruso MR, Garg L, Martinez MW. Cardiac imaging in the athlete: shrinking the "gray zone". Curr Treat Options Cardiovasc Med. 2020;22:5.

12. Quarta G, Papadakis M, Donna PD, Maurizi N, Iacovoni A, Gavazzi A, Senni M, Olivotto I. Grey zones in cardiomyopathies: defining boundaries between genetic and iatrogenic disease. Nat Rev Cardiol. 2017;14:102–12.

13. Martinez MW. Advanced imaging of athletes: added value of coronary computed tomography and cardiac magnetic resonance imaging. Clin Sports Med. 2015;34:433–48.

14. Brosnan M, La Gerche A, Kalman J, Lo W, Fallon K, MacIsaac A, Prior DL. Comparison of frequency of significant electrocardiographic abnormalities in endurance versus nonendurance athletes. Am J Cardiol. 2014;113:1567–73.

15. Sharma S, Drezner JA, Baggish A, Papadakis M, Wilson MG, Prutkin JM, La Gerche A, Ackerman MJ, Borjesson M, Salerno JC, Asif IM, Owens DS, Chung EH, Emery MS, Froelicher VF, Heidbuchel H, Adamuz C, Asplund CA, Cohen G, Harmon KG, Marek JC, Molossi S, Niebauer J, Pelto HF, Perez MV, Riding NR, Saarel T, Schmied CM, Shipon DM, Stein R, Vetter VL, Pelliccia A, Corrado D. International recommendations for electrocardiographic interpretation in athletes. J Am Coll Cardiol. 2017;69:1057–75.

16. Pelliccia A, Maron BJ, Culasso F, Di Paolo FM, Spataro A, Biffi A, Caselli G, Piovano P. Clinical significance of abnormal electrocardiographic patterns in trained athletes. Circulation. 2000;102:278–84.

17. Papadakis M, Basavarajaiah S, Rawlins J, Edwards C, Makan J, Firoozi S, Carby L, Sharma S. Prevalence and significance of T-wave inversions in predominantly Caucasian adolescent athletes. Eur Heart J. 2009;30:1728–35.

18. Papadakis M, Carre F, Kervio G, Rawlins J, Panoulas VF, Chandra N, Basavarajaiah S, Carby L, Fonseca T, Sharma S. The prevalence, distribution, and clinical outcomes of electrocardiographic repolarization patterns in male athletes of African/Afro-Caribbean origin. Eur Heart J. 2011;32:2304–13.

19. Riding NR, Salah O, Sharma S, Carré F, George KP, Farooq A, Hamilton B, Chalabi H, Whyte GP, Wilson MG. ECG and morphologic adaptations in Arabic athletes: are the European Society of Cardiology's recommendations for the interpretation of the 12-lead ECG appropriate for this ethnicity? Br J Sports Med. 2014;48:1138–43.

20. Sharma S, Whyte G, Elliott P, Padula M, Kaushal R, Mahon N, McKenna WJ. Electrocardiographic changes in 1000 highly trained junior elite athletes. Br J Sports Med. 1999;33:319–24.

21. Huston TP, Puffer JC, Rodney WM. The athletic heart syndrome. N Engl J Med. 1985;313:24–32.

22. Sheikh N, Papadakis M, Ghani S, Zaidi A, Gati S, Adami PE, Carré F, Schnell F, Wilson M, Avila P. Comparison of electrocardiographic criteria for the detection of cardiac abnormalities in elite black and white athletes. Circulation. 2014;129:1637–49.

23. Lakdawala NK, Thune JJ, Maron BJ, Cirino AL, Havndrup O, Bundgaard H, Christiansen M, Carlsen CM, Dorval J-F, Kwong RY. Electrocardiographic features of sarcomere mutation carriers with and without clinically overt hypertrophic cardiomyopathy. Am J Cardiol. 2011;108:1606–13.

24. Sheikh N, Papadakis M, Schnell F, Panoulas V, Malhotra A, Wilson M, Carré F, Sharma S. Clinical profile of athletes with hypertrophic cardiomyopathy. Circ Cardiovasc Imaging. 2015;8:e003454.

25. Calore C, Zorzi A, Sheikh N, Nese A, Facci M, Malhotra A, Zaidi A, Schiavon M, Pelliccia A, Sharma S. Electrocardiographic anterior T-wave inversion in athletes of different

ethnicities: differential diagnosis between athlete's heart and cardiomyopathy. Eur Heart J. 2016;37:2515–27.

26. Malhotra A, Dhutia H, Gati S, Yeo T-J, Dores H, Bastiaenen R, Narain R, Merghani A, Finocchiaro G, Sheikh N. Anterior T-wave inversion in young white athletes and nonathletes: prevalence and significance. J Am Coll Cardiol. 2017;69:1–9.

27. Chandra N, Bastiaenen R, Papadakis M, Panoulas VF, Ghani S, Duschl J, Foldes D, Raju H, Osborne R, Sharma S. Prevalence of electrocardiographic anomalies in young individuals: relevance to a nationwide cardiac screening program. J Am Coll Cardiol. 2014;63:2028–34.

28. Pelliccia A, Di Paolo FM, Quattrini FM, Basso C, Culasso F, Popoli G, De Luca R, Spataro A, Biffi A, Thiene G, Maron BJ. Outcomes in athletes with marked ECG repolarization abnormalities. N Engl J Med. 2008;358:152–61.

29. Schnell F, Riding N, O'Hanlon R, Axel Lentz P, Donal E, Kervio G, Matelot D, Leurent G, Doutreleau S, Chevalier L. Recognition and significance of pathological T-wave inversions in athletes. Circulation. 2015;131:165–73.

30. Bent RE, Wheeler MT, Hadley D, Knowles JW, Pavlovic A, Finocchiaro G, Haddad F, Salisbury H, Race S, Shmargad Y. Systematic comparison of digital electrocardiograms from healthy athletes and patients with hypertrophic cardiomyopathy. J Am Coll Cardiol. 2015;65:2462–3.

31. Maron MS, Maron BJ, Harrigan C, Buros J, Gibson CM, Olivotto I, Biller L, Lesser JR, Udelson JE, Manning WJ. Hypertrophic cardiomyopathy phenotype revisited after 50 years with cardiovascular magnetic resonance. J Am Coll Cardiol. 2009;54:220–8.

32. Maron MS, Lesser JR, Maron BJ. Management implications of massive left ventricular hypertrophy in hypertrophic cardiomyopathy significantly underestimated by echocardiography but identified by cardiovascular magnetic resonance. Am J Cardiol. 2010;105:1842–3.

33. Nagueh SF, Bierig SM, Budoff MJ, Desai M, Dilsizian V, Eidem B, Goldstein SA, Hung J, Maron MS, Ommen SR, Woo A. American Society of Echocardiography clinical recommendations for multimodality cardiovascular imaging of patients with hypertrophic cardiomyopathy: endorsed by the American Society of Nuclear Cardiology, Society for Cardiovascular Magnetic Resonance, and Society of Cardiovascular Computed Tomography. J Am Soc Echocardiogr. 2011;24:473–98.

34. Rickers C, Wilke NM, Jerosch-Herold M, Casey SA, Panse P, Panse N, Weil J, Zenovich AG, Maron BJ. Utility of cardiac magnetic resonance imaging in the diagnosis of hypertrophic cardiomyopathy. Circulation. 2005;112:855–61.

35. Link MS, Laidlaw D, Polonsky B, Zareba W, McNitt S, Gear K, Marcus F, Estes NM. Ventricular arrhythmias in the North American multidisciplinary study of ARVC: predictors, characteristics, and treatment. J Am Coll Cardiol. 2014;64:119–25.

36. Marcus FI, McKenna WJ, Sherrill D, Basso C, Bauce B, Bluemke DA, Calkins H, Corrado D, Cox MG, Daubert JP. Diagnosis of arrhythmogenic right ventricular cardiomyopathy/dysplasia: proposed modification of the task force criteria. Circulation. 2010;121:1533–41.

37. Nasir K, Bomma C, Tandri H, Roguin A, Dalal D, Prakasa K, Tichnell C, James C, Jspevak P, Marcus F. Electrocardiographic features of arrhythmogenic right ventricular dysplasia/cardiomyopathy according to disease severity: a need to broaden diagnostic criteria. Circulation. 2004;110:1527–34.

38. Saguner AM, Ganahl S, Kraus A, Baldinger SH, Akdis D, Saguner AR, Wolber T, Haegeli LM, Steffel J, Krasniqi N. Electrocardiographic features of disease progression in arrhythmogenic right ventricular cardiomyopathy/dysplasia. BMC Cardiovasc Disord. 2015;15:4.

39. Prior D. Differentiating athlete's heart from cardiomyopathies – the right side. Heart Lung Circ. 2018;27:1063–71.

40. members ATF, Elliott PM, Anastasakis A, Borger MA, Borggrefe M, Cecchi F, Charron P, Hagege AA, Lafont A, Limongelli G. 2014 ESC Guidelines on diagnosis and management of hypertrophic cardiomyopathy: the task force for the diagnosis and management of hypertrophic cardiomyopathy of the European Society of Cardiology (ESC). Eur Heart J. 2014;35:2733–79.

41. Di Paolo FM, Schmied C, Zerguini YA, Junge A, Quattrini F, Culasso F, Dvorak J, Pelliccia A. The athlete's heart in adolescent Africans: an electrocardiographic and echocardiographic study. J Am Coll Cardiol. 2012;59:1029–36.

42. Baggish AL, Hutter AM, Wang F, Yared K, Weiner RB, Kupperman E, Picard MH, Wood MJ. Cardiovascular screening in college athletes with and without electrocardiography: a cross-sectional study. Ann Intern Med. 2010;152:269–75.
43. Haghjoo M, Mohammadzadeh S, Taherpour M, Faghfurian B, Fazelifar AF, Alizadeh A, Rad MA, Sadr-Ameli MA. ST-segment depression as a risk factor in hypertrophic cardiomyopathy. Europace. 2009;11:643–9.
44. Maron BJ, Wolfson JK, Ciró E, Spirito P. Relation of electrocardiographic abnormalities and patterns of left ventricular hypertrophy identified by 2-dimensional echocardiography in patients with hypertrophic cardiomyopathy. Am J Cardiol. 1983;51:189–94.
45. Etheridge SP, Escudero CA, Blaufox AD, Law IH, Dechert-Crooks BE, Stephenson EA, Dubin AM, Ceresnak SR, Motonaga KS, Skinner JR, Marcondes LD, Perry JC, Collins KK, Seslar SP, Cabrera M, Uzun O, Cannon BC, Aziz PF, Kubuš P, Tanel RE, Valdes SO, Sami S, Kertesz NJ, Maldonado J, Erickson C, Moore JP, Asakai H, Mill L, Abcede M, Spector ZZ, Menon S, Shwayder M, Bradley DJ, Cohen MI, Sanatani S. Life-threatening event risk in children with Wolff-Parkinson-White syndrome: a multicenter international study. JACC Clin Electrophysiol. 2018;4:433–44.
46. Cohen M, Triedman J, Cannon B, Davis A, Drago F, Janousek J, Klein G, Law I, Morady F, Paul T. Pediatric and Congenital Electrophysiology Society (PACES). Heart Rhythm Society (HRS). 2012;9(6):1006–24.
47. Daubert C, Ollitrault J, Descaves C, Mabo P, Ritter P, Gouffalt J. Failure of the exercise test to predict the anterograde refractory period of the accessory pathway in Wolff Parkinson White syndrome. Pacing Clin Electrophysiol. 1988;11:1130–8.
48. Roberts WC, Grayburn PA, Hall SA. Complications of radiofrequency ablation for supraventricular tachycardia in the Wolff-Parkinson-White syndrome associated with noncompaction cardiomyopathy. Am J Cardiol. 2018;121:1442–4.
49. Marek J, Bufalino V, Davis J, Marek K, Gami A, Stephan W, Zimmerman F. Feasibility and findings of large-scale electrocardiographic screening in young adults: data from 32,561 subjects. Heart Rhythm. 2011;8:1555–9.
50. Kim JH, Baggish AL. Electrocardiographic right and left bundle branch block patterns in athletes: prevalence, pathology, and clinical significance. J Electrocardiol. 2015;48:380–4.
51. Le V-V, Wheeler MT, Mandic S, Dewey F, Fonda H, Perez M, Sungar G, Garza D, Ashley EA, Matheson G. Addition of the electrocardiogram to the preparticipation examination of college athletes. Clin J Sport Med. 2010;20:98–105.
52. Platonov PG, Calkins H, Hauer RN, Corrado D, Svendsen JH, Wichter T, Biernacka EK, Saguner AM, Te Riele AS, Zareba W. High interobserver variability in the assessment of epsilon waves: implications for diagnosis of arrhythmogenic right ventricular cardiomyopathy/dysplasia. Heart Rhythm. 2016;13:208–16.
53. Kirchhof P, Fabritz L, Zwiener M, Witt H, Schafers M, Zellerhoff S, Paul M, Athai T, Hiller KH, Baba HA, Breithardt G, Ruiz P, Wichter T, Levkau B. Age- and training-dependent development of arrhythmogenic right ventricular cardiomyopathy in heterozygous plakoglobin-deficient mice. Circulation. 2006;114:1799–806.
54. Zaidi A, Sheikh N, Jongman JK, Gati S, Panoulas VF, Carr-White G, Papadakis M, Sharma R, Behr ER, Sharma S. Clinical differentiation between physiological remodeling and arrhythmogenic right ventricular cardiomyopathy in athletes with marked electrocardiographic repolarization anomalies. J Am Coll Cardiol. 2015;65:2702–11.
55. Marcus FI, McKenna WJ, Sherrill D, Basso C, Bauce B, Bluemke DA, Calkins H, Corrado D, Cox MG, Daubert JP, Fontaine G, Gear K, Hauer R, Nava A, Picard MH, Protonotarios N, Saffitz JE, Sanborn DM, Steinberg JS, Tandri H, Thiene G, Towbin JA, Tsatsopoulou A, Wichter T, Zareba W. Diagnosis of arrhythmogenic right ventricular cardiomyopathy/dysplasia: proposed modification of the Task Force Criteria. Eur Heart J. 2010;31:806–14.
56. Baggish AL, Battle RW, Beckerman JG, Bove AA, Lampert RJ, Levine BD, Link MS, Martinez MW, Molossi SM, Salerno J, Wasfy MM, Weiner RB, Emery MS. Sports cardiology: core curriculum for providing cardiovascular care to competitive athletes and highly active people. J Am Coll Cardiol. 2017;70:1902–18.

57. Singh AM, McGregor RS. Differential diagnosis of chest symptoms in the athlete. Clin Rev Allergy Immunol. 2005;29:87–96.
58. Churchill TW, Disanto M, Singh TK, Groezinger E, Loomer G, Contursi M, DiCarli M, Michaud-Finch J, Stewart KM, Hutter AM, Lewis GD, Weiner RB, Baggish AL, Wasfy MM. Diagnostic yield of customized exercise provocation following routine testing. Am J Cardiol. 2019;123:2044–50.
59. Moya A, Sutton R, Ammirati F, Blanc JJ, Brignole M, Dahm JB, Deharo JC, Gajek J, Gjesdal K, Krahn A, Massin M, Pepi M, Pezawas T, Ruiz Granell R, Sarasin F, Ungar A, van Dijk JG, Walma EP, Wieling W. Guidelines for the diagnosis and management of syncope (version 2009). Eur Heart J. 2009;30:2631–71.
60. Colivicchi F, Ammirati F, Biffi A, Verdile L, Pelliccia A, Santini M. Exercise-related syncope in young competitive athletes without evidence of structural heart disease. Clinical presentation and long-term outcome. Eur Heart J. 2002;23:1125–30.
61. Shen WK, Sheldon RS, Benditt DG, Cohen MI, Forman DE, Goldberger ZD, Grubb BP, Hamdan MH, Krahn AD, Link MS, Olshansky B, Raj SR, Sandhu RK, Sorajja D, Sun BC, Yancy CW. 2017 ACC/AHA/HRS Guideline for the evaluation and management of patients with syncope: a report of the American College of Cardiology/American Heart Association Task Force on clinical practice guidelines and the Heart Rhythm Society. Circulation. 2017;136:e60–e122.
62. Qureshi MY, O'Leary PW, Connolly HM. Cardiac imaging in Ebstein anomaly. Trends Cardiovasc Med. 2018;28:403–9.
63. Porto AG, Brun F, Severini GM, Losurdo P, Fabris E, Taylor MRG, Mestroni L, Sinagra G. Clinical spectrum of PRKAG2 syndrome. Circ Arrhythm Electrophysiol. 2016;9:e003121.
64. Schwartz PJ, Ackerman MJ, Wilde AAM. Channelopathies as causes of sudden cardiac death. Card Electrophysiol Clin. 2017;9:537–49.
65. Ackerman MJ, Priori SG, Willems S, Berul C, Brugada R, Calkins H, Camm AJ, Ellinor PT, Gollob M, Hamilton R, Hershberger RE, Judge DP, Le Marec H, WJ MK, Schulze-Bahr E, Semsarian C, Towbin JA, Watkins H, Wilde A, Wolpert C, Zipes DP. HRS/EHRA Expert consensus statement on the state of genetic testing for the channelopathies and cardiomyopathies this document was developed as a partnership between the Heart Rhythm Society (HRS) and the European Heart Rhythm Association (EHRA). Heart Rhythm. 2011;8:1308–39.
66. Turagam MK, Velagapudi P, Kocheril AG. Atrial fibrillation in athletes. Am J Cardiol. 2012;109:296–302.
67. Boraita A, Santos-Lozano A, Heras ME, González-Amigo F, López-Ortiz S, Villacastín JP, Lucia A. Incidence of atrial fibrillation in elite athletes. JAMA Cardiol. 2018;3:1200–5.
68. Furlanello F, Bertoldi A, Dallago M, Galassi A, Fernando F, Biffi A, Mazzone P, Pappone C, Chierchia S. Atrial fibrillation in elite athletes. J Cardiovasc Electrophysiol. 1998;9:S63–8.
69. Lai E, Chung EH. Management of arrhythmias in athletes: atrial fibrillation, premature ventricular contractions, and ventricular tachycardia. Curr Treat Options Cardiovasc Med. 2017;19:86.
70. Zipes DP, Link MS, Ackerman MJ, Kovacs RJ, Myerburg RJ, Estes NAM 3rd. Eligibility and disqualification recommendations for competitive athletes with cardiovascular abnormalities: task force 9: arrhythmias and conduction defects: a scientific statement from the American Heart Association and American College of Cardiology. J Am Coll Cardiol. 2015;66:2412–23.
71. Parshall MB, Schwartzstein RM, Adams L, Banzett RB, Manning HL, Bourbeau J, Calverley PM, Gift AG, Harver A, Lareau SC, Mahler DA, Meek PM, O'Donnell DE. An official American Thoracic Society statement: update on the mechanisms, assessment, and management of dyspnea. Am J Respir Crit Care Med. 2012;185:435–52.
72. Boulet LP. Cough and upper airway disorders in elite athletes: a critical review. Br J Sports Med. 2012;46:417–21.
73. Tilles SA. Exercise-induced airway dysfunction in athletes. Immunol Allergy Clin N Am. 2018;38:xiii–xiv.

74. Boulet LP, Turmel J, Côté A. Asthma and exercise-induced respiratory symptoms in the ath-lete: new insights. Curr Opin Pulm Med. 2017;23:71–7.
75. Sarma S, Levine BD. Beyond the Bruce protocol: advanced exercise testing for the sports cardiologist. Cardiol Clin. 2016;34:603–8.
76. Watson AM. Sleep and athletic performance. Curr Sports Med Rep. 2017;16:413–8.
77. Meeusen R, Duclos M, Foster C, Fry A, Gleeson M, Nieman D, Raglin J, Rietjens G, Steinacker J, Urhausen A. Prevention, diagnosis, and treatment of the overtraining syndrome: joint con-sensus statement of the European College of Sport Science and the American College of Sports Medicine. Med Sci Sports Exerc. 2013;45:186–205.
78. Goel R, Majeed F, Vogel R, Corretti MC, Weir M, Mangano C, White C, Plotnick GD, Miller M. Exercise-induced hypertension, endothelial dysfunction, and coronary artery disease in a marathon runner. Am J Cardiol. 2007;99:743–4.
79. Möhlenkamp S, Lehmann N, Breuckmann F, Bröcker-Preuss M, Nassenstein K, Halle M, Budde T, Mann K, Barkhausen J, Heusch G, Jöckel KH, Erbel R. Running: the risk of coronary events: prevalence and prognostic relevance of coronary atherosclerosis in marathon runners. Eur Heart J. 2008;29:1903–10.
80. Merghani A, Maestrini V, Rosmini S, Cox AT, Dhutia H, Bastiaenan R, David S, Yeo TJ, Narain R, Malhotra A, Papadakis M, Wilson MG, Tome M, AlFakih K, Moon JC, Sharma S. Prevalence of subclinical coronary artery disease in masters endurance athletes with a low atherosclerotic risk profile. Circulation. 2017;136:126–37.
81. DeFina LF, Radford NB, Barlow CE, Willis BL, Leonard D, Haskell WL, Farrell SW, Pavlovic A, Abel K, Berry JD, Khera A, Levine BD. Association of all-cause and cardiovascular mor-tality with high levels of physical activity and concurrent coronary artery calcification. JAMA Cardiol. 2019;4:174–81.
82. Budoff MJ, Mayrhofer T, Ferencik M, Bittner D, Lee KL, Lu MT, Coles A, Jang J, Krishnam M, Douglas PS, Hoffmann U. Prognostic value of coronary artery calcium in the PROMISE study (Prospective multicenter imaging study for evaluation of chest pain). Circulation. 2017;136:1993–2005.
83. Radford NB, DeFina LF, Barlow CE, Lakoski SG, Leonard D, Paixao AR, Khera A, Levine BD. Progression of CAC score and risk of incident CVD. JACC Cardiovasc Imaging. 2016;9:1420–9.
84. Ekblom-Bak E, Ekblom Ö, Fagman E, Angerås O, Schmidt C, Rosengren A, Börjesson M, Bergström G. Fitness attenuates the prevalence of increased coronary artery calcium in indi-viduals with metabolic syndrome. Eur J Prev Cardiol. 2018;25:309–16.
85. Wilhelm M, Roten L, Tanner H, Schmid JP, Wilhelm I, Saner H. Long-term cardiac remodel-ing and arrhythmias in nonelite marathon runners. Am J Cardiol. 2012;110:129–35.
86. Andersen K, Farahmand B, Ahlbom A, Held C, Ljunghall S, Michaëlsson K, Sundström J. Risk of arrhythmias in 52 755 long-distance cross-country skiers: a cohort study. Eur Heart J. 2013;34:3624–31.
87. Dean PN, Battle RW. Congenital heart disease and the athlete: what we know and what we do not know. Cardiol Clin. 2016;34:579–89.
88. Etheridge SP, Saarel EV, Martinez MW. Exercise participation and shared decision-making in patients with inherited channelopathies and cardiomyopathies. Heart Rhythm. 2018;15:915–20.
89. Van Hare GF, Ackerman MJ, Evangelista JA, Kovacs RJ, Myerburg RJ, Shafer KM, Warnes CA, Washington RL. Eligibility and disqualification recommendations for competitive athletes with cardiovascular abnormalities: task force 4: congenital heart disease: a scientific state-ment from the American Heart Association and American College of Cardiology. Circulation. 2015;132:e281–91.
90. Priori SG, Blomström-Lundqvist C, Mazzanti A, Blom N, Borggrefe M, Camm J, Elliott PM, Fitzsimons D, Hatala R, Hindricks G, Kirchhof P, Kjeldsen K, Kuck KH, Hernandez-Madrid A, Nikolaou N, Norekvål TM, Spaulding C, Van Veldhuisen DJ. 2015 ESC Guidelines for the management of patients with ventricular arrhythmias and the prevention of sudden cardiac

death: the task force for the management of patients with ventricular arrhythmias and the prevention of sudden cardiac death of the European Society of Cardiology (ESC). Endorsed by: Association for European Paediatric and Congenital Cardiology (AEPC). Eur Heart J. 2015;36:2793–867.

91. McKillop A, McCrindle BW, Dimitropoulos G, Kovacs AH. Physical activity perceptions and behaviors among young adults with congenital heart disease: a mixed-methods study. Congenit Heart Dis. 2018;13:232–40.

92. Cohen MS, Eidem BW, Cetta F, Fogel MA, Frommelt PC, Ganame J, Han BK, Kimball TR, Johnson RK, Mertens L, Paridon SM, Powell AJ, Lopez L. Multimodality imaging guidelines of patients with transposition of the great arteries: a report from the American Society of Echocardiography developed in collaboration with the Society for Cardiovascular Magnetic Resonance and the Society of Cardiovascular Computed Tomography. J Am Soc Echocardiogr. 2016;29:571–621.

Chapter 4
Practical Use of Genetic Testing in Athletes

Isha Kalia, Farhana Latif, Muredach P. Reilly, and Marc P. Waase

Introduction

Meet the future of testing and screening athletes: DNA. Meet your genes. What can your DNA say about your health? Understand your risk, so you can understand your options. These are but a few of the many ways that genetic testing companies are strategically marketing their products to consumers. Whether they intend to provide information about your ancestry, determine your athletic potential in a particular sport, or identify your personal health risks, genetic tests are becoming more diverse in their offerings and, notably, more widely accessible to consumers. Genetic testing for health-related purposes is becoming increasingly common in the practice of medicine. As medical providers who work with athletes, we must educate ourselves about current uses of genetic information and appropriate genetic testing practices in athletes in order to best serve our patients and the athletic community.

General Principles of Genetic Testing

Some genetic disorders do confer a known, significant health risk for individuals undertaking strenuous activity/sports. Identification of genetic forms of cardiovascular diseases, including channelopathies, cardiomyopathies, and aortopathies, is becoming more of an important component of sports cardiology practices. Screening for these cardiac disorders that may predispose athletes to sudden cardiac death (SCD) has made identifying these diseases, especially in young athletes, of utmost importance.

I. Kalia · F. Latif · M. P. Reilly · M. P. Waase (✉)
Division of Cardiology, Columbia University Irving Medical Center, New York, NY, USA
e-mail: ik2417@cumc.columbia.edu; fl2203@cumc.columbia.edu; mpr2144@cumc.columbia.edu; mpw2126@cumc.columbia.edu

© Springer Nature Switzerland AG 2021
D. J. Engel, D. M. Phelan (eds.), *Sports Cardiology*,
https://doi.org/10.1007/978-3-030-69384-8_4

53

Genetic testing for athletes can be useful in several ways. First, diagnostic genetic testing can confirm a diagnosis when a specific disease is suspected based on medical history, physical exam findings, symptoms, or imaging test results. Obtaining a definitive diagnosis plays a vital role in a patient's clinical treatment and management. Second, pre-symptomatic genetic testing after obtaining a comprehensive medical and family history can identify genetic variants that place an individual at risk for developing a specific condition. The opportunities afforded by pre-symptomatic genetic testing include targeted surveillance, identification of therapeutic interventions, and a refinement of risk assessment. In addition to medical benefits, there are psychosocial benefits such as reducing anxiety and uncertainty, sharing information among family members, and adjusting life plans according to genetic information. In order for genetic testing to be of clinical utility, it is important to properly identify appropriate candidates within a family for genetic testing.

As with any medical examination, genetic testing should only be performed when clinically indicated after a comprehensive medical history, with particular attention to the family history and a physical examination. The first step in determining whom best qualifies for genetic testing is identifying an individual with a clinical phenotype that fits a specific diagnosis, for instance, an athlete who has aortic root dilation and ecotpia lentis. This clinical phenotype raises suspicion for Marfan syndrome. Therefore, diagnostic genetic testing for Marfan syndrome would be beneficial in this circumstance.

Another factor to consider during the genetic testing process is an individual's family history. A family pedigree evaluation should include a three-generation family tree with an emphasis on premature cardiovascular events (sudden death, heart failure) and associated cardiac (arrhythmias, conduction disease, syncope) and non-cardiac (skeletal myopathy, renal disorder, auditory/visual defects) characteristics. It is important to identify other family members with a similar phenotype. This family history review can assist in recognizing inheritance patterns and narrowing down suspected diagnoses.

Once symptomatic individuals within a family have been identified, it is important to determine who should undergo genetic testing. Typically, the first family member to undergo genetic testing (the proband) should be the youngest symptomatic individual. Diseases with a genetic etiology often manifest early in one's lifespan. Therefore, the most likely person to have a condition caused by a genetic mutation is the individual with the earliest onset of symptoms. If that individual is unavailable for testing, then the next best candidate for testing is another individual in the family with clinical symptoms that support a particular disease phenotype.

Approaches to Genetic Testing

There are several approaches for the performance of genetic testing. If a mutation has previously been identified in the family, then other at-risk family members should be offered testing for that specific familial mutation. The most conservative way to perform this testing is to offer single gene testing. Single gene testing is clinically reasonable if the signs or symptoms are consistent with a particular disease phenotype. This type of testing can be cost-effective, as it reduces the need for the testing of other genes that are not of interest. For example, the sodium channel SCN5A gene would be a candidate for single gene testing in the case for suspected Brugada syndrome, as pathogenic variants in the SCN5A gene account for 15–30% of Brugada syndrome cases [1]. However, this single gene method does not test for all possible genes for a disease that may be associated with a multitude of different genes, thereby missing other potential deleterious gene variants. If single gene testing is negative, repeat testing may be required.

Another approach, called multi-gene panel testing, is to expand the genetic testing to include more rare variants that can be associated with a particular condition. Multi-gene panel testing can include just a few genes or include as many as hundreds of genes. This type of testing can be beneficial when mutations in multiple genes are known to be responsible for a specific condition. For example, genetic testing for long QT syndrome can include the more common genes such as potassium channels, KCNQ1 and KCNH2, and the sodium channel, SCN5A, as well as more rare variants, such as calmodulin 1 and 2 (CALM1 and CALM2), or potassium channels KCNE1, KCNE2, KCNJ2, and KCNJ5.

The final and most liberal approach to genetic testing is to perform whole genome or whole exome sequencing (WGS/WES). While large-scale genetic testing can be cost- and time- effective, it presents several challenges, including limited sensitivity, low prognostic predictive value, low probability to identify pathogenic variants in different genes, and the major risk of noninterpretable results. One of the main limitations toward performing multi-gene panel testing and/or WGS/WES is encountering variants of uncertain significance (VUS). A genetic mutation is classified as a VUS when there is insufficient data to confirm its association with a particular disease [2]. Thus, it is not recommended to use a VUS in an individual's clinical decision-making. As the genetic testing laboratory collects more data on a specific VUS, the laboratory can ultimately reclassify the VUS to pathogenic or benign. However, the timeline for this classification is unknown, ranging from months to years. This obscure timeline creates challenges and questions for providers and patients alike. With high rates of clinician turnover, whose duty is it to recontact families when a VUS is reclassified? Additionally, will families provide clinicians with their updated contact information over the years? Finally, whose responsibility is it to provide cascade screening by genetically testing other at-risk family members, if a variant is reclassified to a pathogenic mutation?

With the simultaneous decrease in the cost of genetic testing and the increase in the number of genes on genetic testing panels, expansive clinical genetic testing, such as WGS/WES, is becoming more commonplace in medical practice. Complicating the genetic testing landscape even further is the issue of incidental or secondary findings. Incidental findings are genetic changes that are not related to the indication for testing but have clinical utility to the provider and patient alike [3]. An example of an incidental finding includes ordering WES for a cardiomyopathy indication and discovering a pathogenic breast cancer gene mutation. While a

Table 4.1 Thirty-one genes for which identified variants should prompt evaluation for heritable cardiovascular disorders, as recommended by the American College of Medical Genetics and Genomics

Phenotype	Genes
ARVC	PKP2, DSP, DSC2, TMEM43, DSG2
HCM or DCM	MYBPC3, MYH7, TNNT2, TNNI3, TPM1, MYL3, ACTC1, PRKAG2, GLA, MYL2, LMNA
CPVT	RYR2
Ehlers-Danlos syndrome, vascular type	COL3A1
Familial hypercholesterolemia	LDLR, ABOB, PCSK9
Marfan syndrome/Loeys-Dietz syndrome/familial thoracic aortic aneurysms and dissections	FBN1, TGFBR1, TGFBR2, SMAD3, ACTA2, MYLK, MYH11
Romano-Ward long QT syndromes Types 1–3/Brugada syndrome	KCNQ1, KCNH2, SCN5A

Adapted from Kalia et al. [32]
ARVC arrhythmogenic right ventricular cardiomyopathy, *CPVT* catecholaminergic polymorphic VT, *DCM* dilated cardiomyopathy, *HCM* hypertrophic cardiomyopathy

hereditary cancer predisposition gene is not related to the cardiomyopathy indication, this information provides the patient with options for future medical decision-making. The American College of Medical Genetics and Genomics issued a policy statement identifying 59 genes that should be disclosed to patients when performing WGS/WES, as these genes are associated to diseases with specific diagnostic tests and medical interventions; 31 of these genes are linked to cardiovascular disease, including cardiomyopathies, heritable arrhythmias, aortopathies, and familial hypercholesterolemia [3], and are shown in Table 4.1.

Another disadvantage to using large-scale genetic testing methods is the issue of penetrance. Penetrance refers to how likely a person is to exhibit the symptoms of a condition when carrying a particular genetic mutation [4]. Penetrance is a significant motivator for clinical decision-making, such that the greater the risk for clinical manifestations (higher penetrance), the more aggressive the medical interventions. As multi-gene panels become more expansive in nature, a significant number of low to moderately penetrant genes are added to these panels. In these cases, it is unclear how the clinical management and treatment would be altered if there were a less penetrant (lower risk of developing clinical manifestations of the disease) gene mutation identified.

Genetic Diseases Associated with Sudden Cardiac Death

As medical professionals, our goal is to help our patients live long and healthy lives. We need to advise our patients on behavioral and lifestyle changes. Exercise is one of the most powerful tools that we encourage our patients to engage in to help improve their health, as it has been associated with improvement in cardiovascular risk factors. Athletes are, by nature, highly fit individuals who exercise daily. However, for a small number of individuals who harbor cardiac conditions, exercise can sometimes be associated with the most feared outcome for our patients, an increased risk of sudden death ("exercise paradox") [5]. The reported incidence of SCD in athletes varies and ranges from 1:30,000 to close to 1:1,000,000 pending methods of data collection and athlete group studied [6–9]. Some population of athletes may be at higher risk than others, and it is crucial for healthcare providers to identify these individuals. The most common congenital/inherited causes of SCD in athletes include structural heart disease such as hypertrophic cardiomyopathy (HCM), arrhythmogenic cardiomyopathy (AC)/arrhythmogenic right ventricular cardiomyopathy (ARVC), dilated cardiomyopathy (DCM), aortopathy, congenital anomalies of coronary arteries, left ventricular noncompaction (LVNC), bilateral mitral valve prolapse, and primary electrical/arrhythmogenic conditions, such as congenital long QT syndrome (LQTS), catecholaminergic polymorphic ventricular tachycardia (CPVT), Brugada syndrome, Wolf-Parkinson-White syndrome, and other ion channelopathies [6, 10] (Tables 4.2 and 4.3).

However, just because a patient has a mutation in a disease-causing gene does not guarantee that the patient suffers from the clinical condition. Phenotypes are highly variable, and genotype does not always predict penetrance, expressivity, age of onset, or severity, all of which can be quite variable. Non-participation is potentially devastating for an athlete, and the risks should be carefully discussed with the patient and family. At present time, there is no evidence basis for disqualification for athletes who are genotype-positive but phenotype-negative for HCM, Marfan, Brugada, CPVT, LQTS, short QT syndrome, DCM, or LVNC. In the United States, the Bethesda Conference and 2015 American Heart Association (AHA)/American College of Cardiology (ACC) Eligibility and Disqualification Recommendations require a threshold of phenotypic expression, except in the case of ARVC, before recommending disqualification [11]. Previously, the European Society of Cardiology recommended disqualification based on the finding of a pathogenic mutation alone,

Table 4.2 Common genetic/congenital cardiovascular conditions associated with sudden cardiac death in athletes

Structurally abnormal heart	Structurally normal heart
Hypertrophic cardiomyopathy	Congenital long QT syndrome
Arrhythmogenic cardiomyopathy/arrhythmogenic right ventricular cardiomyopathy	Catecholaminergic polymorphic ventricular tachycardia
Dilated cardiomyopathy	Wolf-Parkinson-White syndrome and accessory pathway syndromes
Cardiomyopathy (left ventricular noncompaction)	Brugada syndrome
Aortopathy (Marfan syndrome, ascending aortic aneurysm)	Ion channelopathies
Congenital anomalies of coronaries	
Valvular heart disease (congenital aortic stenosis, mitral valve prolapse)	

Adapted from Wasfy et al. [6]

Table 4.3 Principle genes associated with inherited cardiomyopathies

Hypertrophic cardiomyopathy Sarcomeric genes/phenocopy genes	*Frequency (%)*
B-myosin heavy chain (MYH7)	20–30
Myosin-binding protein C (MYBPC3)	30–40
Myosin light chain (MYL2)	2–4
Cardiac troponin T (TNNT2)	3–5
Cardiac troponin I (TNNI3)	<5
A-tropomyosin (TPM1)	<1
A-cardiac actin (ACTC 1)	<1
Essential myosin light chain (MYL3)	<1
Alpha-galactosidase (GLA)	<1 Fabry disease
Lysosomal-associated membrane protein 2 (LAMP2)	<1 Danon disease
Protein kinase, AMP-activated, gamma2 subunit (PRKAG2)	<1 Wolff-Parkinson-White syndrome
Dilated cardiomyopathy Sarcomeric genes/Z-disc genes	*Frequency (%)*
Titin (TTN)	15–25
B-myosin heavy chain (MYH7)	3–4
Cardiac troponin T (TNNT2)	3
A-tropomyosin (TPM1)	1–2
A-cardiac actin (ACTC1)	<1
Cardiac troponin I (TNNI3)	<1
Cardiac troponin C (TNNC1)	<1
Alpha-actinin 2 (ACTN2)	<1
Telethonin TCAP	<1
Cardiac ankyrin repeat protein (ANKRD1)	<1
Cypher/ZASP (LDB3)	<1
Muscle LIM protein (CSRP3)	<1
Other genes (Cytoskeletal, desmosomal, nuclear envelope, dystrophin complex, ion channels, sarcoplasmic reticulum, and cytoplasm)	*Frequency (%)*
Lamin A/C (LMNA/C)	4–8
Type 5 voltage-gated cardiac Na channel (SCN5A)	2–3
Desmoplakin (DSP)	2
RNA-binding protein 20 (RBM20)	2
Metavinculin (VCL)	1
Filamin C (FLNC)	1
Dystrophin (DMD)	<1
Desmin (DES)	<1
Sulfonyl-urea receptor 2A (ABCC9)	<1
Delta-sarcoglycan (SGCD)	<1
Arrhythmogenic right ventricular cardiomyopathy	*Frequency (%)*
Plakopphylin-2 (PKP2)	30–40
Desmoglein-2 (DSG2)	5–20

Table 4.3 (continued)

Desmoplakin (DSP)	10–20
Desmocollin-2 (DSC2)	1–2
Junction plakoglobin (JUP)	1–2
Transmembrane protein 43 (TMEM43)	<1
Transforming growth factor 3 (TGFB3)	<1
Desmin (DES)	<1
Alpha T-catenin (CTNNA3)	<1
Cadherin C (CDH2)	<1

Adapted from Girolami et al. [33]

without phenotypic expression, for certain conditions such as Marfan syndrome or HCM; however, recent guidelines from the European Association of Preventive Cardiology have liberalized these restrictions [12, 13]. Diagnosing and treating athletes with aortopathies secondary to Marfan syndrome, with HCM, and with LQTS will be discussed in detail in subsequent chapters.

Specific Genetic Disorders in Which Competitive Exercise Is Discouraged

Arrhythmogenic Cardiomyopathy

Arrhythmogenic cardiomyopathy (AC) is an inherited cardiac disease characterized by fibrofatty myocardial replacement of the ventricle. Myocardial atrophy is a genetically determined process that occurs progressively with time, starting from the epicardium and extending toward the myocardium. This atrophy leads to life-threatening ventricular arrhythmias and eventual impairment of ventricular systolic function. Originally described as only arrhythmogenic right ventricular cardiomyopathy/dysplasia (ARVC/D), increased recognition of left ventricular involvement (ALVC) has led to adoption of the broader term AC, which incorporates a multitude of cardiac muscle disorders, not explained by ischemic, hypertensive, or valvular heart disease [14]. ARVC and ALVC are genetically and clinically heterogeneous disorders. ARVC is probably the best characterized AC with a prevalence of around 1:2000–1:5000. ARVC is considered one of the major causes of sudden death in young individuals and in athletes, especially in some countries such as Italy and Denmark. ARVC is generally associated with ECG alterations including epsilon waves, negative T-waves in right precordial leads, prolonged S-wave upstroke in precordial leads, progressive conduction disease, and ventricular arrhythmias with a left bundle branch block (LBBB) morphology. Holter and extended rhythm monitoring, echocardiography, and cardiac MRI are useful diagnostic tools. Typically, arrhythmias are the earliest manifestation of this disease. The 2010 Adult Task Force Criteria established diagnostic tools to help identify ARVC [15]. At the present time, similar diagnostic criteria for ALVC have not been established. ARVC is most often autosomal dominant; however recessive forms exist as well. ARVC is frequently caused by mutations in desmosomal genes, which account for 50–60% of all ARVC patients. These mutations lead to alterations in the desmosomal proteins which disturbs cell-to-cell contact. ARVC is often caused by mutations in desmosomal genes such as:

- Desmoplakin (DSP, prevalence ~10%)
- Desmoglein-2 (DSG2, prevalence ~40%)
- Plakophilin-2 (PKP2, prevalence ~40%)
- Desmocollin-2 (DSC2, prevalence ~3%)

In addition, mutations in ion channels such as ryanodine receptor (RYR2) and sodium voltage-gated channel alpha subunit 5 (SCN5a) are associated with ARVC. Meanwhile, ALVC is most often caused by mutations involved in the sarcoplasmic reticulum, sarcomere, ion channels, and mitochondria, such as:

- Lamin A/C (LMNA)
- Transmembrane protein 43 (TMEM43)
- RNA binding motif protein 20 (RBM20)
- Filamin C (FLNC)

Therefore multi-gene panel testing is recommended to identify the genetic etiology for AC. Almost 40% of patients with AC will have no identifiable mutation. These gene-elusive cases may represent oligogenic forms with unknown, low-penetrant genetic variants and/or external factors that lead to disease pathogenesis. The most important objective of clinical treatment of AC is prevention of disease progression and SCD. Current therapeutic options include lifestyle changes, beta-blockers, antiarrhythmic medications, catheter ablation, implantable cardioverter defibrillator (ICD), and heart transplantation. Physical exercise is one of the most important factors which promotes and accelerates the phenotypic expression of ARVC. There is significant evidence that a dose-dependent relationship exists between endurance exercise and likelihood of developing ARVC. In the 2015 AHA/ACC Eligibility and Disqualification Recommendations, athletes with definitive and even borderline ARVC are discouraged from competitive or endurance sports participation [11]. Athletes should be discouraged from high-intensity exercise even if they are phenotype-negative but genotype-positive for ARVC, as exercise may accelerate the development of a cardiomyopathy and may increase the risk of ventricular arrhythmias in otherwise asymptomatic subjects.

Catecholaminergic Polymorphic Ventricular Tachycardia

Catecholaminergic polymorphic ventricular tachycardia (CPVT) is an inheritable cardiac channelopathy with associated symptoms of syncope or catecholamine-mediated ventricular arrhythmias that may result in cardiac arrest. Patients with

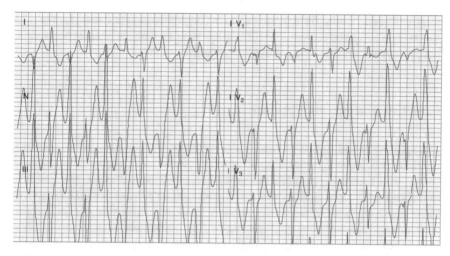

Fig. 4.1 Bidirectional ventricular tachycardia in patient with catecholaminergic polymorphic ventricular tachycardia. (Reprinted with permission. Monteforte et al. [31]. Elsevier Spain)

CPVT present with palpitations or syncope during physical or emotional stress. CPVT is a clinically and genetically heterogeneous disease presenting with a spectrum of polymorphic arrhythmias. CPVT is an uncommon condition with a prevalence as low as around 1:10,000–1:50,000. The diagnosis of CPVT relies on demonstration of ventricular arrhythmias during standard noninvasive exercise treadmill testing or epinephrine drug challenge [16]. A positive test is defined by the development of complex ventricular ectopy, bidirectional ventricular tachycardia (VT), and/or polymorphic VT (Fig. 4.1). Holter monitoring should be used as an adjunctive diagnostic tool. CPVT can be inherited in either an autosomal dominant or autosomal recessive pattern depending on the gene involved. CPVT is caused by mutations in genes responsible for regulating intracellular cardiac calcium. The calcium release from the sarcoplasmic reticulum can lead to calcium overload, which leads to delayed afterdepolarizations and triggered activity. The most common genetic mutations for CPVT are found in the ryanodine receptor (RYR2) which is inherited in autosomal dominant fashion and contributes to approximately 50% of CPVT cases. Alternatively, mutations in the calsequestrin (CASQ2) gene, which is inherited in an autosomal recessive fashion, account for 3% of CPVT cases. Other genes have also been implicated including ankyrin-2 (ANK2), calmodulin (CALM1), trans-2,3-enoyl-CoA reductase (TECRL), and triadin (TRDN), among others, and therefore multi-gene panel testing is recommended. Current therapeutic options include beta-blockers, calcium channel blockers, antiarrhythmic medications, ICD, and left cardiac sympathetic denervation [16]. Although there is some emerging controversy, current recommendations by the Bethesda conference and the 2015 AHA/ACC Eligibility and Disqualification Recommendations discourage athletes with symptomatic CPVT or asymptomatic CPVT with exercise-induced ventricular arrhythmias from participation in competitive sports, except for class 1A sports [17]. However, current guidelines allow athletes who are phenotype-negative but genotype-positive, to participate in competitive sports.

Genetics and Sports Performance

The sporting world, by its nature, is a competitive environment, where athletes, coaches, and trainers are seeking to provide themselves with an advantage, an "edge" over their competition. Participants in competitive sports are susceptible to influence from a rapid expansion of direct-to-consumer services with those services being provided to members of the public without any involvement of a medical practitioner. Direct-to-consumer genetic testing companies have begun offering genetic tests for athletic ability, sports performance, and injury risk. While the research to support this testing is weak, it does not prevent companies from marketing these tests to athletes, coaches, and even parents who aim to determine which sports and how competitive of a sports to place their children. Athletes and coaches are understandably focused on implementing targeted nutritional, training, and recovery strategies in order to optimize athletic performance. For this reason, athletes and coaches may be vulnerable to the allure of direct-to-consumer testing in the belief that the results can help them achieve improved performance. With the advent of direct-to-consumer genetic testing, patients are now confronting providers of all specialties to interpret genetic results. It is our responsibility, as healthcare providers, to understand the clinical utility of genetic testing in the context of athletic performance.

There have been several genes which are weakly associated but have gained traction in many sports cultures, especially in relation to athletic performance and injury, including alpha-actin 3 (ACTN3), apolipoprotein E (Apoe), and angiotensin-converting enzyme II (ACE). ACTN3 is expressed in fast-twitch type II muscle fibers, and specific polymorphisms have been associated with enhanced improvements in strength, protection from eccentric training-induced muscle damage, and sports injury. The ACTN3 R577X allele, which represents a base change in the ACTN3 gene that results in a premature stop codon and a deficiency of the protein, has been associated with improved performance in endurance athletes, while the wildtype normal allele is associated with enhanced performance in sports requiring sprinting or short burst of power [18]. Studies of Apoe have demonstrated an association between Apoe genotype and injury susceptibility, specifically in response to concussion [19]. ACE gene mutations have been associated with improved performance in endurance activities [20]. The I (insertion) allele of the ACE gene, which represents an insertion of 287 bp, has been associated with improved performance in endurance sports, while the deleted form of the variant is associated with enhanced performance in sports requiring sprinting or short burst of power. Furthermore, several single nucleotide polymorphisms (SNPs) in genes COL5A1, TNC, MMP, and GDF-5 have been identified as showing suggestive association with an increased risk of sports-related injuries; however, there is no evidence to demonstrate that they are predictive of injury risk or relevant in all ethnicities and genders [21, 22]. While data for the associations for some of these genes is fairly robust, research is underway to better understand the true impact of ACTN3, Apoe, and ACE genotypes on athletic performance.

Sports genetics as a science is incomplete; it is still hampered by small sample sizes and biased methodology [22]. Sports performance is complex and multifactorial, a result of a combination of many different genes as well as traits including gender and ethnicity, in addition to environmental factors. One of the main limitations to research and studying the genetics of athletic performance is the multifactorial nature of athletic ability. Each sports requires a unique set of physical requirements, such as increased aerobic endurance or muscular strength. Additionally, each sports requires an interaction between various body systems (cardiovascular, respiratory, nervous, musculoskeletal). Genetics is likely only one piece of the puzzle. There is no clear evidence to support routine genetic testing for the abovementioned genes on athletes as they predict only a small proportion of overall athletic performance. Currently available sports genetic tests cannot predict athletic performance with any real accuracy. Therefore, their use for patients is currently dubious at best and possibly dangerous. In 2015, a consensus statement was written by a consortium of world experts in the fields of genomics, exercise, sports performance and injury, and antidoping. The group warned against generalizing the genetic findings from observations in small, underpowered, and unvalidated athlete studies [23]. The panel of experts advocated against the use of direct-to-consumer tests for consumer interpretation or actionability. The lack of evidence-based interpretation of test results may result in aspiring athletes being provided with inappropriate advice about their suitability for specific sports, which could be detrimental to their physical and psychological health. The use of this information should never be used for inclusion or exclusion in predicting performance or in talent identification [23].

Furthermore, while gene therapy has shown a potential promise in the treatment of specific diseases, it is feasible that the same technology will attempt to be adopted by athletes seeking to enhance their performance. The field of gene therapy and, by extension, gene doping is full of unpredictable and dangerous results. In 2018, gene doping was defined and prohibited by the World Anti-Doping Agency (WADA) as the "nontherapeutic use of genes, genetic elements and/or cells that have the capacity to enhance athletic performance" [24].

Concerns Regarding Genetic Testing for Sports Employment

Given the growing use and importance of genetic information in sports and for athletes, there has been rising concerns about privacy and discrimination, especially when it comes to employment. Table 4.4 delineates the global timeline of genetic testing in sports. There is a concern that coaches and team owners may attempt to

Table 4.4 Global timeline of genetic testing in sports

Year	Events
1968	Chromosome testing by the International Olympic Committee designed to identify males potentially disguised as females
2001	Professional Boxing and Martial Arts Board of Victoria considers compulsory genetic screening for APOE4 variant in boxers
2003	World Anti-Doping Agency prohibits methods of gene doping
2005	Eighteen Australian male rugby players were tested and analyzed for 11 genes The Chicago Bulls attempt genetic testing of Eddy Curry for HCM
2009	23andMe conducted the genetic analysis of 100 both former and current NFL players Major League Baseball uses genetic testing with prospective players from the Dominican Republic and other Latin American countries for age and identification
2010	The National Collegiate Athletic Association implements mandatory sickle cell trait screening for Division 1 in 2010, Division II in 2011, and Division III in 2013
2011	Club manager of Premier Football League team has players DNA analyzed to determine how injury-prone they are
2012	The National Football League screens for genetic conditions sickle cell trait and G6PD under the 2011 NFL collective bargaining agreement
2014	English Institute of Sports expresses interest in the integration of genetic technologies to "tailor the training, conditioning, and preparation" of Britain's Olympic and Paralympic athletes
2015	Two Barclays Premier League soccer teams commission tests of their players' DNA for 45 variants
2018	Uzbekistan announced DNA testing on children to determine their physical abilities Ex-NHL player Gary Roberts used genetic testing on his NHL clients to tailor training program at his gym China's Ministry of Science and Technology announced genetic testing of all athletes in Winter Olympics 2022 as part of their evaluation for participation

Adapted from Goodlin et al. [34]

use players' genetic information to predict their medical futures and/or athletic potentials and, accordingly, decide how much or whether to pay the athlete. In 2005, a National Basketball Association team concerned about the health of player, Eddy Curry, required him to submit a genetic test for HCM before they would renew his contract. He refused and signed with another team that did not require genetic testing [25]. Confronted with cases of false identity and age falsification by Latin American baseball prospects, Major League Baseball has conducted genetic testing on some promising young players and their parents. To combat the potential for misuse and discrimination with genetic testing in the United States, the Genetic Information Nondiscrimination Act (GINA), first proposed by Representative Slaughter in 1995, was signed almost unanimously in 2008 to prohibit some types of genetic discrimination for health insurance and employment [26]. The purpose of GINA was to remove the temptation and prohibit employers from asking or receiving genetic information.

Conclusions

Genomics is a rapidly advancing field of medicine. Due to cost reductions and improved technology, genetic research and testing have become widely available outside of the medical community and accessible directly to consumers such as sports organizations, coaches, and athletes. As a result, the international medical community has debated at length regarding the role of cardiovascular genetic screening with respect to sports participation. The dialogue has encompassed medical, ethical, and legal concerns of both the international medical community and sports organizations [27]. Currently, cardiac screening before athletic participation on a national level occurs in the United States, Israel, and Italy, as well as within high-level sports organizations [28]. Directed utilization of genetic screening (whether single gene, multi-gene panel, WGS/WES) has slowly become integrated into this diagnostic armamentarium. With regard to pre-participation screening, the medical community recognizes that there are certain clinical scenarios that warrant genetic scrutiny:

1. Patient that manifests a phenotype suspicious for a possible cardiovascular disorder adversely affected by sports activity
2. Patient who has a family history of an inheritable cardiovascular disorder or sudden death

Interpretation of any genetic results in athletes should be undertaken by a healthcare team composed of genetic counselors and physicians familiar with the care of athletes in order to avoid inconsistent messaging to athletes, as well as to aid in the proper interpretation of disease risk predictions from direct-to-consumer companies, as noted by a report from the US Government Accountability Office [29]. Misinterpretation of genetic data can lead to inappropriate advice about suitability for a specific sporting activity that may adversely impact the physical or psychological health of an individual [30]. In the end, the role of genetic testing in sports medicine is to advance personalized medicine based on validated genetic data to be used for the protection of the health and safety of the athlete.

References

1. Brugada R, Campuzano O, Sarquella-Brugada G, et al. Brugada syndrome. 2005 Mar 31 [Updated 2016 Nov 17]. In: Adam MP, Ardinger HH, Pagon RA, et al., editors. GeneReviews [Internet]. Seattle (WA): University of Washington; 1993–2019. Available from: https://www.ncbi.nih.gov/books/NBK1517.
2. Richards S, Aziz N, Bale S, Laboratory Quality Assurance Committee, et al. Standards and guidelines for the interpretation of sequence variants: a joint consensus recommendation of the American College of Medical Genetics and Genomics and the Association of Molecular Pathology. Genet Med. 2015;17(5):405–24.
3. Green RC, Berg JS, Grody WW, et al. ACMG Recommendations for reporting of incidental findings in clinical exome and genome sequencing. Genet Med. 2013;15(7):565–74.

 4. Cooper DN, Krawczak M, Polychronakos C, Tyler-Smith C, Kehrer-Sawatzk H. Where genotype is not predictive of phenotype: towards an understanding of the molecular basis of reduced penetrance in human inherited disease. Hum Genet. 2013;132(10):1077–130.
 5. Maron BJ. The paradox of exercise. N Engl J Med. 2000;343:1409–11.
 6. Wasfy MM, Hutter AM, Weiner RB. Sudden cardiac death in athletes. Methodist Debakey Cardiovasc J. 2016;12(2):76–80.
 7. Harmon KG, Asif IM, Maleszewski JJ, et al. Incidence, cause, and comparative frequency of sudden cardiac death in National Collegiate Athletic Association Athletes: a decade in review. Circulation. 2015;132(1):10–9.
 8. Roberts WO, Stovitz SD. Incidence of sudden cardiac death in Minnesota high school athletes 1993–2012 screened with a standardized pre-participation evaluation. J Am Coll Cardiol. 2013;62:1298–301.
 9. Steinvil A, Chundadze T, Zeltser D, et al. Mandatory electrocardiographic screening of athletes to reduce their risk for sudden death proven fact or wishful thinking? J Am Coll Cardiol. 2011;57:1291–6.
10. Tiziano FD, Palmieri V, Genuardi M, Zeppilli P. The role of genetic testing in the identification of young athletes with inherited primitive cardiac disorders at risk of exercise sudden death. Front Cardiovasc Med. 2016;3:28.
11. Maron BJ, Udelson JE, Bonow RO, et al. Eligibility and disqualification recommendations for competitive athletes with cardiovascular abnormalities: task force 3. Circulation. 2015;132:e273–80.
12. Pelliccia A, Zipes DP, Maron BJ. Bethesda Conference #36 and the European Society of Cardiology Consensus Recommendations revisited a comparison of U.S. and European criteria for eligibility and disqualification of competitive athletes with cardiovascular abnormalities. J Am Coll Cardiol. 2008;52(24):1990–6.
13. Pellicia A, Solberg EE, Papadakis M, et al. Recommendations for participation in competitive and leisure time sport in athletes with cardiomyopathies, myocarditis, and pericarditis: position statement of the Sport Cardiology Section of the European Association of Preventive Cardiology (EAPC). Eur Heart J. 2019;40:19–33.
14. Towbin JA, McKenna WJ, Abrams DJ, et al. 2019 HRS expert consensus statement on evaluation, risk stratification, and management of arrhythmogenic cardiomyopathy. Heart Rhythm. 2019;16(11):e373–407.
15. Marcus FI, Mckenna WJ, Sherrill D, et al. Diagnosis of arrhythmogenic right ventricular cardiomyopathy / dysplasia proposed modification of the task force criteria. Circulation. 2010;121:1533–41.
16. Lieve KV, van der Werf C, Wilde AA. Wilde catecholaminergic polymorphic ventricular tachycardia. Circ J. 2016;80(6):1285–91.
17. Panhuyzen-Goedkoop NM, Wilde AAM. Athletes with channelopathy may be eligible to play. Neth Heart J. 2018;26(3):146–53.
18. Yang N, MacArthur DG, Gulbin JP, et al. ACTN3 Genotype is associated with human elite athletic performance. Am J Hum Genet. 2003;73(3):627–31.
19. Terrell TR, Bostick RM, Abramson R, et al. Apoe, Apoe promoter and Tau genotypes and risk for concussion in college athletes. Clin J Sport Med. 2008;18(1):10–7.
20. Ma F, Yang Y, Li X, et al. The association of sport performance with ACE and ACTN3 genetic polymorphisms: a systematic review and meta-analysis. PLoS One. 2013;8(1):e54685.
21. Wagner JK. Playing with heart and soul…and genomes: sports implications and applications of personal genomics. PeerJ. 2013;1:e120.
22. Mattsson CM, Wheeler MT, Waggott D, Caleshu C, Ashley EA. Sports genetics moving forward: lessons learned from medical research. Physiol Genomics. 2016;48(3):175–82.
23. Webborn N, Williams A, McNamee M, et al. Direct-to-consumer genetic testing for predicting sports performance and talent identification: consensus statement. Br J Sports Med. 2015;49(23):1486–91.
24. The world antidoping code: international standard 2018. https://www.wada-ama.org/.

25. Beck H. Curry faces tests to evaluate risk factor. The New York Times. 5 Oct 2005.
26. The Genetic Information Nondiscrimination Act of 2008. https://www.eeoc.gov/laws/statutes/gina.cfm.
27. Magavern EF, Badalato L, Finocchiaro G, Borry P. Ethical considerations for genetic testing in the context of mandated cardiac screening before athletic participation. Genet Med. 2017;19(5):493–5.
28. Maron BJ, Friedman R, Caplan A. Ethics of preparticipation cardiovascular screening for athletes. Nat Rev Cardiol. 2015;12:1–4.
29. Direct-to-Consumer genetic tests: misleading test results are further complicated by deceptive marketing and other questionable practices: congressional testimony. US Government Accountability Office. 22 July 2010. https://www.gao.gov/products/GAO-10-847.
30. Vlahovich N, Fricker PA, Brown MA, Hughes D. Ethics of genetic testing and research in sport: a position statement from the Australian Institute of Sport. Br J Sports Med. 2017;51:5–11.
31. Monteforte N, Napolitano C, Priori SG. Genetics and arrhythmias: diagnostic and prognostic applications. Rev Esp Cardiol. 2012;65(3):278–86.
32. Kalia SS, Adelman K, Bale SJ, et al. Recommendations for reporting of secondary findings in clinical exome and genome sequencing, 2016 update (ACMG SF v2.0): a policy statement of the American College of Medical Genetics and Genomics. Genet Med. 2017;19:249–55.
33. Girolami F, Frisso G, Benelli M, et al. Contemporary genetic testing in inherited cardiac disease: tools, ethical issues, and clinical applications. J Cardiovasc Med. 2018;19:1–11.
34. Goodlin GT, Roos TR, Roos AK, Kim SK. The dawning age of genetic testing for sports injuries. Clin J Sport Med. 2015;25(1):1–5.

Chapter 5
Management of Hypertension in Athletes

D. Edmund Anstey and Daichi Shimbo

Introduction

Hypertension is a prevalent condition worldwide and a significant cause of cardiovascular morbidity and mortality [1–3]. Although hypertension prevalence is known to increase with age, its population prevalence may be high even among younger adults [1, 4, 5]. Among adults of ages 20–44 years in the United States, population surveys have found the prevalence of hypertension to be 11.2% for men and 8.7% for women when using a systolic/diastolic blood pressure threshold of 140/90 mmHg [1, 5]. Among children and adolescents, the prevalence of hypertension is approximately 3–6% [6–8]. The high prevalence of hypertension extends to all populations including competitive athletes, for whom hypertension is the most common cardiovascular condition [6]. In an analysis of professional athletes in the National Football League, the prevalence of hypertension was higher among professional football players than in age-matched controls in the US population (13.8% versus 5.5%, respectively) even after adjusting for race and body mass index [9]. In this chapter, we will discuss the implications of hypertension for the competitive athlete and the role of the clinician in the detection and management of high blood pressure.

D. E. Anstey (✉) · D. Shimbo
The Columbia Hypertension Center, Columbia University Irving Medical Center,
New York, NY, USA
e-mail: dea2123@cumc.columbia.edu; ds2231@cumc.columbia.edu

© Springer Nature Switzerland AG 2021
D. J. Engel, D. M. Phelan (eds.), *Sports Cardiology*,
https://doi.org/10.1007/978-3-030-69384-8_5

Hypertension and Cardiovascular Risk

Hypertension has been ranked as the most important risk factor for global mortality and disability adjusted life years [10]. In the general population, hypertension is a leading risk factor for morbidity and mortality, in particular stroke or myocardial infarction [2, 3]. Hypertension is also associated with an increased risk of end-organ damage including arterial stiffening, peripheral vascular disease, retinopathy, proteinuria, chronic kidney disease, and left ventricular hypertrophy [2, 3]. Despite these risks, hypertension is often undertreated and, without appropriate screening, may go undetected until after the onset of subclinical or clinical cardiovascular disease [1]. This is particularly true among young adults as younger individuals with hypertension are less likely to be aware of their hypertension status or be on appropriate treatment. In the United States, an analysis of the 2011–2012 National Health and Nutrition Examination Survey (NHANES) found that adults aged 18–39 had the lowest awareness of their hypertension status compared to those aged 40–59 and ≥60 years (61.8% versus 83.0% and 86.1%, respectively). Similarly, adults with hypertension aged 18–39, compared to those aged 40–59 and ≥60 years, were less likely to be on treatment for hypertension (44.5% versus 73.7% and 82.2%, respectively) or to have attained blood pressure control (34.4% versus 57.8% and 50.5%, respectively) [11]. Recent evidence suggests that hypertension, even at a young age, may be associated with long-term clinical and subclinical cardiovascular disease [12].

This chapter focuses on the detection and management of high blood pressure levels. Less is known about the health implications and appropriate management of acute rises in blood pressure which may occur during exercise. An increase in blood pressure during peak exercise is a normal physiologic response to increased activity. However, extreme rises in intravascular pressure in response to exercise may be pathologic. Some forms of resistance training may lead to temporary, yet significant surges in blood pressure. For example, blood pressure measurements obtained from weight lifters during peak exercise have found that intravascular pressure can reach up to 350–480 mmHg [13]. This raises concern for the potential of acute vascular complications such as aortic dissection or stroke [14]. There is insufficient evidence to know if such short-lived, but severe, rises in intravascular pressure lead to incident hypertension and an increased risk of cardiovascular disease.

Blood Pressure Measurement

A 2015 American College of Cardiology/American Heart Association Scientific Statement on Eligibility and Disqualification Criteria for Athletes with Cardiovascular Abnormalities suggested that the standard pre-participation examination for all athletes includes obtaining an accurate blood pressure [6]. Among individuals without increased blood pressure levels, the frequency with which repeat measurements are obtained is at the discretion of the performing clinician and local guidelines. Given the possible implications of detecting an increased blood pressure level in a competitive athlete – including restriction from participation in sports – recent scientific statements and guidelines have emphasized the importance of obtaining blood pressure using proper and standardized techniques [2, 3, 6]. Failing to use proper technique while measuring blood pressure can result in significant, spurious increases in measured levels. For example, common improperly performed techniques, such as using the wrong cuff size or the blood pressure cuff being placed over clothing, can result in variations of systolic blood pressure from 5 to 50 mmHg [15]. The standard techniques of blood pressure measurement are described in Table 5.1 and should be performed by an appropriately trained clinician. Some considerations of relevance to clinicians caring for athletes is the importance of using an appropriate cuff size – as many athletes may have a larger arm circumference – and avoidance of caffeine or exercise before measurement. Further, in particular for patients less than 30 years of age, if the arm pressure is high, a measurement should be obtained in one leg to evaluate for aortic coarctation [6]. To diagnose hypertension, both the 2017 American College of Cardiology/American Heart Association blood pressure guideline and the 2015 American College of Cardiology/American Heart Association Scientific Statement on Eligibility and Disqualification Criteria for Athletes with Cardiovascular Abnormalities endorsed using an average of ≥2 readings obtained on ≥2 occasions to estimate the individual's blood pressure [2, 6].

Some individuals with high blood pressure levels in the clinic may not have high blood pressure levels when measured outside of the clinic, a phenotype known as "white coat hypertension." There is increasing evidence that this is a prevalent phenotype in the general population, with a population prevalence of 13–35% [2, 3]. The prevalence of white coat hypertension specifically among athletes is unknown. It has been suggested that anxiety may be an important contributor to white coat hypertension. Anxiety may be particularly relevant to the athlete undergoing a pre-participation physical as the physician's findings may directly affect his or her eligibility for competition. When there is a suspicion of white coat hypertension, the presence of out-of-office hypertension can be confirmed using 24-hour ambulatory blood pressure monitoring (ABPM) [6]. As compared to clinic blood pressure measurements, blood pressure levels obtained during ABPM are a better predictor of cardiovascular disease events and subclinical cardiovascular disease in the general population [2, 3, 16]. Further, among individuals with high exercise blood pressure values, ABPM may better predict who will develop left ventricular hypertrophy [17]. Consistent with recent hypertension guidelines [2, 3], the 2015 American College of Cardiology/American Heart Association Scientific Statement on Eligibility and Disqualification Criteria for Athletes with Cardiovascular Abnormalities endorsed that ABPM be used to confirm the diagnosis of hypertension when white coat hypertension is suspected [6]. The 2015 scientific statement on sports eligibility by the American College of Cardiology/American Heart Association does not specifically mention whether home blood pressure monitoring (HBPM) may also be used to evaluate for the presence of white coat hypertension

Table 5.1 Proper steps for blood pressure measurement [30]

Key steps for proper BP measurements	Specific instructions
Step 1: Properly prepare the patient	1. Have the patient relax, sitting in a chair with feet flat on floor and back supported. The patient should be seated for 3–5 min without talking or moving around before recording the first BP reading. A shorter wait period is used for some AOBP devices.
	2. The patient should avoid caffeine, exercise, and smoking for at least 30 min before measurement.
	3. Ensure that the patient has emptied his/her bladder.
	4. Neither the patient nor the observer should talk during the rest period or during the measurement.
	5. Remove clothing covering the location of cuff placement.
	6. Measurements made while the patient is sitting on an examining table do not fulfill these criteria.
Step 2: Use proper technique for BP measurements	1. Use an upper-arm cuff BP measurement device that has been validated and ensure that the device is calibrated periodically.
	2. Support the patient's arm (e.g., resting on a desk). The patient should not be holding his/her arm because isometric exercise will affect the BP levels.
	3. Position the middle of the cuff on the patient's upper arm at the level of the right atrium (midpoint of the sternum).
	4. Use the correct cuff size such that the bladder encircles 75–100% of the arm.
	5. Use either the stethoscope diaphragm or bell for auscultatory readings.
Step 3: Take the proper measurements needed for diagnosis and treatment of elevated BP	1. At the first visit, record BP in both arms.[a] Use the arm that gives the higher reading for subsequent readings.
	2. Separate repeated measurements by 1–2 min.
	3. For auscultatory determinations, use a palpated estimate of radial pulse obliteration pressure to estimate SBP. Inflate the cuff 20–30 mm Hg above this level for an auscultatory determination of the BP level.
	4. For auscultatory readings, deflate the cuff pressure 2 mm Hg/s, and listen for Korotkoff sounds.
Step 4: Properly document accurate BP readings	1. Record SBP and DBP. If using the auscultatory technique, record SBP and DBP as the onset of the first of at least 2 consecutive beats and the last audible sound, respectively.
	2. Record SBP and DBP to the nearest even number.
	3. Note the time that the most recent BP medication was taken before measurements.
Step 5: Average the readings	Use an average of ≥2 readings obtained on ≥2 occasions to estimate the individual's BP.
Step 6: Provide BP readings to patient	Provide patients their SBP/DBP readings both verbally and in writing. Someone should help the patient interpret the results.

Adapted from: Muntner et al. [30]

AOBP Automated Office Blood Pressure, *BP* Blood Pressure, *DBP* Diastolic Blood Pressure, *SBP* Systolic Blood Pressure

[a]When a BP measurement is obtained in one arm followed by the other arm and the BP is substantially lower in the second arm, it is possible that the difference could be caused by acclimation. In this circumstance, BP should be remeasured in the first arm

[6]. However, recent hypertension guidelines have recommended that home blood pressure monitoring (HBPM) be considered as a reasonable alternative to ABPM for cases when ABPM is unavailable or poorly tolerated [2, 3]. Thresholds for defining hypertension on ABPM and HBPM are shown in Table 5.2.

Diagnosing Hypertension

Hypertension is diagnosed when a measured blood pressure exceeds a prespecified blood pressure threshold (Table 5.2) [2, 3]. In children and adolescents, blood pressure may vary by individual characteristics including age, sex, and height [8, 18]. The threshold to establish a diagnosis of hypertension in children is therefore dependent on these variables and is defined by blood pressure level >95% of that predicted by their age, sex, height, and weight. Among adolescents age ≥13 years, hypertension is defined by a systolic/diastolic blood pressure ≥130/80 mmHg [8, 18].

There has been recent debate regarding what threshold should be used to define hypertension among adults. The Seventh Report of the Joint National Committee on Prevention, Detection, Evaluation, and Treatment of High Blood Pressure states that a systolic/diastolic blood pressure threshold of 140/90 mmHg should be used to define hypertension [19]. The 2015 American College of Cardiology/American Heart Association Scientific Statement on Eligibility and Disqualification Criteria for Athletes with Cardiovascular Abnormalities also used the 140/90 mmHg threshold to define hypertension among those ≥18 years of age [6]. However growing evidence has found that a lower blood pressure threshold may be appropriate in order to effectively identify and treat individuals at increased cardiovascular disease risk. The 2017 American College of Cardiology/American Heart Association blood pressure guideline created a new classification system, which defined stage 1 hypertension as a systolic/diastolic blood pressure of 130–139/80–89 mmHg and stage 2 hypertension as systolic/diastolic blood pressure ≥140/90 mmHg [2]. As it relates to the competitive athlete, it is unclear what, if any, implications may result from using the lower 130/80 mmHg threshold. Potential implications for treatment of hypertension using these updated thresholds are discussed further below.

Workup of Hypertension

Any individual in whom hypertension is detected should undergo a subsequent thorough history and physical exam as well as laboratory tests. Key components of the focused history include determining if there is a family history of cardiovascular disease or hypertension. A history should also include an evaluation for symptoms which may reflect secondary causes of hypertension, such as pheochromocytoma (headache, diaphoresis, palpitations, or paroxysms of hypertension), Cushing's

Table 5.2 Thresholds for classifying hypertension on ambulatory blood pressure monitoring and using clinic blood pressure according to major hypertension society guidelines

	Clinic blood pressure thresholds for defining hypertension	Ambulatory blood pressure thresholds for defining hypertension	Home blood pressure thresholds for defining hypertension
ADULTS			
2018 ESC/ESH [3]	Grade 1 hypertension: 140–159/90–99 mmHg Grade 2 hypertension: 160–179/100–109 mmHg Grade 3 hypertension: ≥180/110 mmHg	Daytime ≥135/85 mmHg Nighttime ≥120/70 mmHg 24-hour ≥130/80 mmHg	≥135/85 mmHg
2017 ACC/AHA [2]	Stage 1 hypertension: 130–139/80–89 mmHg Stage 2 hypertension: ≥140/90 mmHg	Daytime ≥135/85 mmHg	≥130/80 mmHg
2017 The Hypertension Canada [31]	AOBP hypertension: ≥135/85 mmHg Non-AOBP hypertension: ≥140/90 mmHg	Daytime ≥135/85 mmHg 24-hour ≥130/80 mmHg	≥135/85 mmHg
2015 ACC/AHA Eligibility and Disqualification Recommendation for Competitive Athletes [6]	Hypertension: ≥140/90 mmHg	*Not specified*	*Not specified*
2011 UK NICE [32]	Hypertension: ≥140/90 mmHg	Daytime ≥135/85 mmHg	≥135/85 mmHg
2003 JNC 7 [19]	Stage 1 hypertension: 140–159/90–99 mmHg Stage 2 hypertension: ≥160/100 mmHg	Daytime ≥135/85 mmHg Nighttime ≥120/70 mmHg	≥130/80 mmHg
CHILDREN/ADOLESCENTS			
2018 AAFP [8]	*Age 1–12 years* Stage 1 hypertension: Blood pressure ≥95 percentile for age, height, and sex OR 130–139/80–89 mmHg (whichever is lower) Stage 2 hypertension: Blood pressure ≥95 percentile for age, height, and sex +12 mmHg or ≥140/90 mmHg (whichever is lower) *Age ≥ 13 years* Stage 1 hypertension: 130–139/80–89 mmHg Stage 2 hypertension: ≥140/90 mmHg	*Not specified*	*Not specified*

| 2017 AAP [18] | *Age 1–12 years*
Stage 1 hypertension: Blood pressure ≥95 percentile to <95th percentile +12 mmHg for age, height, and sex OR 130–139/80–89 mmHg (whichever is lower)
Stage 2 hypertension: Blood pressure ≥95 percentile for age, height, and sex +12 mmHg or ≥140/90 mmHg (whichever is lower)

Age ≥ 13 years
Stage 1 hypertension: 130–139/80–89 mmHg
Stage 2 hypertension: ≥140/90 mmHg | Mean SBP and DBP >95th percentile and SBP and DBP load[a] >25% | *Not Specified* |

AAFP American Academy of Family Physicians, *AAP* American Academy of Pediatrics, *ACC/AHA* American College of Cardiology/American Heart Association, *AOBP* Automated office blood pressure, *ESC/ESH* European Society of Cardiology/European Society of Hypertension, *JNC 7* Seventh Report of the Joint National Committee on Prevention, Detection, Evaluation, and Treatment of High Blood Pressure, *SBP* Systolic Blood Pressure, *DBP* Diastolic Blood Pressure, *UK NICE* United Kingdom National Institute for Health and Care Excellence

[a]Load is defined as the percentage of valid ambulatory SBP and DBP measurements above a set threshold value (e.g., 95th percentile)

syndrome (rapid weight gain, central fat distribution), or hyperthyroidism and hypothyroidism (heat/cold intolerance, dry skin, weight fluctuations) [2]. Athletes should specifically be asked about the use of drugs or behaviors which may increase blood pressure (Table 5.3). Many prescribed, over-the-counter, and illicitly used medications and supplements are known to result in rises in blood pressure. Non-steroidal anti-inflammatory drugs, which may be indicated as an over-the-counter pain killer or anti-inflammatory, are associated with increased blood pressure. Recreational drugs such as cocaine or amphetamines can also increase blood pressure [2, 20]. Athletes should be screened for the use of other substances including caffeine and workout supplements, in particular those containing ephedra. Nicotine and tobacco use should also be evaluated. Performance-enhancing drugs, including human growth hormone and anabolic steroids, may also increase blood pressure levels [21]. Finally, exogenous erythropoietin and erythropoiesis-stimulating agents, which may be used to improve aerobic performance, are a known cause of hypertension among certain populations [22].

A focused physical examination should also be performed to look for signs which may suggest a secondary cause of hypertension. Pulses should be examined in all four extremities as diminished pulses may suggest underlying vascular disease. Younger athletes in particular should have an assessment of upper and lower extremity blood pressure to rule out previously undetected coarctation [6]. An abdominal exam should be performed, including an auscultatory assessment for an abdominal bruit which may be a sign of renovascular hypertension [6]. Patients should be examined for cushingoid features (abdominal striae, moon facies, buffalo hump, thinned skin, etc.) suggestive of elevated adrenocortical hormones. The physical examination should also include a fundoscopic exam, palpation of the thyroid gland, and cardiac auscultation.

A focused laboratory workup should look for evidence of end-organ damage and assess for global cardiovascular risk. This includes testing for diabetes and glucose intolerance, dyslipidemia, hemoglobin, thyroid dysfunction, and proteinuria and chronic kidney disease. A 12-lead electrocardiogram is suggested, but not mandated, by the 2015 American College of Cardiology/American Heart Association Scientific Statement on Eligibility and Disqualification Criteria for Athletes with Cardiovascular Abnormalities to evaluate for left ventricular hypertrophy or conduction abnormalities [6]. If obtained, the electrocardiogram should be interpreted by a physician familiar with evaluating electrocardiograms of athletes and experienced in distinguishing normal physiologic changes in an athlete's electrocardiogram from abnormal changes indicative of pathology [23]. An electrocardiogram in isolation has high specificity but poor sensitivity for left ventricular hypertrophy [6]. The American College of Cardiology/American Heart Association also suggests that an echocardiogram to detect left ventricular hypertrophy may be obtained in some circumstances: in individuals with a systolic blood pressure ≥160 mmHg, diastolic blood pressure ≥100 mmHg, or evidence of hypertensive-related target organ damage. If an echocardiogram is pursued, it is important to distinguish pathologic, hypertension-mediated hypertrophy from physiologic changes that may be present in an athlete's heart [6]. There are special

Table 5.3 Frequently used medications and substances that may cause elevated blood pressure [2]

Agent	Possible management
Alcohol	Limit alcohol to ≤1 drink daily for women and ≤2 drinks for men
Amphetamines (e.g., amphetamine, methylphenidate dexmethylphenidate, dextroamphetamine)	Discontinue or decrease dose Consider behavioral therapies for ADHD
Antidepressants (e.g., MAOIs, SNRIs, TCAs)	Consider alternative agents (e.g., SSRIs) depending on indication Avoid tyramine-containing foods with MAOIs
Atypical antipsychotics (e.g., clozapine, olanzapine)	Discontinue or limit use when possible Consider behavior therapy where appropriate Recommend lifestyle modification Consider alternative agents associated with lower risk of weight gain, diabetes mellitus, and dyslipidemia (e.g., aripiprazole, ziprasidone)
Caffeine	Generally limit caffeine intake to <300 mg/d Avoid use in patients with uncontrolled hypertension Coffee use in patients with hypertension is associated with acute increases in BP; long-term use is not associated with increased BP or CVD
Decongestants (e.g., phenylephrine, pseudoephedrine)	Use for shortest duration possible and avoid in severe or uncontrolled hypertension Consider alternative therapies (e.g., nasal saline, intranasal corticosteroids, antihistamines) as appropriate
Herbal supplements (e.g., Ma Huang [ephedra], St. John's wort [with MAO inhibitors, yohimbine])	Avoid use
Immunosuppressants (e.g., cyclosporine)	Consider converting to tacrolimus, which may be associated with fewer effects on BP
Oral contraceptives	Use low-dose (e.g., 20–30 mcg ethinyl estradiol) agents or a progestin-only form of contraception, or consider alternative forms of birth control where appropriate (e.g., barrier, abstinence, IUD) Avoid use in women with uncontrolled hypertension
Performance-enhancing drugs (e.g., erythropoietin, human growth hormone)	Avoid or limit use when possible
NSAIDs	Avoid systemic NSAIDs when possible Consider alternative analgesics (e.g., acetaminophen, tramadol, topical NSAIDs), depending on indication and risk
Recreational drugs (e.g., "bath salts" [MDPV], cocaine, methamphetamine, etc.)	Discontinue or avoid use
Systemic corticosteroids (e.g., dexamethasone, fludrocortisone, methylprednisolone, prednisone, prednisolone)	Avoid or limit use when possible Consider alternative modes of administration (e.g., inhaled, topical) when feasible
Tyrosine kinase inhibitors (e.g., sunitinib, sorafenib) and angiogenesis inhibitor (e.g., bevacizumab)	Initiate or intensify antihypertensive therapy

Modified from: Whelton et al. [2]

considerations and workup for children who are diagnosed with hypertension. An echocardiogram is suggested for children with a new diagnosis of hypertension when considering pharmacologic treatment of hypertension [8, 18].

Treatment of Hypertension

The decision on whom to treat and when and how to initiate lifestyle modification or antihypertensive therapy is an important decision which should be made collaboratively with both the clinician and the patient. Special circumstances for the competitive athlete which should be taken into consideration include his or her desire to continue training, maintain peak performance, and not be disqualified from competitive sport due to use of a banned substance. Therefore, all treatment options including pharmacologic treatment and lifestyle modifications should be discussed as a means to shared decision-making between the patient and provider.

As previously mentioned, the 2017 American College of Cardiology/American Heart Association blood pressure guideline defined stage 1 hypertension as a systolic/diastolic blood pressure of 130–139/80–89 mmHg and stage 2 hypertension as systolic/diastolic blood pressure ≥140/90 mmHg [2]. According to these guidelines, individuals with stage 2 hypertension should be initiated on antihypertensive medications along with lifestyle modifications, independent of predicted cardiovascular disease risk [2]. Individuals with stage 1 hypertension and an estimated 10-year predicted cardiovascular disease risk ≥10% should also be initiated on antihypertensive medication along with lifestyle modifications. Individuals with stage 1 hypertension who are otherwise not at increased cardiovascular disease risk are recommended lifestyle modification only and do not require initiation of antihypertensive medication.

The treatment implications of applying the lower 130/80 mmHg threshold to athletes is unknown. Using the lower threshold, many individuals will be newly labeled as having stage I hypertension. However, given the younger age and low estimated 10-year cardiovascular disease risk among athletes, it is possible that many athletes with stage 1 hypertension will be recommended lifestyle modification to reduce blood pressure but not recommended to initiate antihypertensive medication [24]. Therefore, while some individuals may be labeled as having hypertension, not all will require pharmacologic treatment [24].

There are many lifestyle modifications which have been shown to effectively reduce blood pressure and prevent or delay the need for initiating antihypertensive therapy (Table 5.4). Practical recommendations for all individuals with hypertension include weight loss, improved diet with particular attention to decreased sodium intake, and increased physical activity. For most athletes with hypertension, regular intense physical activity may already be a part of their daily lives. However, a change in the type of activity performed may result in decreased blood pressure levels among some individuals. There is some evidence to suggest that the effect of exercise on blood pressure may relate to the type of exercise performed [25, 26]. In

Table 5.4 Non-pharmacologic recommendations for blood pressure control for individuals with hypertension [2]

Non-pharmacologic recommendation	Dose/description	Estimated impact on systolic blood pressure (for individuals with hypertension)
Weight loss is recommended for individuals who are overweight or obese	Target ideal body weight, goal of at least 1 kg reduction in body weight but greater weight loss associated with greater reduction in blood pressure	−5 mmHg
Sodium reduction and a low sodium diet	Optimal goal of <1500 mg/d total or reduction of 1000 mg/d	−5/6 mmHg
DASH (Dietary Approaches to Stop Hypertension) diet	Diet rich in whole grain, fruits, vegetables, low-fat dairy products, and reduced saturated and total fats	−11 mmHg
Potassium supplementation if not contraindicated	Goal of 3500–5000 mg/d by eating a diet rich in potassium	−4/5 mmHg
Increased physical activity:		
Aerobic exercise	90–150 min/week 65–75% heart rate reserve	−5/8 mmHg
Dynamic resistance	90–150 min/week 50–80% 1 rep maximum 6 exercises, 3 sets/exercise, 10 repetitions/set	−4 mmHg
Isometric resistance	4 × 2 min (hand grip), 1 min rest between exercises 30–40% maximum voluntary contraction, 3 sessions/week 8–10 weeks	−5 mmHg
Decreased alcohol consumption	In individuals who drink alcohol, reduce alcohol to: Men: ≤2 drinks daily Women: ≤1 drink daily	−4 mmHg

Adapted from: Whelton et al. [2]

an observational study of adult athletes, blood pressure levels were lower in athletes participating in those sports which emphasize "dynamic" exercise (those relying on endurance training such as cycling or swimming) as compared to those engaged in "static" exercise (those relying on heavy resistance training such as weightlifting or body-building) [25]. In a retrospective analysis of the preparticipation physical examinations of male college athletes in the United States, the prevalence of hypertension was significantly higher among football players compared to non-football players (19.2% versus 7.0%, respectively) [27]. Such data have led to a suggestion that athletes with hypertension who perform static sports or exercise should consider performing regular aerobic exercise in order to decrease blood pressure levels [20]. In general, a combination of aerobic and resistance training is considered the optimal exercise strategy to decrease blood pressure [28].

All individuals with hypertension should be advised to avoid substances which may increase blood pressure or cardiovascular disease risk including heavy alcohol use, tobacco or drug abuse, or other substances as elicited from the history. When counseling an athlete, particular attention should be paid to prescribed or over-the-counter medications which may increase blood pressure levels including non-steroidal anti-inflammatory drugs, anabolic steroids, or growth hormones.

In some individuals, either due to the severity of hypertension or failure of lifestyle modifications to adequately reduce blood pressure, it will be necessary to initiate antihypertensive therapy. Regarding the management of hypertension in the general population, the 2017 American College of Cardiology/American Heart Association blood pressure guideline recommended thiazide diuretics, calcium channel blockers, and angiotensin-converting enzyme inhibitors or angiotensin receptor blockers as first-line therapy when initiating antihypertension medication. For individuals with a blood pressure $\geq 160/100$ mmHg, initiating two first-line drugs, of different classes, is also recommended. These strategies should also be effective at reducing blood pressure and decreasing risk for cardiovascular disease events among competitive athletes with hypertension. However, when choosing a treatment regimen for the competitive athlete, there are special considerations which may affect and potentially restrict treatment options. One principle of managing hypertension for the competitive athlete is that clinicians should identify and avoid medications that may limit exercise capacity. Another consideration, of particular relevance to professional athletes, is whether the prescribed medication regimen is banned by the governing body of the athletes' sport. The World Anti-Doping Agency was founded by the International Olympics Committee to standardize and monitor the world anti-doping code and regularly publishes a list of banned substances for competitive sports [29]. While many organizations have adopted the World Anti-Doping Agencies polices, the substance restrictions and/or collective bargaining agreement for each athlete's specific sport should be reviewed prior to initiating any new antihypertensive medication regimen.

For competitive athletes, vasodilator therapies including dihydropyridine calcium channel blockers, angiotensin-converting enzyme inhibitors, and angiotensin receptors blockers are reasonable first-line antihypertensive therapies, specifically for many athletes. In addition to being effective for the treatment of hypertension and reducing blood pressure, these drugs minimally impede athletic performance, do not have to be withheld or dose reduced during competitive training, and are not banned by major regulatory sports agencies. Diuretics may also be very effective for treating hypertension; however, their use in athletes may be limited as these agents can decrease total circulating volume and result in impaired athletic performance. This may be particularly limiting in sports with high aerobic demands. Diuretics are also banned by many governing bodies including the World Anti-doping Agency, the NCAA, the NFL, and the NBA as they are considered "masking agents," which can be used to conceal the presence of anabolic steroids [29]. Beta-blockers are not ideal first-line therapy for many athletes as they can lead to fatigue, blunt an individual's heart rate response, and impair peak physical performance. Beta-blockers are also banned from use in certain precision sports such as archery, golf, and shooting [29]. In some sports, beta-blockers may be allowed for use when not in competition but are prohibited specifically during the time surrounding competitive play. For reference, the World Anti-Doping Agency provides an annual, publicly available banned substance list which can be found at www.wada-ama.org, specifying what substances are prohibited both in- and out-of-competition and which are banned by particular sports. Practitioners who are considering prescribing beta-blockers should consult the banned substances list from the respective governing agencies of their patient's sport prior to treatment. If there are special circumstances which require that an athlete take a banned substance – for example using a beta-blocker as secondary prevention for myocardial infarction – a therapeutic use exemption can be issued by some agencies including the World Anti-Doping Agency through a formalized application and review process.

Protocols for starting dose, subsequent follow-up, and dose titration should be the same for athletes and non-athletes. As is true for the general population, athletes with hypertension on medical therapy should be routinely monitored to follow-up blood pressure responses, to evaluate for any adverse drug effects, and to confirm treatment adherence.

Clearance for Participation in Sport

The 2015 American College of Cardiology/American Heart Association Scientific Statement on Eligibility and Disqualification Criteria for Athletes with Cardiovascular Abnormalities suggested it is reasonable that the presence of a systolic/diastolic blood pressure 140–159/90–99 mmHg in the absence of target organ damage should not limit an individual's eligibility for competitive sports [6]. Individuals with very high blood pressure (systolic blood pressure ≥ 160 mmHg or diastolic blood pressure ≥ 100 mmHg) should be restricted from sports, particularly sports that are considered to be high in static exercise which may further increase blood pressure (weight lifting, boxing, wrestling) until blood pressure is better controlled. As previously discussed, individuals diagnosed as having very high blood pressure or evidence of hypertensive-related target organ damage should undergo a screening echocardiogram. If the echocardiogram shows hypertensive heart disease which, when possible, should be distinguished from the "athlete's heart," involvement in sports should be limited until blood pressure is controlled.

Conclusions

Hypertension is common in the general population and is present among many athletes of all ages. Untreated, hypertension can lead to significant cardiovascular morbidity and mortality. With appropriate screening, hypertension can be effectively detected and managed without necessarily disqualifying an individual from competitive sport. Clinicians caring for athletes should develop treatment strategies in collaboration with their patients to ensure that treatment does not interfere with competitive play, while also helping patients to ensure the best long-term health outcomes.

References

1. Whelton PK. The elusiveness of population-wide high blood pressure control. Annu Rev Public Health. 2015;36:109–30.
2. Whelton PK, Carey RM, Aronow WS, et al. 2017 ACC/AHA/AAPA/ABC/ACPM/AGS/APhA/ASH/ASPC/NMA/PCNA guideline for the prevention, detection, evaluation, and management of high blood pressure in adults: executive summary: a report of the American College of Cardiology/American Heart Association task force on clinical practice guidelines. Hypertension. 2018;71(6):1269–324.
3. Williams B, Mancia G, Spiering W, et al. 2018 ESC/ESH guidelines for the management of arterial hypertension. Eur Heart J. 2018;39(33):3021–104.
4. Go AS, Mozaffarian D, Roger VL, et al. Heart disease and stroke statistics--2013 update: a report from the American Heart Association. Circulation. 2013;127(1):e6–e245.
5. Health, United States, 2013: with special feature on prescription drugs. Hyattsville, MD; 2014.
6. Black HR, Sica D, Ferdinand K, et al. Eligibility and disqualification recommendations for competitive athletes with cardiovascular abnormalities: task force 6: hypertension: a scientific statement from the American Heart Association and the American College of Cardiology. Circulation. 2015;132(22):e298–302.
7. McNiece KL, Poffenbarger TS, Turner JL, Franco KD, Sorof JM, Portman RJ. Prevalence of hypertension and pre-hypertension among adolescents. J Pediatr. 2007;150(6):640–4, 644 e641.
8. Riley M, Hernandez AK, Kuznia AL. High blood pressure in children and adolescents. Am Fam Physician. 2018;98(8):486–94.
9. Tucker AM, Vogel RA, Lincoln AE, et al. Prevalence of cardiovascular disease risk factors among National Football League players. JAMA. 2009;301(20):2111–9.
10. Lim SS, Vos T, Flaxman AD, et al. A comparative risk assessment of burden of disease and injury attributable to 67 risk factors and risk factor clusters in 21 regions, 1990–2010: a systematic analysis for the Global Burden of Disease Study 2010. Lancet. 2012;380(9859):2224–60.
11. Nwankwo T, Yoon SS, Burt V, Gu Q. Hypertension among adults in the United States: National Health and Nutrition Examination Survey, 2011–2012. NCHS data brief, no 133. Hyattsville, MD: National Center for Health Statistics; 2013; https://www.cdc.gov/nchs/data/databriefs/db133.pdf.
12. Yano Y, Reis JP, Colangelo LA, et al. Association of blood pressure classification in young adults using the 2017 American College of Cardiology/American Heart Association blood pressure guideline with cardiovascular events later in life. JAMA. 2018;320(17):1774–82.
13. MacDougall JD, Tuxen D, Sale DG, Moroz JR, Sutton JR. Arterial blood pressure response to heavy resistance exercise. J Appl Physiol (1985). 1985;58(3):785–90.
14. Hatzaras I, Tranquilli M, Coady M, Barrett PM, Bible J, Elefteriades JA. Weight lifting and aortic dissection: more evidence for a connection. Cardiology. 2007;107(2):103–6.
15. Handler J. The importance of accurate blood pressure measurement. Perm J. 2009;13(3):51–4.
16. Banegas JR, Ruilope LM, de la Sierra A, et al. Relationship between clinic and ambulatory blood-pressure measurements and mortality. N Engl J Med. 2018;378(16):1509–20.
17. Zanettini JO, Pisani Zanettini J, Zanettini MT, Fuchs FD. Correction of the hypertensive response in the treadmill testing by the work performance improves the prediction of hyper-

tension by ambulatory blood pressure monitoring and incidence of cardiac abnormalities by echocardiography: results of an eight year follow-up study. Int J Cardiol. 2010;141(3):243–9.

18. Flynn JT, Kaelber DC, Baker-Smith CM, et al. Clinical practice guideline for screening and management of high blood pressure in children and adolescents. Pediatrics. 2017;140(3):e20171904.

19. Chobanian AV, Bakris GL, Black HR, et al. The seventh report of the Joint National Committee on prevention, detection, evaluation, and treatment of high blood pressure: the JNC 7 report. JAMA. 2003;289(19):2560–72.

20. Leddy JJ, Izzo J. Hypertension in athletes. J Clin Hypertens (Greenwich). 2009;11(4):226–33.

21. Achar S, Rostamian A, Narayan SM. Cardiac and metabolic effects of anabolic-androgenic steroid abuse on lipids, blood pressure, left ventricular dimensions, and rhythm. Am J Cardiol. 2010;106(6):893–901.

22. Vaziri ND. Mechanism of erythropoietin-induced hypertension. Am J Kidney Dis. 1999;33(5):821–8.

23. Waase MP, Mutharasan RK, Whang W, et al. Electrocardiographic findings in National Basketball Association athletes. JAMA Cardiol. 2018;3(1):69–74.

24. Muntner P, Carey RM, Gidding S, et al. Potential US population impact of the 2017 ACC/AHA high blood pressure guideline. Circulation. 2018;137(2):109–18.

25. Varga-Pinter B, Horvath P, Kneffel Z, Major Z, Osvath P, Pavlik G. Resting blood pressure values of adult athletes. Kidney Blood Press Res. 2011;34(6):387–95.

26. Whelton SP, Chin A, Xin X, He J. Effect of aerobic exercise on blood pressure: a meta-analysis of randomized, controlled trials. Ann Intern Med. 2002;136(7):493–503.

27. Karpinos AR, Roumie CL, Nian H, Diamond AB, Rothman RL. High prevalence of hypertension among collegiate football athletes. Circ Cardiovasc Qual Outcomes. 2013;6(6):716–23.

28. Sousa N, Mendes R, Abrantes C, Sampaio J, Oliveira J. A randomized 9-month study of blood pressure and body fat responses to aerobic training versus combined aerobic and resistance training in older men. Exp Gerontol. 2013;48(8):727–33.

29. World anti-doping agency prohibited list. 2019. https://www.wada-ama.org/. Accessed 1 Feb 2019.

30. Muntner P, Shimbo D, Carey RM, et al. Measurement of blood pressure in humans: a scientific statement from the American Heart Association. Hypertension. 2019;73(5):e35–66.

31. Leung AA, Daskalopoulou SS, Dasgupta K, et al. Hypertension Canada's 2017 guidelines for diagnosis, risk assessment, prevention, and treatment of hypertension in adults. Can J Cardiol. 2017;33(5):557–76.

32. National Clinical Guideline Center (UK). Hypertension: the clinical management of primary hypertension in adults: update of clinical guidelines 18 and 34. London: Royal College of Physicians; 2011.

Chapter 6
Valvular Heart Disease

Tamanna K. Singh

Introduction

Valvular heart disease (VHD) affects approximately 1–2% of young individuals, many of whom choose to participate in competitive sports or maintain highly active lifestyles [1]. The pathologic changes in valve structure and function inherent in intrinsic valve disease may progress with sports participation; however, the effects of exercise intensity on the progression of valve disease have not been investigated extensively. A potential contributing etiology for progression of valve disease in athletes is the adrenergic surge associated with exercise that places an increased hemodynamic load on a heart that has pre-existing valve impairment. This added stress on the heart can result in the development of secondary cardiac abnormalities including acceleration in aortopathy from increased aortic wall stress and pressure, pulmonary hypertension, atrial or ventricular arrhythmias, adverse cardiac remodeling (ventricular hypertrophy or enlargement), myocardial ischemia, and eventual functional deterioration [1].

VHD can be categorized, or staged, based on the severity of valve dysfunction, the presence of associated symptoms, and the status of ventricular function. The 2014 American Heart Association/American College of Cardiology (AHA/ACC) classification for the progression of valve disease is summarized [2]:

- *Stage A*: Asymptomatic individuals who are at risk for developing clinically significant valve stenosis or regurgitation
- *Stage B*: Patients with mild to moderate VHD who are asymptomatic with preserved left or right ventricular systolic function

T. K. Singh (✉)
Sports Cardiology Center, Heart, Vascular and Thoracic Institute, Cleveland Clinic Foundation, Cleveland, OH, USA

© Springer Nature Switzerland AG 2021
D. J. Engel, D. M. Phelan (eds.), *Sports Cardiology*,
https://doi.org/10.1007/978-3-030-69384-8_6

85

- *Stage C1*: Asymptomatic patients with severe VHD and preserved left or right ventricular systolic function
- *Stage C2*: Asymptomatic patients with severe VHD and impaired left or right ventricular systolic function
- *Stage D*: Symptomatic patients with severe VHD with or without left or right ventricular systolic dysfunction

To date, no prospective trial investigating asymptomatic VHD in athletes has been published. As a result, recommendations for management of VHD in asymptomatic athletes (stages A to C2) are limited to AHA/ACC expert and consensus opinion, based upon cohort analyses of the nonathletic population [3]. Athletes who have stage D VHD are *not* eligible for competitive sports participation and should be referred for valve repair or replacement, similar to management guidelines in the general population. However, athletes who remain asymptomatic, irrespective of valve lesion severity and status of ventricular function, may be eligible for sports participation after completing an exercise stress test and demonstrating tolerance to the exertional intensity required for the specific sports type. An algorithm for performing an exercise tolerance test based on valve lesion and severity is provided in Table 6.1. Based on clinical findings and results of stress testing, a shared decision should be made between provider and the athlete with VHD to determine the appropriate degree of sports participation [1, 2].

This chapter will review and outline strategies for evaluation and surveillance, and recommendations for sports participation, for athletes with stages A to D VHD, with a focus on aortic valve disease (aortic stenosis, aortic regurgitation) and mitral valve disease (mitral stenosis, mitral regurgitation).

Aortic Valve Disease

Acquired aortic valve disease is characterized by valve calcification and degeneration with the former a more common etiology in masters athletes and the latter common across all ages [5]. Congenital aortic valve disease, including bicuspid aortic valve disease, is seen in approximately 1.5–2.0% of younger athletes.

Aortic Stenosis

Aortic stenosis (AS) is a valve lesion seen in both young and masters athletes that has been reported to be responsible for nearly 4% of sudden cardiac deaths in athletes [6]. Common symptoms elucidated in a medical history suggestive of AS include dyspnea, dizziness, or chest pain with exertion, as well as decreased exercise tolerance. Physical exam findings suggestive of AS include a crescendo-decrescendo systolic murmur and a delayed and diminished upstroke of the carotid

Table 6.1 AHA/ACC recommendations for exercise testing in asymptomatic athletes with valvular heart disease

Valve disease	Eligibility for competitive sports	Exercise tolerance testing[a]
Aortic valve		
Aortic stenosis		
Severe	None except possibly low-intensity sports: class IA sports (class III)	No
Moderate	Low and moderate static/dynamic sports: classes IA, IB, IIA sports (class IIa)	Yes (class IIa)
Mild	All sports (class IIa)	Yes (class IIa)
Aortic regurgitation		
Severe[b]	All sports (class IIb)	Yes (class IIb)
LVEF <50% or severe LV dilation[c]	None (class III)	No
Mild to moderate	All sports (class I)	Yes (class I)
Moderate LV dilation[d]	All sports (class IIa)	Yes (class IIa)
Mitral valve		
Mitral stenosis		
Severe	None except possibly low-intensity sports: class IA sports (class III)	Yes (class I)
Moderate	No specific recommendation given	Yes (class I)
Mild	AH sports (class IIa)	Yes (class 1)
Mitral regurgitation[e]		
Severe	No specific recommendation given; recommend same as below	Yes (class I)
Mild LV enlargement[f]	Low- and some moderate-intensity sports: class IA, IIA, IB (class IIb)	Yes (class I)
Moderate with mild LV enlargement[f]	All sports (class IIa)	Yes (class I)
Mild to moderate[g]	All sports (class I)	Yes (class I)
LV enlargement[h], PHTN, or LVEF <60%	None except possibly low-intensity class IA sports (class III)	No
Anticoagulation	None with risk of bodily contact (class III)	No

ACC American College of Cardiology, *AHA* American Heart Association, *LV* left ventricle, *LVEF, LV* ejection fraction, *PHTN* pulmonary hypertension
[a]Exercise tolerance testing performed to the level achieved in competition or training without symptoms, ST segment depression, abnormal blood pressure response, or ventricular tachyarrhythmias
[b]If normal exercise tolerance, LVEF >50%, LV end-systolic diameter (LVESD) <50 mm (men) or <40 mm (female) or indexed LVESD <25 mm/m^2, and without evidence of progression of aortic regurgitation severity or severity of LV dilatation
[c]LVEF <50%, LVESD >50 mm or indexed LVESD 25 mm/m^2, or severe increase in LV end-diastolic diameter (LVEDD) (>70 mm or 35.3 mm/m^2 for men; >65 mm or >40.8 mm/m^2 for women)
[d]LVESD <50 mm for males or <40 mm for females or indexed LVESD <25 mm/m^2
[e]Sustained increases in LV systolic pressures are theorized to potentiate further damage in patients with prior infective endocarditis or rupture chordae; therefore, the above recommendations should be tempered in these patients
[f]LVEDD <60 mm or 35.3 mm/m^2 in men or <40 mm/m^2 in women
[g]Sinus rhythm, normal LV size and function, and normal pulmonary artery pressure
[h]LVEDD >65 mm or 35.3 mm/m^2 for men or >40 mm/m^2 for women
Reprinted with permission from Gentry et al. [4], Karger Publishers

Table 6.2 Echocardiographic quantification of aortic stenosis severity in patients with normal left ventricular systolic function

Aortic stenosis severity	Jet velocity (m/s)	Mean gradient (mmHg)	Aortic valve area (cm^2)
Mild	2.6–2.9	<20	>1.5
Moderate	3.0–3.9	20–39	1.0–1.5
Severe	≥4.0	≥40	<1.0

Adapted from Nishimura et al. [2]

pulse. Transthoracic echocardiography (TTE) will provide supplemental information on the degree of AS and is the current standard for quantifying the severity of stenosis. Table 6.2 outlines the quantification of AS and TTE parameters for classification of the severity of AS based upon current AHA/ACC valvular heart disease guidelines [2].

Annual echocardiographic evaluation is recommended in athletes with AS to monitor progression of stenosis and to monitor left ventricular function and structure. Exercise stress testing provides additional information regarding the athlete's exercise tolerance, the presence or absence of exercise-induced myocardial ischemia, and the blood pressure response to exercise (Table 6.1).

Recommendations for competitive sports participation for athletes with AS are dependent upon the severity of AS as well as the presence of symptoms. Asymptomatic athletes with mild AS and preserved left ventricular function (jet velocity <3 m/s or aortic valve area >1.5 cm^2, *stage B*) may participate in competitive sports without restriction provided the athlete continues with annual physical exams and TTE imaging to assess for progression of stenosis. Yearly exercise testing is also required to assess for exercise-induced hypotension or myocardial ischemia and to objectively assess maximal exercise tolerance. Asymptomatic athletes with moderate AS (jet velocity 3.0–3.9 m/s, aortic valve area 1.0–1.5 cm^2, *stage B*) are advised to participate in low-moderate static or dynamic competitive sports provided that satisfactory exercise tolerance is demonstrated on exercise stress testing without evidence of a blunted or dropped blood pressure response with exercise or without evidence of exercise-induced myocardial ischemia. Asymptomatic athletes with severe AS (jet velocity ≥4.0 m/s, aortic valve area <1.0 cm^2, *stage C*) are advised to participate in low-intensity sports only. Symptomatic athletes with any degree of AS (*stage D*) are advised to refrain from all competitive sports participation [1, 3]. These recommendations for AS are summarized in Fig. 6.1.

Aortic Regurgitation

Aortic regurgitation (AR) commonly occurs with congenital aortic valve disease (e.g., bicuspid aortic valve disease) and genetic connective tissue disorders with aortopathy (e.g., Marfan syndrome). AR may also be seen in association with rheumatic valve disease or aortic dilatation resulting from hypertensive heart disease [3]. Physical exam findings that may suggest AR include a systolic flow murmur due to

	Valve severity (stage)	Surveillance recommendations	Sports participation recommendations
Asymptomatic	Mild (Stage B) Jet velocity <3 m/s AVA >1.5 cm²	Annual physical exam, echocardiography, exercise stress testing	Unrestricted
Asymptomatic	Moderate (Stage B) Jet velocity 3.0–3.9 m/s AVA 1.0–1.5 cm²	Annual physical exam, echocardiography, exercise stress testing	Low-moderate static or dynamic⁺
Asymptomatic	Severe (Stage C) Jet velocity ≥4 m/s AVA <1.0 cm²	Annual physical exam, echocardiography, exercise stress testing	Low-intensity (class IA)
Symptomatic	Any severity (Stage D)		No competitive sports participation

Fig. 6.1 Recommendations for competitive sports participation in athletes with aortic stenosis. *AVA* aortic valve area
⁺If satisfactory exercise tolerance is demonstrated on exercise stress testing without evidence of a blunted or dropped blood pressure response with exercise or without evidence of exercise-induced myocardial ischemia

increased stroke volume and/or a decrescendo diastolic murmur appreciated along the left or right sternal border.

Many athletes with AR remain asymptomatic for years, tolerating the gradual increase in left ventricular dimension, volume, and pressure arising from progressive increases in aortic regurgitant volume. Symptom onset typically ensues when pathologic left ventricular remodeling begins. This process is marked by a decline in left ventricular compliance resulting from interstitial fibrosis, leading to an increase in both end-systolic and end-diastolic pressures that further dilate the left ventricle, inevitably leading to left ventricular dysfunction, increased intracardiac pressures, and heart failure [7]. The challenge in athletes lies in differentiating early pathologic left ventricular dilatation associated with chronic AR from physiologic left ventricular enlargement seen as part of the spectrum of exercise-induced cardiac remodeling (EICR, athlete's heart) [8, 9].

Data from Italy suggests that there is an overlap between left ventricular end-diastolic and end-systolic dimensions in athletes with EICR, predominately in dynamic and mixed dynamic-static athletes, and nonathletes with chronic AR [10, 11]. In Italian mixed-sports elite male athletes, left ventricular end-diastolic dimension (LVEDD) >55 mm was observed in nearly 50% of athletes, but LVEDD >60 mm was uncommon, and LVEDD >70 mm was exceedingly rare [10, 11]. In highly trained Italian mixed-sports female athletes, LVEDD >55 mm was present in <10% of athletes, and LVEDD exceeding 60 mm was rare, present in just 1% of athletes [10, 11]. Reported upper limits of normal for left ventricular end-systolic dimension (LVESD) in Italian elite male and female athletes were 49 mm and 38 mm, respectively [11].

Athletes with AR and LVESD and/or LVEDD greater than these reference values should first have these dimensions indexed for body surface area to determine an accurate assessment of chamber size [12]. If indexed dimensions remain above reference values, then further evaluation with exercise stress testing should be performed to assess exercise capacity and exercise hemodynamics (Table 6.1). TTE evaluation should also include Doppler evaluation of AR severity, assessment of left ventricular function, aortic valve morphology, and aortic dimensions and morphology [3].

Current AHA/ACC guideline recommendations suggest that asymptomatic athletes with AR should have annual echocardiographic and exercise stress testing at or beyond the level of sports intensity achieved in competition to assess symptom burden and the blood pressure response to exercise to determine whether competitive sports participation should remain unrestricted. Athletes with mild to moderate AR with normal left ventricular systolic function and dimensions (*stage B*) may continue to participate in unrestricted competitive sports provided exercise tolerance during stress testing is normal. Athletes with stage B AR with preserved left ventricular systolic function and mild-moderate left ventricular dilatation (LVESD <50 mm in men, LVESD <40 mm in women, or LVESD <25 mm/m^2 for either sex) may continue to participate in competitive sports without restriction if exercise tolerance is normal during exercise stress testing. Athletes with *stage C1* AR classified by:

- Severe AR
- Left ventricular ejection fraction (LVEF) >50%
- LVESD <50 mm in men, <40 mm in women, or <25 mm/m^2 for either sex
- Normal exercise tolerance on exercise stress testing
- No progression of AR or LV dilatation by echocardiography

May continue to participate in competitive sports without restriction. Finally, asymptomatic athletes with *stage C2* AR (LVEF <50%; LVESD >50 mm, LVEDD >70 mm or >35.3 mm/m^2 in men; LVEDD >65 mm or >40.8 mm/m^2 in women) should not participate in competitive sports. Similarly, symptomatic athletes with severe AR (*stage D*) are advised not to participate in competitive sports. Of note, athletes with AR and aortic dimensions between 41 and 45 mm may participate in competitive sports where there is expected to be a low risk of bodily collision [1, 3]. These recommendations for AR are summarized in Fig. 6.2.

Mitral Valve Disease

Acquired causes of mitral valve disease include rheumatic heart disease, mitral annular calcification, infective endocarditis, radiation valvulitis, valvulitis from systemic inflammatory disease processes (e.g., rheumatoid arthritis, lupus

	Valve severity (stage)	Surveillance recommendations	Sports participation recommendations
Asymptomatic	Mild-moderate (Stage B) ± LV dilatation[+]	Annual physical exam, echocardiography, exercise stress testing	Unrestricted
	Severe (Stage C1)[++]		
	Mild-severe Aortic dimensions 41–45 mm		Competitive sports without bodily contact
	Severe (Stage C2)[+++]		No competitive sport participation
Symptomatic	Severe (Stage D)		

Fig. 6.2 Recommendations for competitive sports participation in athletes with aortic regurgitation. *AVA* aortic valve area

[+]LVESD <50 mm in men, <40 mm in women, or <25 mm/m^2 for either sex[++]LVEF >50%, LVESD <50 mm in men, <40 mm in women, or <25 mm/m^2 for either sex, normal exercise tolerance on exercise stress testing, no progression of AR or LV dilatation[+++]LVEF <50%, LVESD >50 mm, LVEDD >70 mm or >35.3 mm/m^2 in men; LVEDD >65 mm or >40.8 mm/m^2 in women

erythematous), obstructive lesions (e.g., atrial myxoma), and left ventricular (LV) chamber dysfunction with both LV and mitral annular dilatation leading to mitral leaflet tethering with restricted leaflet closure and functional mitral regurgitation [13]. Genetically mediated causes of mitral valve disease include myxomatous mitral valve disease and prolapse, as well as connective tissue diseases (e.g., Marfan syndrome).

Mitral Stenosis

Mitral stenosis (MS) is most commonly caused by rheumatic heart disease and is most prevalent in developing countries [13]. Rheumatic MS is a consequence of cross-reactivity between mitral valve tissue and a streptococcal antigen, leading to immune activation on mitral valve tissue and morphologic valve changes that include leaflet thickening, commissural fusion, a "fish-mouth" appearance of the valve orifice, and chordal shortening and fusion [13]. As MS increases, left atrial pressure rises and forward flow into the LV decreases, leading to an increase in transmitral gradients that increase with tachycardia [13]. Additional sequelae of progressive MS include an increased risk of atrial arrhythmias (e.g., atrial fibrillation), secondary pulmonary hypertension, tricuspid regurgitation, right ventricular failure, and low cardiac output [13].

MS is a rare cause of sudden cardiac death in athletes. Athletes are often asymptomatic even with hemodynamically significant MS but can develop sudden increases in intracardiac pressures with exercise-induced tachycardia and increased cardiac output that can cause acute pulmonary edema [14]. Athletes are also at risk for developing atrial tachyarrhythmias, including atrial fibrillation as a consequence of left atrial dilatation. As a result, anticoagulation for stroke prophylaxis is advised for patients with MS. Although there is a risk of systemic embolization with atrial fibrillation, there is no current evidence to suggest that exercise poses an increase in the risk for embolization [3].

Similar to AS, athletes with MS should undergo physical exam, electrocardiogram, TTE with Doppler assessment, and exercise stress testing to assess exercise tolerance and intracardiac pressures noninvasively (Table 6.1). Mild MS correlates with a mitral valve area (MVA) between 1.6 and 2.0 cm^2, moderate MS with MVA between 1.1 and 1.5 cm^2, and severe MS with MVA ≤ 1.0 cm^2 [2]. Additionally, a mean transmitral gradient >10 mmHg with pulmonary artery systolic pressure >50 mmHg suggests severe MS [3].

All athletes with MS should undergo annual evaluation to determine whether they may continue to participate in competitive sports. Athletes with mild MS (mean transmitral gradient <5 mmHg at rest) in sinus rhythm (*stage B*) may continue with unrestricted competitive sports participation. Asymptomatic athletes with mild to moderate MS and who demonstrate preserved exercise tolerance on exercise stress testing and resting pulmonary artery systolic pressure <35 mmHg (*stage B*) may continue to participate in unrestricted competitive sports. Athletes with severe MS, regardless of the presence or absence of symptoms, and whether in sinus rhythm or atrial fibrillation (*stages C and D*), are advised against competitive sports participation with the exception of low-intensity class IA sports. Athletes in atrial fibrillation with mild, moderate, or severe MS are advised to take anticoagulation for stroke prophylaxis and thus avoid participation in competitive sports where bodily collision is expected [3]. These recommendations for MS are summarized in Fig. 6.3.

Mitral Regurgitation

Mitral valve prolapse is the most common etiology of mitral regurgitation (MR) in athletes. Athletes with MR should undergo annual physical and TTE evaluation with Doppler, specifically assessing mitral regurgitant volume, left ventricular chamber size and function, left atrial size and volume, and intracardiac pressures. Exercise stress testing is also advised to assess exercise tolerance and hemodynamics (Table 6.1) [2, 3]. Caution should be taken when evaluating athletes with MR associated with prior endocarditis and torn/ruptured chordae, as maximal exercise stress testing in individuals with vulnerable valve integrity could possibly lead to acute on chronic valvular insufficiency.

	Valve severity	Surveillance recommendations	Sports participation recommendations
Asymptomatic	Mild (Stage B) MTG <5 mmHg	Annual physical exam, echocardiography, exercise stress testing	Unrestricted (in sinus rhythm)
	Mild-Moderate (Stage B) MTG <10 mmHg		Unrestricted+
	Severe (Stage C) MTG >10 mmHg		Low-intensity (Class IA) regardless of rhythm++
Symptomatic	Mild-Severe (Stage D)		No competitive sports participation

Fig. 6.3 Recommendations for competitive sports participation in athletes with mitral stenosis. *MTG* mean transmitral gradient
+Intact exercise tolerance on exercise stress testing with resting pulmonary artery systolic pressure <35 mmHg++Athletes in atrial fibrillation with mild, moderate, or severe MS are advised to take anticoagulation for stroke prophylaxis and thus avoid participation in competitive sports where bodily collision is expected

Exercise does not generally appear to cause a significant increase in MR above resting conditions; however, athletes with significantly elevated heart rate and/or blood pressure with exercise may develop prominent increases in pulmonary artery pressure [3]. Similar to AR, it can be challenging in athletes with significant MR to distinguish athletic physiologic LV dilatation from pathologic LV dilatation related to MR when the LVEDD is <60 mm (<40 mm/m^2). LVEDD >60 mm in the presence of significant MR is highly suggestive of pathologic cardiac remodeling and need for surgical mitral valve repair [3].

With regard to exercise recommendations, athletes with mild to moderate MR in sinus rhythm with normal LV size and function (LVEDD <60 mm, LVEF >60%) and normal pulmonary artery pressures (*stage B*) may participate in competitive sports without restriction. Athletes with moderate MR in sinus rhythm and with mild LV dilatation within parameters consistent with athletic remodeling (LVEDD <60 mm or <35 mm/m^2 in males, LVEDD <40 mm/m^2 in females, *stage B*) may participate in competitive sports without restriction. Athletes with severe MR in sinus rhythm and with normal LV function, and with mild LV dilatation within parameters associated with athletic remodeling (*stage C1*), are advised to participate in low-intensity and moderate-intensity sports (classes IA, IIA, IB) only. Athletes with MR and LV dilatation greater than that which is expected with

	Valve severity (stage)	Surveillance recommendations	Sports participation recommendations
Asymptomatic	Mild-moderate (Stage B)[+]	Annual physical exam, echocardiography, exercise stress testing	Unrestricted
	Moderate (Stage B)[++]		Unrestricted (in sinus rhythm)
	Severe (Stage C1)[++]		Low-intensity or moderate-intensity (classes IA, IIA, IB)
	Severe (Stage C2)[+++]		Low-intensity (class IA) regardless of rhythm[++++]
Symptomatic	Stage D		No competitive sports participation

Fig. 6.4 Recommendations for competitive sports participation in athletes with mitral regurgitation [+]In sinus rhythm, normal LV size and systolic function (LVEDD <60 mm, LVEF >60%), normal pulmonary artery pressure[++]Mild LV dilatation within parameters consistent with athletic remodeling (LVEDD <60 mm or <35 mm/m^2 in males, LVEDD <40 mm/m^2 in females)[+++]LV dilatation greater than that which is expected with training (LVEDD >65 mm or >35.5 mm/m^2 in men, >40 mm/m^2 in women, LVESD >40 mm), pulmonary hypertension, or LV systolic dysfunction at rest (LVEF <60%)[++++] Athletes with MR and atrial fibrillation on chronic anticoagulation are advised against participating in competitive sports where bodily collision is expected

training (LVEDD >65 mm or >35.5 mm/m^2 in men, >40 mm/m^2 in women, LVESD >40 mm), pulmonary hypertension, or LV systolic dysfunction at rest (LVEF <60%) (*stage C2*) are advised against competitive sports participation, though they may participate in low-intensity class IA sports. Finally, athletes with MR and atrial fibrillation on chronic anticoagulation are advised against participating in competitive sports where bodily collision is expected [3]. These recommendations for MR are summarized in Fig. 6.4.

Tricuspid and Pulmonary Valve Disease

Tricuspid and pulmonary valve disease are most commonly associated with congenital and genetic abnormalities though they may be secondary sequelae of progressive left heart failure, pulmonary hypertension, and eventual right-sided chamber dilation and dysfunction. Athletes with secondary tricuspid or pulmonary valve disease should undergo serial evaluation by TTE and exercise stress testing similar to recommendations for aortic and mitral valve disease. At the present time,

AHA/ACC guidelines for valve disease in competitive athletes do not provide recommendations for tricuspid and pulmonary valve disease [3]. Clinical judgment, plus strategies and algorithms applied to athletes with aortic and mitral valve disease, should be utilized in determining physical activity guidelines for athletes with tricuspid and pulmonary valve disorders.

Valvular Interventions and Recommendations for Return to Play

Symptomatic athletes with severe valvular heart disease should be referred for surgical and/or percutaneous treatment for valve repair or replacement in a similar manner to nonathletes [2]. A shared decision-making model is advised when discussing surgical strategies, timing of intervention, and expectations regarding competitive sports participation after valve intervention. Implantation of valve prostheses have specific implications for athletes. Prosthetic transvalvular gradients may increase with exercise more prominently than with native valves [2, 15]. Additionally, athletes with implanted mechanical prostheses are relegated to chronic anticoagulation and thus are advised to avoid competitive sports where bodily collision can be expected. Athletes who have undergone aortic or mitral valve repair and who are at risk of physical trauma from sports participation are advised to discuss risks and benefits of participation prior to return to play [3].

A thorough evaluation of prosthetic valve function and the hemodynamic results of valve repair by TTE and exercise testing should be conducted to assess symptoms with exercise, resting and exercise valve function, exercise capacity prior to return to competitive sports participation, and serially thereafter. Exercise capacity should meet the level required for the intended sports intensity. To date, there are no large retrospective or prospective studies evaluating outcomes of surgical valvular interventions in competitive athletes with respect to return of preoperative exercise capacity. A shared decision-making model should be employed to ensure that an appropriate discussion of the athlete's goals for sports participation, along with potential risks associated with that participation, is held.

The current AHA/ACC guidelines suggest it is reasonable for athletes with aortic or mitral bioprosthetic valves, not requiring anticoagulation, with preserved valvular and left ventricular function to participate in low- and moderate-intensity competitive sports (classes IA, IB, IC, and IIA sports). Athletes with mechanical aortic and mitral prosthetic valves on chronic anticoagulation with preserved valvular and left ventricular function may participate in low-intensity competitive sports where bodily collision is not expected (classes IA, IB, IIA). Athletes who have undergone surgical aortic or mitral valve repair for regurgitant valve disease without residual AR or MR, and with intact left ventricular function, are advised to follow a shared decision-making model to determine whether they may safely participate in competitive sports where there is expected to be a low likelihood of bodily collision (classes IA, IB, IIA) [3].

Conclusion

Athletes with VHD require careful initial and serial evaluations to guide recommendations regarding sports participation on an ongoing basis given that valve disease can be progressive. Many asymptomatic athletes with VHD, even in the presence of moderate-severe VHD, can continue to participate in competitive sports with close monitoring by TTE and assessment of clinical status. With regurgitant valve disease, it can be challenging to differentiate cardiac changes seen as part of the spectrum of exercise-induced cardiac remodeling from pathologic remodeling associated with valve regurgitation. Using the provided algorithms and clinical judgment, safe participation in competitive sports for athletes with VHD can continue, and shared decision-making between athlete and physician will ultimately be required regarding the timing and need to discontinue competitive sports and consider valve intervention when and if valve disease progresses to an advanced stage.

References

1. Gati S, Malhotra A, Sharma S. Exercise recommendations in patients with valvular heart disease. Heart. 2019;105(2):106–10.
2. Nishimura RA, et al. 2014 AHA/ACC Guideline for the management of patients with valvular heart disease: executive summary: a report of the American College of Cardiology/American Heart Association task force on practice guidelines. J Am Coll Cardiol. 2014;63(22):2438–88.
3. Bonow RO, et al. Eligibility and disqualification recommendations for competitive athletes with cardiovascular abnormalities: task force 5: valvular heart disease: a scientific statement from the American Heart Association and American College of Cardiology. J Am Coll Cardiol. 2015;66(21):2385–92.
4. Gentry Iii JL, et al. The role of stress echocardiography in valvular heart disease: a current appraisal. Cardiology. 2017;137(3):137–50.
5. Siu SC, Silversides CK. Bicuspid aortic valve disease. J Am Coll Cardiol. 2010;55(25):2789–800.
6. Maron BJ. Sudden death in young athletes. N Engl J Med. 2003;349(11):1064–75.
7. Akinseye OA, Pathak A, Ibebuogu UN. Aortic valve regurgitation: a comprehensive review. Curr Probl Cardiol. 2018;43(8):315–34.
8. Beaudry R, et al. A modern definition of the athlete's heart-for research and the clinic. Cardiol Clin. 2016;34(4):507–14.
9. Prior DL, La Gerche A. The athlete's heart. Heart. 2012;98(12):947–55.
10. Pelliccia A, et al. Physiologic left ventricular cavity dilatation in elite athletes. Ann Intern Med. 1999;130(1):23–31.
11. Pelliccia A, et al. Long-term clinical consequences of intense, uninterrupted endurance training in Olympic athletes. J Am Coll Cardiol. 2010;55(15):1619–25.
12. Dujardin KS, et al. Mortality and morbidity of aortic regurgitation in clinical practice. A long-term follow-up study. Circulation. 1999;99(14):1851–7.
13. Harb SC, Griffin BP. Mitral valve disease: a comprehensive review. Curr Cardiol Rep. 2017;19(8):73.
14. Rahimtoola SH, et al. Current evaluation and management of patients with mitral stenosis. Circulation. 2002;106(10):1183–8.
15. Rahimtoola SH. Choice of prosthetic heart valve for adult patients. J Am Coll Cardiol. 2003;41(6):893–904.

Chapter 7
Hypertrophic Cardiomyopathy

Dermot M. Phelan and John Symanski

Introduction

Hypertrophic cardiomyopathy (HCM) is an inheritable myocardial disease caused primarily by mutations in genes encoding the sarcomeric contractile proteins. The diagnosis is predicated on demonstrating thickening of at least one segment of the left ventricular (LV) wall >15 mm in a non-dilated ventricle and in the absence of potentially causative loading conditions [1, 2]. For LV wall thicknesses less than 15 mm, the diagnosis requires other features including a family history of HCM or identification of a causative gene mutation, electrocardiographic abnormalities, or other typical features on cardiac imaging. Some individuals may be genotype positive and phenotypically negative. The prevalence of HCM in the general population is estimated to be approximately 1:500 [3]; however the prevalence of HCM in highly trained athletes is likely lower as the structural and functional changes associated with HCM naturally select out many individuals with HCM from competing at elite levels [4].

D. M. Phelan (✉) · J. Symanski
Sports Cardiology Center, Hypertrophic Cardiomyopathy Center,
Sanger Heart & Vascular Institute, Atrium Health, Charlotte, NC, USA
e-mail: dermot.phelan@atriumhealth.org; john.symanski@atriumhealth.org

© Springer Nature Switzerland AG 2021
D. J. Engel, D. M. Phelan (eds.), *Sports Cardiology*,
https://doi.org/10.1007/978-3-030-69384-8_7

Differentiating Athlete's Heart from Hypertrophic Cardiomyopathy

Over the past decade, prodigious advances have been made in defining the normal physiological adaptations of the heart in athletes. The so-called athlete's heart manifests through electrical, morphological, and functional adaptations to improve the efficiency of cardiac function. Frequently, a 10–20% increase in LV wall thickness can be expected in well-trained athletes, resulting in the potential for crossover with HCM. Thankfully, in most instances there are clear distinctions between phenotypically expressed HCM and athlete's heart; however in a small minority of athletes, it can be challenging to differentiate these entities. Unfortunately, with rare exceptions, most of the literature in this regard compares athletes to patients with clearly expressed HCM who are often nonathletes. These data are not helpful in differentiating the true, "gray-zone" individuals. The following is a proposed algorithm for differentiating these entities.

Understanding the pretesting probability of the disease is of paramount importance. Concerning symptoms of exertional chest pain or syncope, a provocable LV outflow tract murmur or a family history of HCM should prompt a thorough evaluation for HCM. Establishing the diagnosis of HCM in the absence of any of these features should mandate a high burden of proof.

The second step in the evaluation should be the 12-lead electrocardiogram (ECG). The majority of patients with HCM will express abnormalities on the ECG beyond what would be deemed normal adaptation in an athlete. Left ventricular hypertrophy (LVH) in isolation is considered a normal variant in athletes while T wave abnormalities, prominent Q waves, and ST segment depression are the most commonly seen abnormalities in HCM [1, 2, 5]. However, ~5–10% of young people with morphologically expressed HCM will have a normal ECG [6, 7]. Furthermore, up to 4% of black athletes will manifest lateral T wave changes that are considered pathological and suggestive of HCM [8, 9]. The recent International Recommendations for ECG interpretation in the athlete have optimized the sensitivity and specificity of the test [5]. Knowledge of expected electrical changes in the athlete obviates the need for further testing in many individuals while guiding more extensive evaluation in others. For example, T wave inversion extending out to V4, when preceded by J point elevation and convex ST elevation, is considered a normal variant in a black athlete, while T wave inversion in the lateral leads is highly associated with HCM (Fig. 7.1). In a study by Schnell et al., this ECG pattern was associated with HCM 35% of the time, and echocardiography missed the diagnosis almost 50% of the time primarily due to poor visualization of the apex [8]. As a result, the current guidelines recommend exercise ECG, a 24-hour Holter monitor, and cardiac magnetic resonance (CMR) imaging as a routine in the evaluation of this ECG pattern if the echocardiogram does not clearly visualize all segments, in particular, the apex [5].

For individuals presenting for evaluation as a result of documented LVH, practitioners must have knowledge of the expected range of LV wall thickness for that

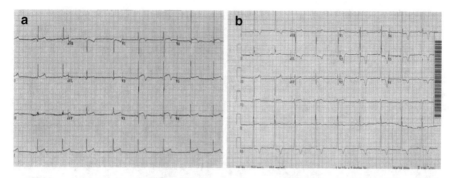

Fig. 7.1 (a) 12-lead electrocardiogram demonstrating T wave inversion to V4 preceded by J point elevation and coved ST segment elevation is a normal variant seen in black athletes. (**b**) 12-lead electrocardiogram demonstrating deep T wave inversion V2–V6, I, and aVL has been associated with HCM in almost one third of athletes

particular athlete. Factors which influence LV wall thickness include the type and intensity of sport, race, sex, age, and body size. For example, a LV wall thickness of >12 mm was reported by Basavarajaiah et al. in 18% of black male athletes but only <2% in white male athletes [10]. Indeed 3% of black athletes in this study had a wall thickness >15 mm. In females, it is rare for a white female athlete to have a LV wall thickness of >11 mm, and LV wall thickness of >11 mm is only seen in 3% of black female athletes. It is also rare for a female athlete to express concentric hypertrophy. Mixed endurance and static sports, such as rowing or cycling, tend to have the most profound effect on LV wall thickness.

Careful evaluation of imaging is required to ensure the accuracy of measurements. Overestimation of septal wall thickness due to inclusion of right ventricular (RV) trabeculation can be avoided by correlation with short axis imaging and, when necessary, CMR (Fig. 7.2).

LVH in the athlete's heart is usually eccentric (balanced increase in chamber size with wall thickness) with <2 mm difference in LV wall thickness between adjacent segments. By contrast, LVH in HCM is usually asymmetric, frequently with >2 mm difference in adjacent segments. Further, the chamber cavity size in HCM is usually smaller than expected; even in individuals with HCM who are very athletic, the LV end diastolic diameter is rarely >5.5 cm. Contrary to traditional teaching, athletic individuals with HCM can often have normal parameters of diastolic function including normal tissue Doppler velocities of the mitral annulus [6]. Global longitudinal strain is usually normal in athletes but reduced in HCM, particularly at the site of greatest hypertrophy. However, these data were reported in HCM patients with severe LVH, and its applicability to differentiating "gray-zone" athletes with mild LVH is not well defined. One study which compared sedentary patients with HCM to athletic individuals with HCM and athletes without HCM, all matched for LV wall thickness, showed no difference in global longitudinal strain between the latter two groups but a significant reduction in strain in the sedentary HCM group.

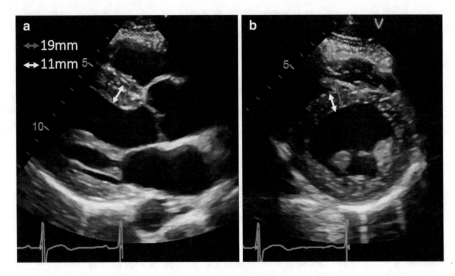

Fig. 7.2 Parasternal long-axis (**a**) and short-axis (**b**) two-dimensional echocardiographic views of a professional athlete initially referred for concern of HCM based on septal wall measurement of 19 mm (red arrows). Careful evaluation and comparison with the short-axis image show that this measurement includes a large section of right ventricular trabeculation. The true compacted left ventricular septum measured 11 mm (white arrows)

A novel technique using mechanical dispersion did differentiate the athletic HCM from the athletic non-HCM, but this technique requires further validation [11].

Fewer athletes with HCM have resting left ventricular outflow tract obstruction (LVOTO) than sedentary patients with HCM, but a thorough evaluation of the mitral valve apparatus is mandatory in the evaluation of the "gray-zone" athlete. Up to 70% of patients with HCM have abnormalities of the mitral valve apparatus (elongated mitral valve leaflets, displaced papillary muscles, multiheaded and mobile papillary muscles) which predisposes to LVOTO. Evaluation for LVOTO should be performed using stress echocardiography, particularly in individuals with exertional symptoms.

Along with optimal evaluation of LV wall thickness, LV chamber size and function, and the mitral valve apparatus, CMR has the additional advantage of evaluating for myocardial scar. Late gadolinium enhancement (LGE) is seen in ~65% of patients with HCM [12] usually at the site of RV insertion or the site of greatest wall thickness. While some studies have described LGE in athletes, these studies are of middle-aged and older, long-term, endurance athletes. LGE should always be considered an abnormal finding in young athletes with the possible exception of LGE at the RV insertion point.

Cardiopulmonary exercise testing in patients with HCM often reveals abnormalities including reduced peak VO_2 and anaerobic threshold, low O_2 pulse with plateauing of the O_2P/VO_2 relation; however on rare occasions, these parameters can be normal in athletes with HCM.

Occasionally, detraining has been advised to document regression of LV wall thickness. This technique has been validated in only very small numbers of athletes, but the degree to which LV wall thickness may regress in an athlete with HCM has not been evaluated; therefore, the utility of this strategy remains unclear.

Finally, genetic testing should be performed in individuals with a family history of HCM where the index family member has an identified disease-causing gene mutation. Genetic testing outside of this context in an athlete with mild LVH is controversial and should only be undertaken under the guidance of a cardiovascular geneticist.

Clinical Course and Management

HCM is a heterogeneous disease in terms of morphological expression, clinical course, and prognosis. Most individuals with HCM are asymptomatic and experience few major complications although some individuals can develop severe symptoms and experience a complex clinical course. The pathophysiology of exercise limitation in individuals with HCM is complex and relates to multiple factors including diastolic dysfunction, LVOTO, mitral regurgitation, autonomic dysregulation, and subendocardial ischemia. Approximately, one third of patients will have LVOTO at rest with a further third developing LVOTO with provocation. Stress echocardiography with a focus on identifying and quantifying LVOTO should be performed in athletes with concern for HCM and exertional symptoms. Treatment strategies for LVOTO include lifestyle advice (including the avoidance of dehydration, excess alcohol intake, and certain provoking medications), medications (most commonly non-vasodilating beta-blockers, verapamil, or occasionally disopyramide), or septal reduction therapy (alcohol septal ablation or surgical myectomy). It is important to note that none of these strategies have been shown to reduce the incidence of sudden cardiac death (SCD) in a randomized control trial and advice regarding sporting activity should not be affected by these treatments [13]. Other complications, including heart failure, atrial fibrillation, and cardioembolic stroke, rarely affect athletes with HCM.

Ventricular arrhythmias with associated SCD are the most feared complication in young athletes with HCM and can occur in the absence of prior symptoms. Those deemed at highest risk should receive a primary preventative implantable cardioverter defibrillator (ICD); however only a small number of those who have an ICD implanted ever receive an appropriate shock [14].

Prognosis

The US National Registry of Sudden Death in Athletes from the Minneapolis Heart Institute Foundation has reported that HCM is the number one cause of SCD in athletes in the United States. However, this finding was not reproduced in other populations, and more recent studies have indicated that 30–40% of SCD events in children and adults <35 years of age occur the absence of any identifiable pathology even after extensive autopsy with toxicology and histological examination. A recent meta-analysis found that a structurally normal heart was more a common postmortem finding in young individuals than was HCM. While there was some regional variability, HCM was not a more common cause of death in any patient subgroup analyzed, including athletes [15].

It is important, when discussing risk of SCD with young athletes with HCM, to note that most individuals with the disease have a normal life expectancy [16]. Furthermore, the majority of individuals with HCM die of causes unrelated to HCM [17]. For those that do die from causes related to HCM, death usually occurs during non-exercise-related activities. In the general adult HCM population, the annual incidence of SCD is estimated to be ~1%, while the estimated risk of SCD in young athletes with HCM is comparable to the general HCM population [13].

Unfortunately, prediction for those with HCM at highest risk of SCD remains imperfect. A history of prior resuscitated cardiac arrest, ventricular fibrillation, or ventricular tachycardia (VT) are the strongest predictors of a subsequent event, with an annualized event rate of ~10%. Other factors which have been associated with an increased risk of SCD have been felt to have a low positive predictive value, and ICDs placed for one or more of these risk factors have an annual discharge rate of ~4%. In a recent longitudinal observational study by Maron et al., 2094 patients with HCM were followed over 17 years to assess reliability of SCD prediction models leading to prophylactic ICD implantation [18]. ICDs were implanted in the presence of one or more risk factors based on a combination of traditionally described risk factors for SCD including:

1. A family history of SCD judged to definitely or likely be related to HCM in a first-degree relative 50 years or younger
2. Massive LVH with LV wall thickness ≥30 mm
3. Unexplained syncope unlikely to be neurocardiogenic within 5 years
4. Non-sustained ventricular tachycardia (NSVT) (defined as three or more runs of three or more beats of NSVT at a rate of >130 bpm or one run of NSVT greater than ten beats over a 24–48 hour monitoring period)

And newer risk factor markers including:

1. LGE >15% of the LV mass by CMR
2. LV ejection fraction <50%
3. LV apical aneurysm

Using this algorithm 15.6% of individuals with an ICD implanted experienced an appropriate device therapy. Only five individuals who did not have an ICD placed died suddenly; two of these had refused an ICD, two had no risk factors, and one had an apical aneurysm before this was recognized as a risk factor for SCD. Overall, only 2 of 2094 individuals (0.2%) experienced SCD in the absence of risk factors, a rate similar to that of the general population [18]. While differentiation between athletes and nonathletes was not a part of the study, it would be safe to assume that in such a large cohort there were some individuals that continued to exercise, and this risk factor algorithm identified almost all individuals at risk of SCD. Of note, the European Society of Cardiology 5-year risk score for SCD in HCM was much less sensitive at identifying high-risk patients in this study. This study supports the concept that the risk of SCD is not uniform and individuals with HCM can be reasonably classified into a "low-risk" category absent the aforementioned risk factors.

Benefits of Exercise in HCM

Most of the focus regarding exercise in individuals with HCM has been on avoidance of potential triggers of ventricular arrhythmias with little focus on the benefits of exercise. This has translated into increased levels of a sedentary lifestyle in HCM patients and increased body mass index when compared to controls, with over 50% of HCM patients not meeting minimum physical activity guidelines [19]. These exercise restrictions have been shown to negatively affect emotional well-being and social integration. Yet exercise has been shown to improve outcomes in almost every cardiac condition. The exercise paradox describes the fact that in normal individuals and those with heart disease, the risk of cardiac arrest is transiently increased, to a very small degree, during vigorous exercise, but habitual exercise is associated with a significant overall decreased mortality. Does this apply to individuals with HCM? In a study of 426 patients with HCM who underwent stress testing at the Cleveland Clinic and were followed for 8.7 ± 3 years, the group who achieved >100% of their maximal age-predicted heart rate had a 1% event rate versus a 12% rate in those who achieved <85% [20]. Higher functional capacity is achieved and maintained by regular exercise. Further, a sedentary lifestyle in individuals with HCM leads to a reduction in functional capacity and reduced VO2 max which has been strongly associated with worse long-term outcomes [21, 22].

One frequently expressed concern is that exercise may accelerate hypertrophy and fibrosis and worsen diastolic dysfunction and overall disease expression. However, there is extensive evidence showing the benefits of exercise on ventricular compliance in healthy individuals which also appears to apply to individuals with HCM [23, 24]. A murine model of HCM has shown that exercise training reduces fibrosis and myocyte disarray suggesting that exercise can prevent and even partially reverse the pathological phenotype in HCM [25]. Observational studies of athletes with HCM have consistently shown a mild phenotypic expression with less hypertrophy, improved and often normal diastolic function, normal longitudinal strain, less outflow tract obstruction, and larger LV cavity sizes [6, 11, 26]. While it is certainly possible that this mild phenotype permits athletic performance, the above data would also suggest that regular exercise positively impacts disease expression.

Recently, a number of studies have highlighted the beneficial effects of exercise in HCM. A prospective, non-randomized control trial enrolled 20 individuals with HCM to a structured exercise program over an average of 41 hours of moderate-intensity exercise and showed a significant improvement in functional capacity (4.7 ± 2.2 to 7.2 ± 2.8 metabolic equivalents) [27]. The RESET-HCM trial was a multicenter, randomized control trial of 136 patients with HCM who underwent 16 weeks of moderate-intensity exercise training or usual activity [24]. Those in the exercise arm experienced a modest improvement in exercise capacity associated with an improvement of quality of life without any adverse effects compared to the control group. While these data do not address the question of safety of intense competitive sports in patients with HCM, they do highlight the importance of counselling patients with HCM on the safety and significant benefits of regular moderate- and low-intensity exercise.

Current Recommendations for Sports Participation in HCM

Exercise, in particular high-intensity exercise, results in increased myocardial oxygen demand, alterations in autonomic tone, blood volume and electrolyte levels, and induction of catecholamine surges. Exercise-induced exacerbation of LVOTO will further increase LV wall stress, which may exacerbate demand ischemia in the thickened myocardium with coronary arteriole dysplasia. In the context of a pro-arrhythmic substrate due to myocyte disarray and fibrosis, the concern is that these physiological stressors may precipitate a malignant arrhythmia and SCD. Data identifying HCM as the number one cause of SCD in athletes in the United States serve to heighten concern [28]. The current American Heart Association (AHA)/ American College of Cardiology (ACC) eligibility and disqualification recommendations for competitive athletes with cardiovascular abnormalities note that "in the presence of underlying (and often unsuspected) HCM, participation in high-intensity competitive sports may itself promote ventricular tachycardia/ventricular fibrillation and act as a potent (yet modifiable) independent risk factor, even in the absence of conventional risk markers intrinsic to the disease process"; however there is little objective evidence to support that statement, particularly in low-risk individuals.

In 1994 Maron et al. first described a group of 14 athletes with HCM most of whom competed at a national, collegiate, or professional level for an average of 15 years without difficulties [29]. In a registry of athletes with ICD, Lampert et al. noted that athletes with HCM who had an ICD in place who continued to participate in sports had similar rates of ICD discharge during competition as during recreational activities [30]. Pelliccia et al. followed 35, mostly low-risk, athletes with HCM over a 9-year follow-up, 20 of whom suspended exercise participation after their diagnosis and 15 choose to remain physically active and even compete and showed no difference in outcomes between the two groups [31]. One death occurred in this cohort, unrelated to exercise. Furthermore, patients with HCM that have high functional capacity have the lowest event rates. Two further observational studies have demonstrated physiological benefits to high-intensity exercise in athletes [6, 26]. Taken together, these data suggest that not all individuals with HCM are at high risk of SCD despite participation in sports.

Despite these data, the current 2015 ACC/AHA eligibility and disqualification recommendations for competitive athletes with cardiovascular abnormalities recommend that "athletes with a probable or unequivocal clinical expression and diagnosis of HCM (ie, with the disease phenotype of LV hypertrophy) should not participate in most competitive sports, with the exception of those of low intensity (class IA sports) (Class III; Level of Evidence C)." The recommendations do note that they do not strictly exclude sporting participation "as long as such a decision is ultimately made in concert with their physician and third-party interests" [32].

The more recently published European guidelines have challenged this more indiscriminatory approach and attempted to be more patient specific [33]. They recognize that the "systematic restriction from competitive sport in all affected individuals is probably unjustified and a more liberal approach to sport participation may be reasonable after considering the age of the athlete, duration in competitive sport prior to diagnosis and the presence of conventional risk factors for SCD." Accordingly, they recommend that athletes with a mild expression of HCM, low-risk score, and adult age may participate in sports following a complete shared decision-making process. However, they do recommend restriction from sports participation in certain clinical scenarios (Table 7.1).

The 2020 AHA/ACC guidelines for the diagnosis and treatment of patients with HCM have followed a similar trajectory to the Europeans and have given a class 2a recommendation for participation in high-intensity recreational or moderate-high-intensity competitive sports after "comprehensive evaluation and shared discussion, repeated annually with an expert provider who conveys that the risk of sudden death and ICD shocks may be increased, and with the understanding that eligibility decisions for competitive sports participation often involve third parties (e.g., team physicians, consultants, and other institutional leadership) acting on behalf of the schools or teams" [34]. These recommendations should supplant the 2015 recommendations.

Shared Decision-Making

Recognizing the nuances in decisions regarding competitive sporting participation in individuals with HCM, there has been an evolution from a paternalistic approach using a binary "yes-no" framework toward a patient-clinician collaboration in a shared decision-making model [33, 34]. The clinician's role is to present the known facts and uncertainties regarding the risk and benefits of sporting participation in the context of the individual's disease. The patient's symptoms, risk factors for SCD, and sporting discipline should be considered while recognizing the personal importance placed on ongoing sporting participation for that individual. Key stakeholders, including parents/guardians/family and representatives from the team/college/club/sports organization, should be included, and if the decision is made to allow participation in sports, clear guidance for an emergency action plan must be established along with criteria for re-evaluation and follow-up.

Table 7.1 Comparison of American and European cardiology societies recommendations for competitive sporting participation in athletes with hypertrophic cardiomyopathy. Recent evolution of recommendations for exercise and participation in competitive sports in individuals with HCM

	2015 Task Force 3 American Heart Association/American College of Cardiology (AHA/ACC) [32]	2018 European Society of Cardiology (ESC) [33]	2020 AHA/ACC Guideline for the diagnosis and treatment of HCM [34]
Permit to compete	All individuals with HCM may only participate in class IA sports	Individuals may participate in all sports (except those where occurrence of syncope may be associated with harm or death) if they: 1. Have a mild clinical expression of HCM 2. Have a low ESC risk score 3. Are of adult age 4. Do not fulfill any of the exclusion criteria below and only after a complete shared decision-making process	Class 1: For most patients with HCM, mild- to moderate-intensity recreational exercise is beneficial Class 2a recommendation: For most patients with HCM, participation in low-intensity competitive sports is reasonable Class 2b recommendation: All athletes with HCM participation in high-intensity recreational activities or moderate- to high-intensity competitive sports activities may be considered after a comprehensive evaluation and shared discussion, repeated annually with an expert provider who conveys that the risk of sudden death and ICD shocks may be increased, and with the understanding that eligibility decisions for competitive sports participation often involve third parties (e.g., team physicians, consultants, and other institutional leadership) acting on behalf of the schools or teams
Restricted	All athletes with the probable or unequivocal clinical expression and diagnosis of HCM in all competitive sports except for class IA	Absolute contraindication to sporting participation: 1. History of aborted SCD/CA 2. Symptoms, particularly unheralded syncope 3. Exercise-induced ventricular tachycardia 4. High ESC 5-year risk score 5. Significant increase in LV outflow gradient (>50 mmHg) 6. Abnormal blood pressure response to exercise	

CA cardiac arrest, *ESC* European Society of Cardiology, *HCM* hypertrophic cardiomyopathy, *LV* left ventricle, *SCD* sudden cardiac death

Conclusion

HCM is a heterogeneous disease with significant variations in phenotypic expression and clinical outcomes. Occasionally, the expression of the disease can overlap with the physiological adaptation of intense athletic training. An understanding of the expected ranges of hypertrophy for the individual athlete, along with a critical appraisal of testing, can help the clinician differentiate these two entities.

The most feared complication of HCM is SCD in athletes and nonathletes. However, there are identifiable risk factors for SCD in HCM, and most individuals without these risk factors have a normal life expectancy. Due to concerns about the potential for exercise to be a trigger for SCD, recommendations regarding exercise and sporting participation have been restrictive and have not differentiated low- and high-risk individuals. This has resulted in higher rates of sedentary lifestyles, lower quality of life, and increased risk of obesity, with all the inherent risks, in patients with HCM. Newer data highlight the safety and benefit of regular low- and moderate-intensity exercise in patients with HCM, and there has been an evolution in the approach to high-intensity exercise to an individualized, shared decision-making model.

References

1. Gersh BJ, Maron BJ, Bonow RO, et al. 2011 ACCF/AHA Guideline for the diagnosis and treatment of hypertrophic cardiomyopathy: a report of the American College of Cardiology Foundation/American Heart Association Task Force on Practice Guidelines. Developed in collaboration with the American Association for Thoracic Surgery, American Society of Echocardiography, American Society of Nuclear Cardiology, Heart Failure Society of America, Heart Rhythm Society, Society for Cardiovascular Angiography and Interventions, and Society of Thoracic Surgeons. J Am Coll Cardiol. 2011;58(25):e212–60.
2. Elliott PM, Anastasakis A, Borger MA, et al. 2014 ESC Guidelines on diagnosis and management of hypertrophic cardiomyopathy: the task force for the diagnosis and management of hypertrophic cardiomyopathy of the European Society of Cardiology (ESC). Eur Heart J. 2014;35(39):2733–79.
3. Maron BJ, Gardin JM, Flack JM, Gidding SS, Kurosaki TT, Bild DE. Prevalence of hypertrophic cardiomyopathy in a general population of young adults. Echocardiographic analysis of 4111 subjects in the CARDIA Study. Coronary artery risk development in (young) adults. Circulation. 1995;92(4):785–9.
4. Basavarajaiah S, Wilson M, Whyte G, Shah A, McKenna W, Sharma S. Prevalence of hypertrophic cardiomyopathy in highly trained athletes: relevance to pre-participation screening. J Am Coll Cardiol. 2008;51(10):1033–9.
5. Sharma S, Drezner JA, Baggish A, et al. International recommendations for electrocardiographic interpretation in athletes. J Am Coll Cardiol. 2017;69(8):1057–75.
6. Sheikh N, Papadakis M, Schnell F, et al. Clinical profile of athletes with hypertrophic cardiomyopathy. Circ Cardiovasc Imaging. 2015;8(7):e003454.
7. Rowin EJ, Maron BJ, Appelbaum E, et al. Significance of false negative electrocardiograms in preparticipation screening of athletes for hypertrophic cardiomyopathy. Am J Cardiol. 2012;110(7):1027–32.

8. Schnell F, Riding N, O'Hanlon R, et al. Recognition and significance of pathological T-wave inversions in athletes. Circulation. 2015;131(2):165–73.
9. Papadakis M, Carre F, Kervio G, et al. The prevalence, distribution, and clinical outcomes of electrocardiographic repolarization patterns in male athletes of African/Afro-Caribbean origin. Eur Heart J. 2011;32(18):2304–13.
10. Basavarajaiah S, Boraita A, Whyte G, et al. Ethnic differences in left ventricular remodeling in highly-trained athletes relevance to differentiating physiologic left ventricular hypertrophy from hypertrophic cardiomyopathy. J Am Coll Cardiol. 2008;51(23):2256–62.
11. Schnell F, Matelot D, Daudin M, et al. Mechanical dispersion by strain echocardiography: a novel tool to diagnose hypertrophic cardiomyopathy in athletes. J Am Soc Echocardiogr. 2017;30(3):251–61.
12. Rudolph A, Abdel-Aty H, Bohl S, et al. Noninvasive detection of fibrosis applying contrast-enhanced cardiac magnetic resonance in different forms of left ventricular hypertrophy relation to remodeling. J Am Coll Cardiol. 2009;53(3):284–91.
13. Alpert C, Day SM, Saberi S. Sports and exercise in athletes with hypertrophic cardiomyopathy. Clin Sports Med. 2015;34(3):489–505.
14. Catto V, Dessanai MA, Sommariva E, Tondo C, Russo AD. S-ICD is effective in preventing sudden death in arrhythmogenic cardiomyopathy athletes during exercise. Pacing Clin Electrophysiol. 2019;42(9):1269–72.
15. Ullal AJ, Abdelfattah RS, Ashley EA, Froelicher VF. Hypertrophic cardiomyopathy as a cause of sudden cardiac death in the young: a meta-analysis. Am J Med. 2016;129(5):486–496.e482.
16. Cannan CR, Reeder GS, Bailey KR, Melton LJ 3rd, Gersh BJ. Natural history of hypertrophic cardiomyopathy. A population-based study, 1976 through 1990. Circulation. 1995;92(9):2488–95.
17. Maron BJ, Rowin EJ, Casey SA, Garberich RF, Maron MS. What do patients with hypertrophic cardiomyopathy die from? Am J Cardiol. 2016;117(3):434–5.
18. Maron MS, Rowin EJ, Wessler BS, et al. Enhanced American College of Cardiology/American Heart Association strategy for prevention of sudden cardiac death in high-risk patients with hypertrophic cardiomyopathy. JAMA Cardiol. 2019;4(7):644–57.
19. Reineck E, Rolston B, Bragg-Gresham JL, et al. Physical activity and other health behaviors in adults with hypertrophic cardiomyopathy. Am J Cardiol. 2013;111(7):1034–9.
20. Masri A, Pierson LM, Smedira NG, et al. Predictors of long-term outcomes in patients with hypertrophic cardiomyopathy undergoing cardiopulmonary stress testing and echocardiography. Am Heart J. 2015;169(5):684–692 e681.
21. Sharma S, Elliott PM, Whyte G, et al. Utility of metabolic exercise testing in distinguishing hypertrophic cardiomyopathy from physiologic left ventricular hypertrophy in athletes. J Am Coll Cardiol. 2000;36(3):864–70.
22. Sorajja P, Allison T, Hayes C, Nishimura RA, Lam CS, Ommen SR. Prognostic utility of metabolic exercise testing in minimally symptomatic patients with obstructive hypertrophic cardiomyopathy. Am J Cardiol. 2012;109(10):1494–8.
23. Bhella PS, Hastings JL, Fujimoto N, et al. Impact of lifelong exercise "dose" on left ventricular compliance and distensibility. J Am Coll Cardiol. 2014;64(12):1257–66.
24. Saberi S, Wheeler M, Bragg-Gresham J, et al. Effect of moderate-intensity exercise training on peak oxygen consumption in patients with hypertrophic cardiomyopathy: a randomized clinical trial. JAMA. 2017;317(13):1349–57.
25. Konhilas JP, Watson PA, Maass A, et al. Exercise can prevent and reverse the severity of hypertrophic cardiomyopathy. Circ Res. 2006;98(4):540–8.
26. Dejgaard LA, Haland TF, Lie OH, et al. Vigorous exercise in patients with hypertrophic cardiomyopathy. Int J Cardiol. 2018;250:157–63.
27. Klempfner R, Kamerman T, Schwammenthal E, et al. Efficacy of exercise training in symptomatic patients with hypertrophic cardiomyopathy: results of a structured exercise training program in a cardiac rehabilitation center. Eur J Prev Cardiol. 2015;22(1):13–9.

28. Maron BJ, Doerer JJ, Haas TS, Tierney DM, Mueller FO. Sudden deaths in young competitive athletes: analysis of 1866 deaths in the United States, 1980–2006. Circulation. 2009;119(8):1085–92.
29. Maron BJ, Klues HG. Surviving competitive athletics with hypertrophic cardiomyopathy. Am J Cardiol. 1994;73(15):1098–104.
30. Lampert R, Olshansky B, Heidbuchel H, et al. Safety of sports for athletes with implantable cardioverter-defibrillators: results of a prospective, multinational registry. Circulation. 2013;127(20):2021–30.
31. Pelliccia A, Lemme E, Maestrini V, et al. Does sport participation worsen the clinical course of hypertrophic cardiomyopathy? Clinical outcome of hypertrophic cardiomyopathy in athletes. Circulation. 2018;137(5):531–3.
32. Maron BJ, Udelson JE, Bonow RO, et al. Eligibility and disqualification recommendations for competitive athletes with cardiovascular abnormalities: task force 3: hypertrophic cardiomyopathy, arrhythmogenic right ventricular cardiomyopathy and other cardiomyopathies, and myocarditis: a scientific statement from the American Heart Association and American College of Cardiology. J Am Coll Cardiol. 2015;66(21):2362–71.
33. Pelliccia A, Solberg EE, Papadakis M, et al. Recommendations for participation in competitive and leisure time sport in athletes with cardiomyopathies, myocarditis, and pericarditis: position statement of the Sport Cardiology Section of the European Association of Preventive Cardiology (EAPC). Eur Heart J. 2019;40(1):19–33.
34. Writing Committee M, Ommen SR, Mital S, et al. AHA/ACC Guideline for the diagnosis and treatment of patients with hypertrophic cardiomyopathy: a report of the American College of Cardiology/American Heart Association Joint Committee on clinical practice guidelines. J Am Coll Cardiol. 2020;76(25):3022–55.

Chapter 8
Other Cardiomyopathies

Bradley Lander and David J. Engel

Introduction

Cardiac structural adaptation that commonly develops in athletes in response to the hemodynamic demands of long-term and intensive athletic training is referred to as exercise-induced cardiac remodeling (EICR) and is often described as "the athlete's heart." These cardiac structural changes in athletes can resemble cardiac structural changes associated with many forms of cardiomyopathy. Hypertrophic cardiomyopathy (HCM) was described in detail in Chap. 7. This chapter will review the core anatomic and physiologic characteristics of EICR and then highlight areas of overlap between EICR and structural features of several other cardiomyopathies. Finally, this chapter will review the available evidence and current expert recommendations to guide the care of athletes with these conditions.

EICR and Basic Physiologic Principles

Exercise involves a combination of "static" and "dynamic" physical activity. Static or isometric exercise, such as weight lifting and track and field throwing events, can be described by short, forceful skeletal muscle contractions and quantified by estimating the percentage of maximal voluntary contraction by the involved groups [1]. This type of activity leads to acute increases in systemic vascular resistance and arterial blood pressure. In response, the cardiac system adapts over time to maintain cardiac output in light of an increased left ventricular (LV) afterload [1]. In contrast, dynamic exercise, also known as isotonic or endurance exercise, such as running, is

B. Lander · D. J. Engel (✉)
Division of Cardiology, Columbia University Irving Medical Center, New York, NY, USA
e-mail: bl2276@cumc.columbia.edu; de165@cumc.columbia.edu

© Springer Nature Switzerland AG 2021
D. J. Engel, D. M. Phelan (eds.), *Sports Cardiology*,
https://doi.org/10.1007/978-3-030-69384-8_8

characterized by repetitive contraction and relaxation of large skeletal muscle groups which requires an increase in oxidative metabolism and is quantified by measuring oxygen uptake (VO_2) [1]. The cardiovascular system increases cardiac output during this type of exercise in proportion to the intensity of the activity and manages cardiac output by both increasing heart rate and stroke volume and by reducing systemic vascular resistance [1]. As a consequence of these adaptations to an increased workload, regular exercise can lead to an increase in right and left heart chamber sizes with increased LV mass arising from both increased wall thickness and cavity size [2–7]. These adaptations are most pronounced in athletes whose sports have significant static and endurance components (rowers) as compared to endurance alone (runners) [1, 8–11].

While LV chamber enlargement is a common adaptation to training, some degree of athletic remodeling can be reversible with cessation of systemic conditioning [11–14]. This method of "detraining" is often cited as a mechanism to distinguish athletic physiologic adaptation from cardiac pathology associated with cardiomyopathies. Among individuals with cardiomyopathies, left ventricular hypertrophy (LVH) and cavity enlargement are less likely to regress with athletic detraining, though some degree of regression is possible. Unfortunately, at the present time, no prospective study has been performed to address this question in subjects with genetically confirmed HCM or dilated cardiomyopathy, though there have been a few case reports of some degree of reverse remodeling in athletes with HCM [8, 15]. In healthy athletes who cease intense physical activity, small studies have shown that LV wall thickness and mass regress toward normal limits in a time frame of 6 weeks to 6 months [11, 12, 16].

Differing Characteristics of EICR Associated with Strength Versus Endurance Athletics

Cardiac remodeling, determined by the intensity, duration, and frequency of training, is typically more pronounced in endurance athletes [10]. This may be due, in part, to the athletes' prolonged exposure to increased hemodynamic stress [10]. Isotonic, or endurance, exercise training increases the LV end-diastolic chamber size as a principal cardiac adaptation and is associated with a balanced increase in LV mass with resultant eccentric left ventricular hypertrophy and often normal wall thickness [16, 17]. Conversely, isometric, or strength-based training is characterized predominantly by an increased pressure load on the LV which leads to concentric and typically symmetric LVH without a significant increase in LV cavity size [16, 17]. Overall, the physiology associated with increased volume in endurance exercise can lead to chamber dilation in both atria and ventricles, whereas the pressure load associated with static activity leads to LV wall thickening with less effect on the other three chambers [1]. These adaptive changes associated with endurance and strength training are depicted and summarized in Fig. 8.1.

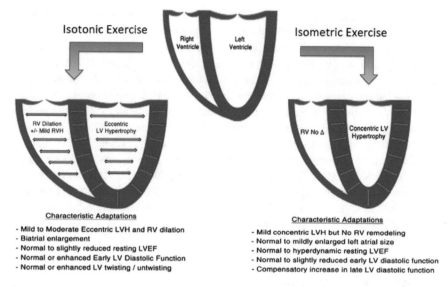

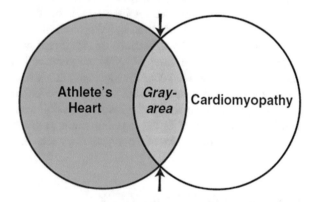

Fig. 8.1 Summary and features of exercise-induced cardiac remodeling by the type of exercise. (Reprinted with permission from Kim and Baggish [59], Elsevier)

Fig. 8.2 The gray area: overlap exists between features of the athlete's heart and cardiomyopathy. (Adapted from Maron et al. [54])

Distinguishing EICR from Cardiomyopathy: The Gray Zone

Distinguishing EICR from a potential cardiomyopathy can at times present clinical challenges as there can be structural overlap between these two processes; this overlap is typically referred to as the "gray area" or "gray zone" (Fig. 8.2). For example, approximately 2% of athletes with LVH have LV wall thickness that is above the expected measurements but less than the diagnostic threshold for HCM, 13–15 mm in men and 12–13 mm in women [6–8, 13, 14, 18–21]. In these cases, imaging should be reviewed to ensure that papillary muscles, trabeculae, and the RV moderator band were not included in original measurements [8]. In addition to increases in LV wall thickness, for those endurance athletes with significant ventricular dilation, a "gray zone" also exists for the distinction of EICR with forms of dilated cardiomyopathy [1]. As Baggish et al. note that physiologic LV and right ventricular (RV) dilation are often seen in conjunction with enlargement of the other ventricle, biatrial dilation, and normal to low-normal resting systolic function that appropriately augments during exercise. Isolated LV or RV dilation with other structural or functional abnormalities should be considered pathological unless proven otherwise [1]. Further distinctions between physiologic adaptations and cardiomyopathies will be described in the subsequent sections of this chapter.

Hypertrophic cardiomyopathy was described in detail in Chap. 7. This chapter will focus on several other cardiomyopathies affecting the left and right ventricles. Where applicable, data will be presented supporting the appropriate use of 12-lead electrocardiograms (ECG), echocardiography/strain imaging, stress testing, and cardiac magnetic resonance imaging (CMR) to aid in the distinction between each cardiomyopathy and EICR.

Dilated Cardiomyopathy

Dilated cardiomyopathy (DCM) is a recognized cause of sudden cardiac death (SCD) in athletes and has been defined as dilation of the LV associated with impaired systolic function and a reduction in LV ejection fraction (LVEF) without evidence of coronary disease, hypertension, or significant valvular disease [8, 22, 23]. Approximately 40% of cases of DCM are genetically determined [24], with titin and lamin A/C (LMNA) being the most commonly implicated genes, though there are over 50 genes reportedly associated with the condition [23]. Since an increase in left and right chamber sizes, with associated small decreases in LVEF, can be seen within the spectrum of EICR, it is important to distinguish between appropriate adaptations seen in athletes and true pathology seen in DCM.

Distinction of DCM from EICR

The main overlapping features between DCM and the athlete's heart can be LV cavity enlargement along with low-normal to mildly reduced LVEF [8]. Unfortunately, most parameters to distinguish between the two entities were validated in sedentary DCM patients and thus are less applicable to athletes who may have co-existing DCM [8].

12-Lead ECG Although there are limited data on ECG findings in asymptomatic DCM, atrioventricular (AV) block or conduction delays are seen in a large proportion of cases [8, 25–27]. First-degree AV block and type 1 second-degree AV block (Wenckebach) can be seen in about 7% of healthy athletes, but higher-degree AV block is uncommon and always abnormal [8, 28, 29]. Other ECG findings seen in

DCM include low QRS voltages, abnormal T-wave inversions, left atrial enlargement, left axis deviation, pathological Q waves, left and right bundle-branch blocks (LBBB, RBBB), premature ventricular contractions, and atrial fibrillation [8]. Many of these findings are uncommon in healthy athletes.

Echocardiography Current guidelines suggest that the combination of a left ventricular end-diastolic dimension (LVEDD) $\geq$60 mm and reduced resting LVEF should raise the suspicion of DCM in athletes [8, 30]. However, LV cavity dimensions may exceed this in healthy endurance athletes, such as rowers, cross-country skiers, and road cyclists. In a study of 1309 healthy elite athletes, Pelliccia et al. showed that LVEDD >60 mm was present in 14% of all athletes and LVEDD reached up to 66 mm in females and 70 mm in males [31]. It is important to note that all subjects in this study had normal LV ejection fraction [31]. In a study of National Basketball Association (NBA) basketball players, Engel et al. showed that LVEDD $\geq$59 mm was present in 36.5% of athletes and LVEDD $\geq$65 mm was seen in 4.4% of athletes [32].However, LV cavity sizes were normal in comparison to reference adults when LVEDD was indexed to the extreme height and body surface area (BSA) of these athletes [32]. This study also demonstrated that 1% of the NBA athletes had an LVEF <50% (lowest LVEF was 45%) and the athletes with this reduced LVEF had larger LVEDD (62.4 mm vs 56.8 mm) when compared with those with LVEF $\geq$50% [32]. The finding of a small proportion of athletes with low normal to mildly reduced LVEF has been similarly reported in other athlete groups, such as professional football players and cyclists [33, 34], but LVEF <50% is highly uncommon in athletes and should warrant further investigation to exclude the possibility of a cardiomyopathy. While resting global longitudinal strain (GLS) has been proposed as an additive echocardiographic analysis to help distinguish DCM and the EICR, a reduction in GLS values can be seen in both healthy athletes and individuals with DCM [35, 36]. In a study of 650 elite mixed-sport athletes, 37% of healthy, asymptomatic athletes who had below-normal LVEF had normal GLS, whereas 58% of athletes with normal LVEF had abnormal GLS, thus showing that GLS has uncertain utility in clarifying LV contractile function [37].

Cardiac Magnetic Resonance Imaging (CMR) Late gadolinium enhancement (LGE) on contrast-enhanced CMR is not a feature of EICR. However, nonspecific LGE, often in the interventricular septum and RV insertion point, has occasionally been observed in asymptomatic endurance athletes [8, 38]. It is important to note that while nonspecific LGE may be present in middle-aged and older athletes, it is never normal in young athletes. LGE that is observed in DCM is more often present in the mid wall of the ventricle, though LGE is not necessary for diagnosis of DCM given that it is absent in 68% of patients with genetically proven disease [39]. T1 mapping techniques have shown some potential to distinguish between DCM and EICR, but more studies are needed [40].

Stress Testing Healthy athletes and individuals with DCM may both have borderline resting LVEF, but the ability to increase cardiac output during exercise has been proposed as a useful way to distinguish between these two groups despite the lack of significant evidence to support this seemingly logical proposal [8]. Stress echocardiography has shown that healthy athletes with a low-normal resting LVEF will augment LVEF with exercise [34], whereas individuals with DCM fail to appropriately augment their LVEF [41]. Claessen et al. compared ten healthy endurance athletes to five endurance athletes with arrhythmias and subepicardial fibrosis on CMR and nine patients with mild DCM. All patients had a borderline resting LVEF. Exercise CMR was used to assess changes in exercise capacity (VO_2 max) and cardiac contractility in response to maximal exercise. Healthy athletes and athletes with fibrosis had better exercise capacity than the sedentary participants with mild DCM, unsurprisingly. However, the athletes with fibrosis and individuals with mild DCM both had blunted augmentation in LVEF when compared with the healthy athletes ($14 \pm 3\%$ improvement in LVEF in healthy athletes versus $5 \pm 6\%$ in DCM and $4 \pm 3\%$ in athletes with fibrosis) [42]. Exercise capacity alone did not distinguish between healthy athletes and those athletes with myocardial fibrosis and arrhythmias, but reduced contractile reserve with exercise did help with the distinction [42]. More data is needed in this area, but there is a promise that functional cardiac evaluation during exercise may be the best discriminatory test for DCM and EICR. Still, supranormal exercise capacity does not exclude potential underlying pathology in an athlete with suspected DCM [8].

Guidelines for Established Dilated Cardiomyopathy

The 2015 AHA/ACC Scientific Statement on Eligibility and Disqualification Recommendations for Competitive Athletes with Cardiovascular Abnormalities Task Force 3 recommended that symptomatic athletes with DCM should not participate in most competitive sports, with the possible exception of low intensity (class 1A sports) in selected cases (Class III, Level of Evidence C) [21]. Of note, an absolute number for LVEF was not used as a determining factor for guiding recommendations regarding the intensity of sports participation. The panel did note, consistent with cardiac studies of large athlete populations, that it is uncommon for an athlete to have a resting LVEF of <45% [21].

Left Ventricular Non-compaction

Left ventricular non-compaction (LVNC) is an inherited cardiomyopathy resulting from an embryological abnormality in which the trabecular meshwork with intertrabecular recesses, predominantly at the ventricular mid-portion and apex, persist after birth into childhood and adulthood [8, 21]. As a result, there are numerous excessively prominent trabeculations which can lead to heart failure and arrhythmias in a subset of patients [43].

Echocardiography and Cardiac MRI

Conventional diagnostic criteria by echocardiography are based on the ratio of compacted to non-compacted myocardium. The Chin criteria (Fig. 8.3a) require a compacted myocardium/non-compacted plus compacted myocardium ratio of ≤0.5 at end-diastole as seen on short-axis parasternal or apical views [44]. The Jenni criteria (Fig. 8.3b) require a ratio of non-compacted/compacted myocardium >2 at end-systole on short-axis parasternal views [45]. Other criteria (Petersen) have suggested an end-diastole compacted/non-compacted myocardium ratio of >2.3 on CMR [46] or a detailed analysis of trabecular structure using two-dimensional and color Doppler echocardiography (Stollberger criteria) [47]. In general, CMR is superior to echocardiography for the identification of regions of non-compacted myocardium and may provide a more accurate and definitive diagnosis of LVNC than echocardiography [21]. Importantly, because these measurements and diagnostic criteria have been derived from nonathletic cohorts, the generalizability to athletic cohorts may be limited.

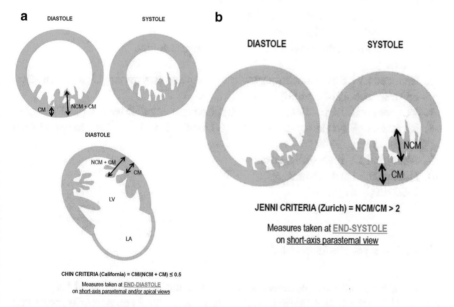

Fig. 8.3 Echocardiographic criteria for the diagnosis of LV non-compaction (LVNC) (**a**). Chin criteria (**b**). Jenni criteria. CM compacted myocardium, LA left atrium, LV left ventricle, NCM non-compacted myocardium. (Hotta et al. [60]. http://creativecommons.org/licenses/by/4.0/)

Distinguishing LVNC and EICR

Complicating the definitive diagnosis of LVNC in highly trained athletes is the observation that prominent LV trabeculations are relatively common in elite athletes and may represent a component of the adaptive physiological response to training [44]. In one study of 1146 healthy European athletes, prominent LV trabeculations were seen in 18.3% of athletes (29% in African American athletes versus 16% in white athletes), with 8.1% of total athletes fulfilling traditional criteria for LVNC [48]. A 2014 study of a population-representative cohort by Zemrak et al. demonstrated that while 25% met the Petersen criteria for LVNC, these individuals did not have an increased incidence of adverse events or reduced ejection fraction over approximately 10 years of follow-up [49]. Thus, it is important to approach a diagnosis of LVNC in an athlete with caution and avoid using hypertrabeculation alone as a marker to recommend exercise restriction. Currently, there are no specific criteria to distinguish features of the athlete's heart from LVNC, but the presence of any of the following findings may favor a diagnosis of LVNC:

1. Inferolateral T-wave inversions on ECG
2. The presence of cardiac symptoms
3. Confirmed family history of LVNC
4. A first-degree relative with a similar cardiac phenotype
5. LBBB
6. Reduced LVEF on echocardiography or failure of appropriate LV augmentation on stress echocardiography
7. VO_2 max <100% predicted on cardiopulmonary exercise testing (CPET)
8. Reduced tissue velocity on echo tissue Doppler imaging (E' at the lateral wall <9 cm/s)
9. Abnormal LV myocardial strain
10. Documented arrhythmias
11. LGE on CMR [8, 50]

Guidelines for Established LVNC

With respect to athletic participation for individuals with established LVNC, the AHA/ACC Task Force guidelines state that participation in competitive sports can be considered for individuals with LVNC who are asymptomatic, have normal LV systolic function, who are without important ventricular tachyarrhythmias on ambulatory monitoring or exercise testing, and who have no prior history of unexplained syncope (Class IIb, Level of Evidence C). However, athletes with an unequivocal diagnosis of LVNC and impaired systolic function or important atrial or ventricular tachyarrhythmias on ambulatory monitoring or exercise testing (or with a history of syncope) should not participate in competitive sports, except for possibly low-intensity class 1A sports, until further clinical information is available (Class III, Level of Evidence C) [21].

Arrhythmogenic Right Ventricular Cardiomyopathy

Arrhythmogenic right ventricular cardiomyopathy (ARVC) is a predominantly autosomal dominant disorder of the myocardium characterized pathologically by fibrofatty replacement of the right ventricular myocardium which can lead to segmental or diffuse wall thinning [21, 51]. Establishing the clinical diagnosis of ARVC can be challenging. General diagnostic criteria include a known family history of the disorder, left bundle-branch pattern ventricular arrhythmias, T-wave inversions in precordial leads V_1–V_3, epsilon waves, RV dilation or RV segmental wall motion abnormalities, RV aneurysm formation, and fatty deposition in the RV wall identified by CMR [21].

The 2010 revised criteria include the following components: global or regional RV dysfunction and structural alterations identified by echocardiography or CMR, tissue changes that include fibrofatty replacement as detected by endomyocardial biopsy, ECG depolarization or repolarization abnormalities, ventricular arrhythmias, and family history [51]. Each of these components is composed of major and minor criteria and is summarized in Table 8.1 [52].

A definite diagnosis of ARVC is fulfilled with two major criteria, one major and two minor criteria, or four minor criteria from different categories. A borderline diagnosis of ARVC requires one major and one minor criteria or three minor criteria from different categories; a possible diagnosis of ARVC requires one major criteria or two minor criteria from different categories.

ARVC is characterized by a broad phenotypic spectrum, and some individuals may be genotype positive but phenotype negative. These individuals should be followed serially over time as they may progress phenotypically [21]. There is some data to suggest that exercise increases the penetrance and arrhythmic risk in mutation carriers of ARVC without overt phenotypic expression, thus raising concern in these individuals regarding participation, not only in competitive sports but also in moderate to extreme recreational physical activity [53]. A 2015 study by Ruwald et al. showed that competitive athletics were associated with a twofold increased risk of ventricular arrhythmias/death and earlier presentation of symptoms when compared with recreational athletes or inactive subjects; however, this increased risk was not seen when recreational athletes were compared to inactive individuals [54].

Table 8.1 2010 Task Force major and minor criteria for arrhythmogenic RV cardiomyopathy. Current 2010 TFC Diagnosis

	Major	Minor
I. Global or regional dysfunction and structural alterations	By 2D echocardiogram: Regional RV akinesia, dyskinesia, or aneurysm _and_ 1 of the following (end-diastole): PLAX RVOT $\geq$32 mm (PLAX/BSA $\geq$19 mm/m^2) PSAX RVOT $\geq$36 mm (PSAX/BSA $\geq$21 mm/m^2) Or RFAC $\leq$33%	By 2D echocardiogram: Regional RV akinesia or dyskinesia, _and_ 1 of the following (end-diastole): 29$\leq$PLAX RVOT <32 mm (16 $\leq$PLAX/BSA <19 mm/m^2) 32 $\leq$PSAX RVOT <36 mm (18 $\leq$PSAX/BSA <21 mm/m^2) Or 33% <RFAC $\leq$40%
	By MRI: Regional RV akinesia or dyskinesia or dyssynchronous RV contraction _and_ 1 of the following: RV end-diastolic volume/ BSA $\geq$110 ml/m^2 (male) Or $\geq$100 ml/m^2 (female) Or RV ejection fraction $\leq$40%	By MRI: Regional RV akinesia or dyskinesia or dyssynchronous RV contraction _and_ 1 of the following (end-diastole): 100 ml/m^2 $\leq$ RV end-diastolic volume/BSA M110 ml/m^2 (male) or 90 ml/m^2 $\leq$ RV end-diastolic volume/ BSA <100 ml/m^2 (female) Or 40% < RV ejection fraction $\leq$45%
	By RV angiography: Regional RV akinesia, dyskinesia, or aneurysm	
II. Tissue characterization of wall	Residual myocytes <60% by morphometric analysis (or <50% if estimates), with fibrous replacement of the RV free wall myocardium in $\geq$1 sample, with or without fatty replacement of tissue on endomyocardial biopsy	Residual myocytes 60% to 75% by morphometric analysis (or 50% to 65% if estimated), with fibrous replacement of the RV free wall myocardium in $\geq$1 sample, with or without fatty replacement of tissue on endomyocardial biopsy
III. Repolarization abnormalities	Inverted T waves in right precordial leads (V_1, V_2, and V_3) or beyond in individuals >14 years of age (in the absence of complete RBBB QRS $\geq$120 ms)	Inverted T waves in leads V_1 and V_2 in individuals >14 years of age (in the absence of complete RBBB) or in V_4, V_5, or V_6 Inverted T waves in leads V_1, V_2, V_3, and V_4 in individuals >14 years of age in the presence of complete RBBB

Table 8.1 (continued)

	Major	Minor
IV. Depolarization/ conduction abnormalities	Epsilon wave in the right precordial leads (V_1 to V_3)	Late potentials by SAECG in ≥1 of 3 parameters in the absence of an ORS duration ≥110 ms on the standard ECG Filtered QRS duration ≥114 ms Duration of terminal QRS <40 µV (low-amplitude signal duration) ≥38 ms Root mean square voltage of terminal 40 ms ≤20 µV Terminal activation duration of QRS ≥55 ms measured from the nadir of the S-wave to the end of the QRS, including R', in V_1, V_2, or V_3, in the absence of complete RBBB
V. Ventricular arrhythmias	Nonsustained or sustained VT of LBBB morphology with superior axis (negative or indeterminate QRS in leads, II, III, and aVF and positive in lead aVL)	Nonsustained or sustained RVOT VT of LBBB morphology with inferior axis (positive QRS in leads II, III, and aVF and negative in lead aVL) or with unknown axis >500 ventricular extrasystoles 24 h (Holter)
VI. Family history	ARVC/D confirmed in a first-degree relative with meets current TFC ARVC/D confirmed pathologically at autopsy or surgery in a first-degree relative Identification of a pathogenic mutation categorized as associated or probably associated with ARVC/D in the patient	History of ARVC/D in a first-degree relative in whom it is not possible or practical to determine whether the family member meets current TFC Premature sudden death (<35 years of age) due to suspected ARVC/D in a first-degree relative ARVC/D confirmed pathologically or by current TFC in a second-degree relative

Adapted with permission form Marcus et al. [4]

2D two-dimensional, *ARVC/D* arrhythmogenic right ventricular cardiomyopathy/dysplasia, *ECG* electrocardiography, *BSA* body surface area, *LBBB* left bundle branch block, *MRI* magnetic resonance imaging, *PLAX* parasternal long-axis view, *PSAX* parasternal short-axis view, *RBBB* right bundle branch block, *RFAC* right fractional area change, *RV* right ventricular, *RVOT* right ventricular outflow tract, *SAECG* signal-averaged electrocardiography, *TFC* task force criteria, *VT* ventricular tachycardia

Reprinted with permission from Gandjbakhch et al. [51], Elsevier

Distinction Between Pathology and RV Adaptation in Athletes

Despite rigorous data, as represented by D'Ascenzi et al. [55], there are no clear criteria to distinguish morphologic changes seen in ARVC from similar appearing RV remodeling that can occur in association with EICR. The extent of athletic RV remodeling correlates with the type of exercise: endurance athletics (swimming, running) are often characterized by RV elongation and dilation, while isometric athletics (weight lifting, rowing) cause little change in RV structure [56, 57]. The underlying mechanisms are not entirely understood, but sustained increased cardiac output during high-intensity aerobic exercise expands end-diastolic RV volume [56]. The RV, when compared with the LV, is a non-compacted structure with more compliance, thus making its shape more sensitive to loading conditions [57]. RV enlargement is more common in trained athletes than in the general population [58]; thus RV size criterion alone cannot be a reliable distinguishing factor between elite athletes and ARVC [56]. In addition, a proportion of elite endurance athletes will additionally manifest a rounded RV apex and have prominent RV trabeculations and moderator bands [52], findings that may also be present in individuals with ARVC. A high false-positive rate for diagnosing ARVC in athletes can be expected given this overlap in RV structure and dimensions. However, because ARVC is associated with RV akinesia, dyskinesia, or aneurysm formation, the combination of RV dilation and these abnormalities can be useful in characterizing ARVC [56].

Guidelines for ARVC

The 2015 AHA/ACC Scientific Statement on Eligibility and Disqualification Recommendations for Competitive Athletes with Cardiovascular Abnormalities Task Force 3 recommended that athletes with a definite, borderline, or possible diagnosis of ARVC not participate in most competitive sports, with the possible exception of low-intensity class 1A sports (Class III, Level of Evidence C). Prophylactic ICD placement in athlete-patients with ARVC for the sole or primary purpose of permitting participation in high-intensity sports is not recommended because of the possibility of device-related complications (Class III, Level of Evidence C) [21].

Infiltrative Cardiomyopathies

There is a paucity of data on infiltrative cardiomyopathies in relation to athletes. The clinical principles guiding the care of athletes with other forms of cardiomyopathy should be applied to this cohort of patients until further data is generated. It stands to reason that athletes are at higher risk of sports-related cardiac complications if they have symptoms consistent with congestive heart failure, a reduced LVEF, documented arrhythmias, or other comorbidities.

It is important for medical personnel caring for athletes to be familiar with published reference literature describing the upper limits of cardiac dimensions associated with EICR, detailed in this chapter and throughout this book. If athletes fall into the gray area by traditional measurements, or if clinical concerns are present, additional imaging should be considered. With respect to infiltrative cardiomyopathies, CMR can be especially useful to distinguish athletic hypertrophy from an infiltrative process. The degree of left ventricular infiltration influences the risk for catecholamine-induced (exercise-triggered) arrhythmias.

Guidelines for Infiltrative Cardiomyopathies

The 2015 AHA/ACC Scientific Statement on Eligibility and Disqualification Recommendations for Competitive Athletes with Cardiovascular Abnormalities Task Force 3 recommended that symptomatic athletes with infiltrative cardiomyopathies should not participate in most competitive sports, with the possible exception of low intensity (class 1A sports) in selected cases, at least until more information is available (Class III, Level of Evidence C) [21].

Conclusion

This chapter has reviewed the basic physiologic principles of exercise-induced cardiac remodeling and described how these expected and adaptive athletic changes can overlap (gray zone) with features of several forms of cardiomyopathy including dilated cardiomyopathy, left ventricular non-compaction, arrhythmogenic right ventricular cardiomyopathy, and infiltrative cardiomyopathy. Clinical approaches, and uses of cardiac imaging tests and procedures, have been presented to help aid in the recognition of athletes who may unknowingly harbor these cardiomyopathies and be at risk for exercise-triggered cardiac emergencies. Similarly, the information provided in this chapter will hopefully assist to lessen unnecessary disqualifications and delays in return to play for athletes found to have cardiac changes consistent with EICR alone, without the clinical or imaging factors that raise concern for the presence of cardiomyopathy. Finally, the current expert recommendations to guide the care of athletes with these cardiomyopathies have been summarized, though it must be reiterated that limited prospective data keeps the majority of current recommendations as consensus recommendations only.

References

1. Baggish AL, Battle RW, Beckerman JG, et al. Sports cardiology: core curriculum for providing cardiovascular care to competitive athletes and highly active people. J Am Coll Cardiol. 2017;70(15):1902–18. https://doi.org/10.1016/j.jacc.2017.08.055.
2. Huston TP, Puffer JC, Rodney WM. The athletic heart syndrome. N Engl J Med. 1985;313(1):24–32. https://doi.org/10.1056/NEJM198507043130106.

3. Pluim BM, Zwinderman AH, van der Laarse A, van der Wall EE. The athlete's heart. A meta-analysis of cardiac structure and function. Circulation. 2000;101(3):336–44. https://doi.org/10.1161/01.cir.101.3.336.

4. Hauser AM, Dressendorfer RH, Vos M, Hashimoto T, Gordon S, Timmis GC. Symmetric cardiac enlargement in highly trained endurance athletes: a two-dimensional echocardiographic study. Am Heart J. 1985;109(5 Pt 1):1038–44. https://doi.org/10.1016/0002-8703(85)90247-9.

5. Maron BJ. Structural features of the athlete heart as defined by echocardiography. J Am Coll Cardiol. 1986;7(1):190–203. https://doi.org/10.1016/s0735-1097(86)80282-0.

6. Pelliccia A, Maron BJ, Spataro A, Proschan MA, Spirito P. The upper limit of physiologic cardiac hypertrophy in highly trained elite athletes. N Engl J Med. 1991;324(5):295–301. https://doi.org/10.1056/NEJM199101313240504.

7. Maron BJ, Pelliccia A. The heart of trained athletes: cardiac remodeling and the risks of sports, including sudden death. Circulation. 2006;114(15):1633–44. https://doi.org/10.1161/CIRCULATIONAHA.106.613562.

8. Brosnan M, Rakhit D. Differentiating athlete's heart from cardiomyopathies — the left side. Hear Lung Circ. 2018;27:1052–62. https://doi.org/10.1016/j.hlc.2018.04.297.

9. Kooreman Z, Giraldeau G, Finocchiaro G, et al. Athletic remodeling in female college athletes, the "Morganroth hypothesis" revisited. Clin J Sport Med. 2018. https://doi.org/10.1097/JSM.0000000000000501.

10. Beaudry R, Haykowsky MJ, Baggish A, La Gerche A. A modern definition of the athlete's heart-for research and the clinic. Cardiol Clin. 2016;34(4):507–14. https://doi.org/10.1016/j.ccl.2016.06.001.

11. Spence AL, Naylor LH, Carter HH, et al. A prospective randomised longitudinal MRI study of left ventricular adaptation to endurance and resistance exercise training in humans. J Physiol. 2011;589(Pt 22):5443–52. https://doi.org/10.1113/jphysiol.2011.217125.

12. Pelliccia A, Maron BJ, De Luca R, Di Paolo FM, Spataro A, Culasso F. Remodeling of left ventricular hypertrophy in elite athletes after long-term deconditioning. Circulation. 2002;105(8):944–9. https://doi.org/10.1161/hc0802.104534.

13. Caselli S, Maron MS, Urbano-Moral JA, Pandian NG, Maron BJ, Pelliccia A. Differentiating left ventricular hypertrophy in athletes from that in patients with hypertrophic cardiomyopathy. Am J Cardiol. 2014;114(9):1383–9. https://doi.org/10.1016/j.amjcard.2014.07.070.

14. Maron BJ, Pelliccia A, Spirito P. Cardiac disease in young trained athletes. Insights into methods for distinguishing athlete's heart from structural heart disease, with particular emphasis on hypertrophic cardiomyopathy. Circulation. 1995;91(5):1596–601. https://doi.org/10.1161/01.cir.91.5.1596.

15. de Gregorio C, Speranza G, Magliarditi A, Pugliatti P, Andò G, Coglitore S. Detraining-related changes in left ventricular wall thickness and longitudinal strain in a young athlete likely to have hypertrophic cardiomyopathy. J Sports Sci Med. 2012;11(3):557–61. https://www.ncbi.nlm.nih.gov/pubmed/24149368.

16. Weiner RB, Wang F, Berkstresser B, et al. Regression of "gray zone" exercise-induced concentric left ventricular hypertrophy during prescribed detraining. J Am Coll Cardiol. 2012;59(22):1992–4. https://doi.org/10.1016/j.jacc.2012.01.057.

17. Wasfy MM, Weiner RB. Differentiating the athlete's heart from hypertrophic cardiomyopathy. Curr Opin Cardiol. 2015;30(5):500–5. https://doi.org/10.1097/HCO.0000000000000203.

18. Basavarajaiah S, Boraita A, Whyte G, et al. Ethnic differences in left ventricular remodeling in highly-trained athletes relevance to differentiating physiologic left ventricular hypertrophy from hypertrophic cardiomyopathy. J Am Coll Cardiol. 2008;51(23):2256–62. https://doi.org/10.1016/j.jacc.2007.12.061.

19. Rawlins J, Carre F, Kervio G, et al. Ethnic differences in physiological cardiac adaptation to intense physical exercise in highly trained female athletes. Circulation. 2010;121(9):1078–85. https://doi.org/10.1161/CIRCULATIONAHA.109.917211.

20. Pelliccia A, Maron MS, Maron BJ. Assessment of left ventricular hypertrophy in a trained athlete: differential diagnosis of physiologic athlete's heart from pathologic hypertrophy. Prog Cardiovasc Dis. 2012;54(5):387–96. https://doi.org/10.1016/j.pcad.2012.01.003.

21. Maron BJ, Udelson JE, Bonow RO, et al. Eligibility and disqualification recommendations for competitive athletes with cardiovascular abnormalities: task force 3: hypertrophic cardiomyopathy, arrhythmogenic right ventricular cardiomyopathy and other cardiomyopathies, and myocarditis: a scientific statement from the American Heart Association and American College of Cardiology. Circulation. 2015;132(22):e273–80. https://doi.org/10.1161/CIR.0000000000000239.

22. Maron BJ, Doerer JJ, Haas TS, Tierney DM, Mueller FO. Sudden deaths in young competitive athletes: analysis of 1866 deaths in the United States, 1980–2006. Circulation. 2009;119(8):1085–92. https://doi.org/10.1161/CIRCULATIONAHA.108.804617.

23. Pinto YM, Elliott PM, Arbustini E, et al. Proposal for a revised definition of dilated cardiomyopathy, hypokinetic non-dilated cardiomyopathy, and its implications for clinical practice: a position statement of the ESC working group on myocardial and pericardial diseases. Eur Heart J. 2016;37(23):1850–8. https://doi.org/10.1093/eurheartj/ehv727.

24. Merlo M, Cannatà A, Gobbo M, Stolfo D, Elliott PM, Sinagra G. Evolving concepts in dilated cardiomyopathy. Eur J Heart Fail. 2018;20(2):228–39. https://doi.org/10.1002/ejhf.1103.

25. Drezner JA, Ashley E, Baggish AL, et al. Abnormal electrocardiographic findings in athletes: recognising changes suggestive of cardiomyopathy. Br J Sports Med. 2013;47(3):137–52. https://doi.org/10.1136/bjsports-2012-092069.

26. Dec GW, Fuster V. Idiopathic dilated cardiomyopathy. N Engl J Med. 1994;331(23):1564–75. https://doi.org/10.1056/NEJM199412083312307.

27. Grünig E, Tasman JA, Kücherer H, Franz W, Kübler W, Katus HA. Frequency and phenotypes of familial dilated cardiomyopathy. J Am Coll Cardiol. 1998;31(1):186–94. https://doi.org/10.1016/s0735-1097(97)00434-8.

28. Brosnan M, La Gerche A, Kalman J, et al. Comparison of frequency of significant electrocardiographic abnormalities in endurance versus nonendurance athletes. Am J Cardiol. 2014;113(9):1567–73. https://doi.org/10.1016/j.amjcard.2014.01.438.

29. Sharma S, Drezner JA, Baggish A, et al. International recommendations for electrocardiographic interpretation in athletes. J Am Coll Cardiol. 2017;69(8):1057–75. https://doi.org/10.1016/j.jacc.2017.01.015.

30. Galderisi M, Cardim N, D'Andrea A, et al. The multi-modality cardiac imaging approach to the Athlete's heart: an expert consensus of the European Association of Cardiovascular Imaging. Eur Heart J Cardiovasc Imaging. 2015;16(4):353. https://doi.org/10.1093/ehjci/jeu323.

31. Pelliccia A, Culasso F, Di Paolo FM, Maron BJ. Physiologic left ventricular cavity dilatation in elite athletes. Ann Intern Med. 1999;130(1):23–31. https://doi.org/10.7326/0003-4819-130-1-199901050-00005.

32. Engel DJ, Schwartz A, Homma S. Athletic cardiac remodeling in US professional basketball players. JAMA Cardiol. 2016;1(1):80–7. https://doi.org/10.1001/jamacardio.2015.0252.

33. Abergel E, Chatellier G, Hagege AA, et al. Serial left ventricular adaptations in world-class professional cyclists: implications for disease screening and follow-up. J Am Coll Cardiol. 2004;44(1):144–9. https://doi.org/10.1016/j.jacc.2004.02.057.

34. Abernethy WB, Choo JK, Hutter AM. Echocardiographic characteristics of professional football players. J Am Coll Cardiol. 2003;41(2):2–6.

35. D'Andrea A, Cocchia R, Riegler L, et al. Left ventricular myocardial velocities and deformation indexes in top-level athletes. J Am Soc Echocardiogr. 2010;23(12):1281–8. https://doi.org/10.1016/j.echo.2010.09.020.

36. Tarando F, Coisne D, Galli E, et al. Left ventricular non-compaction and idiopathic dilated cardiomyopathy: the significant diagnostic value of longitudinal strain. Int J Cardiovasc Imaging. 2017;33(1):83–95. https://doi.org/10.1007/s10554-016-0980-3.

37. Flannery MD, Beaudry R, Prior D, et al. P1535Global longitudinal strain does not help differentiate between athlete's heart and pathology in athletes with low LVEF. Eur Heart J. 2017;38(Suppl_1). https://doi.org/10.1093/eurheartj/ehx502.P1535.

38. La Gerche A, Burns AT, Mooney DJ, et al. Exercise-induced right ventricular dysfunction and structural remodelling in endurance athletes. Eur Heart J. 2012;33(8):998–1006. https://doi.org/10.1093/eurheartj/ehr397.

39. Tayal U, Newsome S, Buchan R, et al. Phenotype and clinical outcomes of titin cardiomyopathy. J Am Coll Cardiol. 2017;70(18):2264–74. https://doi.org/10.1016/j.jacc.2017.08.063.
40. Mordi I, Carrick D, Bezerra H, Tzemos N. T1 and T2 mapping for early diagnosis of dilated non-ischaemic cardiomyopathy in middle-aged patients and differentiation from normal physiological adaptation. Eur Heart J Cardiovasc Imaging. 2016;17(7):797–803. https://doi.org/10.1093/ehjci/jev216.
41. Ennezat PV, Maréchaux S, Huerre C, et al. Exercise does not enhance the prognostic value of Doppler echocardiography in patients with left ventricular systolic dysfunction and functional mitral regurgitation at rest. Am Heart J. 2008;155(4):752–7. https://doi.org/10.1016/j.ahj.2007.11.022.
42. Claessen G, Schnell F, Bogaert J, et al. Exercise cardiac magnetic resonance to differentiate athlete's heart from structural heart disease. Eur Heart J Cardiovasc Imaging. 2018;19(9):1062–70. https://doi.org/10.1093/ehjci/jey050.
43. Arbustini E, Favalli V, Narula N, Serio A, Grasso M. Left ventricular noncompaction: a distinct genetic cardiomyopathy? J Am Coll Cardiol. 2016;68(9):949–66. https://doi.org/10.1016/j.jacc.2016.05.096.
44. Chin TK, Perloff JK, Williams RG, Jue K, Mohrmann R. Isolated noncompaction of left ventricular myocardium. A study of eight cases. Circulation. 1990;82(2):507–13. https://doi.org/10.1161/01.cir.82.2.507.
45. Jenni R, Oechslin E, Schneider J, Attenhofer Jost C, Kaufmann PA. Echocardiographic and pathoanatomical characteristics of isolated left ventricular non-compaction: a step towards classification as a distinct cardiomyopathy. Heart. 2001;86(6):666–71. https://doi.org/10.1136/heart.86.6.666.
46. Petersen SE, Selvanayagam JB, Wiesmann F, et al. Left ventricular non-compaction: insights from cardiovascular magnetic resonance imaging. J Am Coll Cardiol. 2005;46(1):101–5. https://doi.org/10.1016/j.jacc.2005.03.045.
47. Stöllberger C, Gerecke B, Finsterer J, Engberding R. Refinement of echocardiographic criteria for left ventricular noncompaction. Int J Cardiol. 2013;165(3):463–7. https://doi.org/10.1016/j.ijcard.2011.08.845.
48. Gati S, Chandra N, Bennett RL, et al. Increased left ventricular trabeculation in highly trained athletes: do we need more stringent criteria for the diagnosis of left ventricular non-compaction in athletes? Heart. 2013;99(6):401–8. https://doi.org/10.1136/heartjnl-2012-303418.
49. Zemrak F, Ahlman MA, Captur G, et al. The relationship of left ventricular trabeculation to ventricular function and structure over a 9.5-year follow-up: the MESA study. J Am Coll Cardiol. 2014;64(19):1971–80. https://doi.org/10.1016/j.jacc.2014.08.035.
50. Gati S, Sharma S. CardioPulse: the dilemmas in diagnosing left ventricular non-compaction in athletes. Eur Heart J. 2015;36(15):891–3. https://www.ncbi.nlm.nih.gov/pubmed/26052607.
51. Marcus FI, Mckenna WJ, Sherrill D, et al. Diagnosis of arrhythmogenic right ventricular cardiomyopathy / dysplasia proposed modification of the Task Force criteria. Circulation. 2010;121:1533–41. https://doi.org/10.1161/CIRCULATIONAHA.108.840827.
52. Gandjbakhch E, Redheuil A, Pousset F, Charron P, Frank R. Clinical diagnosis, imaging, and genetics of arrhythmogenic right ventricular cardiomyopathy/dysplasia: JACC State-of-the-Art review. J Am Coll Cardiol. 2018;72(7):784–804. https://doi.org/10.1016/j.jacc.2018.05.065.
53. James CA, Bhonsale A, Tichnell C, et al. Exercise increases age-related penetrance and arrhythmic risk in arrhythmogenic right ventricular dysplasia/cardiomyopathy-associated desmosomal mutation carriers. J Am Coll Cardiol. 2013;62(14):1290–7. https://doi.org/10.1016/j.jacc.2013.06.033.
54. Ruwald A-C, Marcus F, Estes NAM 3rd, et al. Association of competitive and recreational sport participation with cardiac events in patients with arrhythmogenic right ventricular cardiomyopathy: results from the North American multidisciplinary study of arrhythmogenic right ventricular cardiomyopathy. Eur Heart J. 2015;36(27):1735–43. https://doi.org/10.1093/eurheartj/ehv110.

55. D'Ascenzi F, Pisicchio C, Caselli S, Di Paolo FM, Spataro A, Pelliccia A. RV Remodeling in Olympic athletes. JACC Cardiovasc Imaging. 2017;10(4):385–93. https://doi.org/10.1016/j.jcmg.2016.03.017.
56. Maron BJ, Maron BA. Revisiting athlete's heart versus pathologic hypertrophy. JACC Cardiovasc Imaging. 2017;10(4):394–7. https://doi.org/10.1016/j.jcmg.2016.05.011.
57. Weiner RB, Baggish AL. Exercise-induced cardiac remodeling. Prog Cardiovasc Dis. 2012;54(5):380–6. https://doi.org/10.1016/j.pcad.2012.01.006.
58. Kawut SM, Barr RG, Lima JAC, et al. Right ventricular structure is associated with the risk of heart failure and cardiovascular death: the Multi-Ethnic Study of Atherosclerosis (MESA)--right ventricle study. Circulation. 2012;126(14):1681–8. https://doi.org/10.1161/CIRCULATIONAHA.112.095216.
59. Kim JH, Baggish AL. Differentiating exercise-induced cardiac adaptations from cardiac pathology: the "grey zone" of clinical uncertainty. Can J Cardiol. 2016;32(4):429–37.
60. Hotta VT, Tendolo SC, Rodrigues ACT, Fernandes F, Nastari L, Mady C. Limitations in the diagnosis of noncompaction cardiomyopathy by echocardiography. Arq Bras Cardiol. 2017;109(5):483–8.

Chapter 9
Inflammatory Cardiac Disorders in the Athlete

Kenneth G. Zahka, Nishant P. Shah, and Kara Denby

Introduction

Inflammatory disorders of the heart are associated with significant morbidity and mortality. Inflammation can affect both the outer protective layer of the heart (pericardium) and the actual muscular layers of the heart (myocardium). Inflammation of these layers result in conditions known as pericarditis and myocarditis, respectively. In addition, there can also be overlap or extension of inflammation in disorders known as perimyocarditis or myopericarditis. Myopericarditis is predominately a pericardial inflammatory disorder that fulfills pericarditis diagnostic criteria but also has concurrent myocardial involvement [1]. Conversely, perimyocarditis is primarily a myocardial inflammatory disorder with concurrent pericardial involvement [1]. Regardless of the type, inflammatory disorders of the heart can lead to severe complications such as severe chest pain, pericardial effusion, cardiac tamponade, congestive heart failure, cardiogenic shock, electrical instability, or sudden cardiac death (SCD). Therefore, early detection of signs and symptoms of these disorders is critical for timely treatment and monitoring.

Physical activity restriction is recommended for inflammatory cardiac disorders to promote recovery. However, restriction of activity can be distressing to the athlete or to those for whom competitive sport is a major part of their lives. Currently, both the American Heart Association (AHA) and European Association of Preventive Cardiology (EAPC) guidelines recommend activity restriction in athletes diagnosed with inflammatory disorders of the heart until there is evidence of resolution of

K. G. Zahka (✉)
Department of Pediatric Cardiology, Cardiovascular Medicine, Cleveland Clinic, Cleveland, OH, USA
e-mail: zahkak@ccf.org

N. P. Shah · K. Denby
Department of Cardiovascular Medicine, Cleveland Clinic, Cleveland, OH, USA
e-mail: shahn2@ccf.org; denbyk@ccf.org

© Springer Nature Switzerland AG 2021
D. J. Engel, D. M. Phelan (eds.), *Sports Cardiology*,
https://doi.org/10.1007/978-3-030-69384-8_9

inflammation [2, 3]. While the evidence for this recommendation is more established in cases of myocarditis, the data for pericarditis is limited and based on expert consensus. In this chapter we will review the etiologies and clinical symptoms, current sport participation guidelines and the evidence behind the guidelines for both myocarditis and pericarditis.

Myocarditis

Myocarditis is a nonischemic inflammatory disease of the myocardium that can result in heart failure and arrhythmias [4]. Myocarditis with preserved ejection fraction is also well described. The etiologies of myocarditis fall broadly into three categories: infectious, toxic, and autoimmune. Viral myocarditis is the most common etiology in the developed world and the most studied. However, in the context of young athletes, toxins such as amphetamines and cocaine should be inquired about during medical history intake [5]. The pathophysiology of myocarditis is mediated primarily through myocardial inflammatory infiltrates and necrosis [4].

The diagnostic evaluation of myocarditis typically begins with a clinical history and physical exam. The clinical presentation of myocarditis can be highly variable as patients can present with chest pain, exertional dyspnea, and fatigue or overtly decompensated heart failure, cardiogenic shock, or electrical instability [6–8]. The initial electrocardiogram (ECG) can be variable with ST segment deviations, ectopic beats, conduction abnormalities, sustained arrhythmias, or QRS low voltages. Transthoracic echocardiography (TTE) may show global left ventricular dysfunction; however, localized wall motion abnormalities with pericardial effusions are also common, as well as evidence of dilated cardiomyopathy (DCM). The gold standard to establish a diagnosis of myocarditis is an endomyocardial biopsy; however, this test is limited by inherent risk and low sensitivity if the inflammation has a patchy distribution [8]. The diagnosis is more commonly based on the clinical history, elevation in cardiac enzymes, and a nonischemic pattern of late gadolinium enhancement (LGE) on cardiac magnetic resonance imaging (CMR). Often DCM can form in later phases of the disease and can take up to 6–12 weeks to resolve. CMR can also often confirm a diagnosis of perimyocarditis or myopericarditis [1]. Therefore, taking both clinical and diagnostic information into consideration, there is expert consensus that the diagnosis of probable myocarditis can be made by the following [2]:

1. A clinical syndrome that includes acute heart failure, angina-type chest pain (often preceded by a viral prodrome), or myopericarditis of <3 months duration.
2. An otherwise unexplained elevation in serum troponin with associated findings that can include:

   - Electrocardiographic features of cardiac ischemia
   - Otherwise unexplained high-degree atrioventricular (AV) block or arrhythmias
   - Ventricular wall motion abnormalities
   - Pericardial effusion on echocardiography or CMR imaging

3. Additional CMR findings that suggest myocarditis in the acute clinical setting include characteristic alterations in tissue signal on T2- or T1-weighted images and the presence of LGE.

Once diagnosed with myocarditis, treatment depends on the underlying etiology and whether or not there is left ventricular (LV) dysfunction [4]. For instance, in rare types of viral etiologies such as giant cell myocarditis or eosinophilic myocarditis, corticosteroids or other immunosuppressants (e.g., intravenous immunoglobulin) are important for treatment [7]. For cases that occur as a result of an underlying systemic disorder such as systematic lupus erythematosus, treatment of the underlying cause can aid in myocardial recovery [4]. If there is LV dysfunction with an ejection fraction <40%, then guideline-directed medical therapy (GDMT) for heart failure is also recommended [4]. GDMT includes angiotensin-converting enzyme inhibitors or angiotensin II receptor blockers, beta-blockers, or mineralocorticoid receptor antagonists. In cases of severe myocarditis, also known as fulminant myocarditis, that results in acute heart failure, cardiogenic shock, or malignant arrhythmias, inotropes or cardiac mechanical circulatory support measures may be needed for support during the acute phase of illness [8].

It is also important for clinicians to be familiar with the current guidelines regarding participation in competitive sports with respect to myocarditis [9] as physical activity has been linked to SCD [10]. It remains unclear whether or not physical activity is also primarily responsible for recurrence. Activity restriction also pertains to patients with perimyocarditis and myopericarditis due to the risk for SCD [11]. Serial follow-up and imaging (especially if low ejection fraction) is often needed for evaluation of recovery. The frequency of follow-up should be determined on an individualized basis.

Current Guideline Recommendations for Athletes with Myocarditis

American Heart Association (AHA)/American College of Cardiology (ACC) Guidelines

The most recent eligibility and disqualification task force recommendations for competitive athletes recommend that any athlete with probable or definite myocarditis should not participate in competitive sports during a time of active inflammation independent of age, gender, or LV function (Class III, level of evidence (LOE) C) [2]. Before returning to competitive sport, individuals with myocarditis should have a resting echocardiogram, 24-hour Holter monitor, and exercise ECG stress test no earlier than 3–6 months after the initial illness (Class I, LOE C) [2]. It is reasonable for athletes to resume sport if the following criteria are met (Class IIa, LOE C) [2]:

(a) Ventricular systolic function has normalized.
(b) Serum markers of inflammation, injury, or heart failure have normalized.
(c) Clinically relevant arrhythmias are absent on Holter monitoring or graded exercise ECG.

European Association of Preventive Cardiology (EAPC) Guidelines

Guidelines from the EAPC recommend that athletes with myocarditis restrict vigorous exercise and competition for 3–6 months to allow adequate time to heal (Class IIb, LOE C) [3]. The extent of time depends on the clinical severity of disease including duration of illness, extent of LV dysfunction, or extent of LGE on CMR. Athletes with a previous history of myocarditis should have periodic reassessment for silent progression of disease within the first 2 years (Class IIa, LOE C) [3]. Similar to the AHA/ACC guidelines, return to sport may be reasonable if LV function has normalized, biomarkers for injury have normalized, and there is no clinically relevant arrhythmias on exercise ECG or Holter monitoring (Class IIa, LOE C) [3]. Additionally, if there is evidence of LGE on CMR in an otherwise asymptomatic athlete, then annual clinical surveillance is warranted.

The American and European guidelines are summarized and compared in Table 9.1.

Table 9.1 Comparison of the American Heart Association/American College of Cardiology (AHA/ACC) and European Association of Preventive Cardiology (EAPC) guidelines for sport participation in athletes with myocarditis

	Activity restriction	Reassessment testing	Criteria for return to play
AHA/ACC guidelines	Athletes with probable or definite myocarditis should not participate in competitive sports while inflammation is present independent of age, gender, and LV function	Echocardiogram, 24-hour Holter monitoring, exercise ECG stress test Testing should be performed at least 3–6 months after initial illness	LV systolic function has returned to normal range Serum markers of myocardial injury, inflammation, and heart failure have normalized Clinically relevant arrhythmias absent on exercise ECG and Holter monitoring
	Class III, LOE C	Class I, LOE C	Class IIa, LOE C
EAPC guidelines	Athletes with myocarditis should be restricted from exercise programs for 3–6 months according to the clinical severity and duration of the illness, LV function at onset, and extent of inflammation on CMR	Echocardiogram, 24-hour Holter monitoring, exercise ECG stress test If LGE is present on CMR but no arrhythmias are present, it is reasonable for athletes to resume a training program Annual surveillance is recommended while LGE is present	LV systolic function has returned to normal range Serum biomarkers of myocardial injury have normalized Clinically relevant arrhythmias are absent on exercise ECG and Holter monitoring
	Class IIa, LOE C	Class III, LOE C	Class IIa, LOE C

Adapted from Maron et al. [2] and Pelliccia et al. [3]
CMR cardiac magnetic resonance imaging, *ECG* electrocardiogram, *LOE* level of evidence, *LGE* late gadolinium enhancement, *LV* left ventricle

Evidence for the Guidelines

Myocarditis is responsible for up to 5–22% of cases of SCD [12–22]. Many cases of SCD associated with myocarditis also appear to be in the context of exercise based on early autopsy data [14, 17–23]. In an early retrospective study evaluating Swedish orienteers who experienced SCD, of the 15 men and 1 woman studied, myocarditis was the most common histopathological diagnosis after autopsy. Most of the cases of myocarditis were associated with exercise [19]. Another analysis looked at autopsy data of 126 military recruits who experienced non-traumatic sudden death. A total of 108 deaths were related to exercise, and 64 deaths were due to cardiac causes of which myocarditis made up 20% [20]. In another 10-year observational study of 162 subjects under 40 years of age who experienced SCD, myocarditis was discovered on autopsy in 22% of cases, and 23% of cases of SCD were associated with exercise [21]. Thus, even though these early analyses were small and observational, an association with SCD was established in cases of myocarditis. This risk of SCD was further increased with exercise, especially in younger patients, which is of particular concern to athletes where training and competitive sport is a significant component of their life.

Pathologic Mechanism of Myocarditis

The natural history of myocarditis is hypothesized to begin with an acute phase triggered by a stimulus (i.e., viral replication), followed by a subacute immune response phase, and finally a chronic phase. The chronic phase can range from complete recovery to mechanical failure of the heart. It is unclear whether most SCDs in athletes occur in the early (acute and subacute) or late (chronic) phases in the disease course.

Based on early animal models, the mechanism of increased SCD with exercise in the early phases of disease is felt to result from an accelerated and progressive inflammatory response leading to an unstable myocardial substrate [24–27]. Many of these early studies focused on viral etiologies of myocarditis, but they provided insight into how exercise can affect the immune system [11, 28–30]. Excessive physical exertion results in a period of immune suppression mediated by T lymphocytes, interleukins, and the natural killer cell system [29]. This period can predispose the patient to upper respiratory infections and also allow an already infected myocardium to be more susceptible during a time when a virus can replicate at rapid rates [24, 27].

This immunosuppressant phase is followed by a surge of inflammation, which can be enhanced given the extent of the myocardium already affected by the earlier phase. This surge allows for necrosis, fibrosis, and subsequently a pro-arrhythmic myocardium, thus increasing the risk of SCD. Even in models that studied noninfectious myocarditis, exercise was associated with a pronounced inflammatory response that led to structural changes in the heart [28]. Moreover, an exaggerated inflammatory response leads to increased catabolism and degradation of the myocardium and skeletal muscle due to high demand for energy sources. This response can delay recovery due to deconditioning, as well as lead to poor athletic performance predisposing an athlete to injury [30].

Many of the persistent structural changes of the heart occur in the chronic phase of the disease. Whereas edema from myocardial inflammation is a predominant source of cardiac dysfunction in the earlier phases, myocardial fibrosis, or scar, is the predominant cause of dysfunction in the later phase. Scar can also serve as a stimulus for arrhythmias and increase the risk of SCD. CMR can be used to determine the extent of scar by evaluating the presence of LGE (Fig. 9.1). However, it is currently unclear if the presence of LGE should disqualify an otherwise asymptomatic athlete without evidence of active inflammation from competitive sports. As noted earlier, EAPC guidelines recommend close surveillance if there is evident LGE [3].

The role of follow-up CMR to evaluate for resolution of LGE remains unresolved and controversial. In human observational studies of SCD related to myocarditis, many subjects did not report symptoms, but were later discovered to have myocarditis on autopsy. This raises the question of the significance of residual scar formation after an episode of myocarditis. The literature is limited in this area, but available data suggests a possible prognostic role for residual scar. In one study, 35 athletes with ventricular arrhythmias and LGE on CMR were compared to athletes with ventricular arrhythmias without LGE and healthy control athletes. Of the athletes with LGE, 77% had a LGE predominance in a stria pattern on the lateral wall compared to healthy controls ($p < 0.001$) [31]. Subsequently, at 38-month

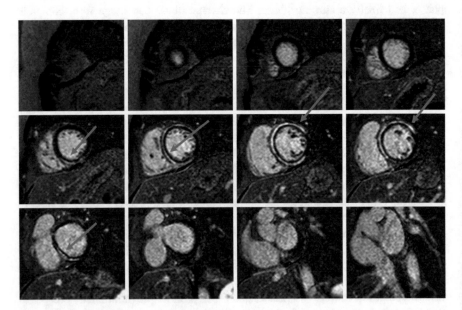

Fig. 9.1 Late gadolinium enhancement observed with cardiac magnetic resonance imaging. Blue arrows demonstrate enhancement in a mid-myocardial distribution, consistent with myocarditis

follow-up, six athletes with a stria pattern had malignant arrhythmic events including a shock from an implantable defibrillator, sustained ventricular tachycardia, or sudden death [30]. Additionally, five of the six athletes had events that occurred during exercise. In another smaller study that followed seven athletes with lateral wall LGE over 3 years, six of the seven athletes were prohibited from participating in competitive sports due to either ventricular arrhythmias or progressive LV dysfunction [32]. Larger studies have also supported the prognostic role of LGE. These studies included all patients with myocarditis and were not specific to athletes. In a study of 670 patients with myocarditis, the presence of LGE was significantly associated with major adverse cardiac events (MACE) in a multivariate model (HR, 2.22; $p < 0.001$) [33]. This finding was replicated in a second study of 374 patients with acute myocarditis and preserved ejection fraction where the authors also demonstrated that the presence of LGE was an independent predictor of MACE (OR 2.73; $p = 0.01$) [34].

Pericarditis

Acute pericarditis is the most common pericardial disease with a reported incidence of about 27.7 cases per 100,000 individuals per year [35]. Acute pericarditis accounts for 0.1% of hospital admissions and 5% of emergency department visits for chest pain [35–37]. Unfortunately, recurrences of pericarditis can affect up to about 30% of patients within 18 months after the initial diagnosis and can be associated with significant morbidity [38, 39].

Etiologies of pericarditis largely fall into three categories: idiopathic, infectious, and noninfectious. In the developed world, the most common etiologies are idiopathic and viral [40], whereas in the developing world, tuberculosis is the leading cause [41]. The diagnosis of pericarditis is based on a constellation of clinical symptoms, physical exam findings, ECG changes, laboratory abnormalities, and imaging findings. Typically, there is a history of characteristic chest pain that is worse with inspiration and supine positioning, diffuse concave ST segment elevation and PR deviation on ECG (Fig. 9.2), and a pericardial friction rub with or without a pericardial effusion [37, 42].

Presentations of pericarditis include acute, incessant, chronic, and recurrent pericarditis. The incessant form is defined by symptoms lasting for approximately 4–6 weeks but less than 3 months without remission. The chronic form is defined by symptoms that exceed 3 months. Finally, the recurrent form of pericarditis is defined by a recurrence of symptoms after the first episode of pericarditis and a symptom-free interval of 4–6 weeks or longer [43].

The medical treatment of pericarditis consists of anti-inflammatory agents like nonsteroidal anti-inflammatory drugs and colchicine [44–46]. Treatment with steroids and immune modulators is usually reserved for incessant, chronic, or recurrent cases. However, there are also non-pharmacologic measures, such as physical activity restriction, that can aid in recovery [3, 47]. As mentioned previously, activity

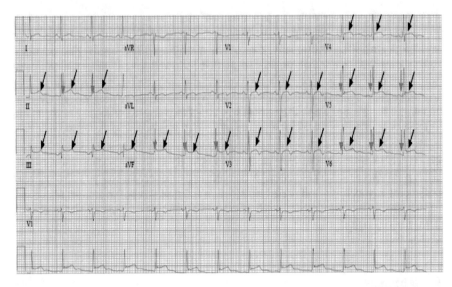

Fig. 9.2 12-lead electrocardiogram in a patient with acute pericarditis. There are diffuse ST seg-ment elevations (black arrows) and PR segment depressions (red arrows)

restriction can significantly impact the life of an athlete, but the evidence for activity restriction in pericarditis is limited [48, 49].

Current Guideline Recommendations for Athletes with Pericarditis

AHA/ACC Guidelines

Guidelines for athletes are primary based on expert consensus, as the data for physi-cal activity restriction is limited. Currently, athletes in the acute phase of pericarditis should not participate in competitive sports and can return to full activity when there is complete absence of evidence of active disease (Class III, LOE C) [2]. This absence of disease includes resolution of pericardial effusion by echo or normaliza-tion of serum inflammatory markers. If there is extension of inflammation into the myocardium, then recommendations for myocarditis must be followed. If an athlete has evidence of constrictive pericarditis, then he or she is disqualified from all com-petitive sport activity (Class III, LOE C) [2].

EAPC Guidelines

EAPC guidelines are similar to the AHA/ACC guidelines and recommend that ath-letes in the acute phase of pericarditis should not participate in competitive sports until resolution of inflammation (Class III, LOE C) [3]. However, the EAPC

Table 9.2 Comparison of the American Heart Association/American College of Cardiology (AHA/ACC) and European Association of Preventive Cardiology (EAPC) guidelines for sport participation in athletes with pericarditis

	Activity restriction	Reassessment testing	Criteria for return to play
ACC/AHA guidelines	Athletes with pericarditis, regardless of etiology, should not participate in competitive sports during the acute phase. If myocardial involvement is present, guidelines for myocarditis should be followed. Constrictive disease disqualifies from all athletes from competitive sports	Echocardiography to assess for effusion. Inflammatory markers	Complete absence of evidence for active disease. Normalized inflammatory markers. Resolution of pericardial effusion
	Class III, LOE C		Class III, LOE C
EAPC guidelines	Athletes with pericarditis should not participate in competitive sports during the acute phase. Athletes should abstain from exercise for at least 3 months after resolution of acute illness. A 1-month period of exercise can be considered in mild cases. If myocardial involvement is present, use guidelines for myocarditis	Echocardiography to assess LV function. Inflammatory markers. Exercise ECG stress test. 24-hour Holter monitoring	Complete resolution of active disease. Normalized LV function. Normal inflammatory markers. No arrhythmias on exercise ECG stress test or Holter
	Class IIa, LOE C	Class IIa, LOE C	Class IIa, LOE C

Adapted from Maron et al. [2] and Pelliccia et al. [3]
ECG electrocardiogram, *LOE* level of evidence, *LV* left ventricle

guidelines suggest a time period of at least 1 (in mild cases) to 3 months to allow adequate healing. Resolution of inflammation includes normalization of biomarkers and LV function and no resting or exercise-induced ventricular arrhythmias (Class IIa, LOE C) [3]. Athletes with concomitant myocarditis should follow recommendations for myocarditis (Class IIa, LOE C) [3].

A summary and comparison of the AHA/ACC and EAPC guidelines can be found in Table 9.2.

Evidence for the Guidelines

The literature is limited regarding the role of exercise in pericarditis. Guideline recommendations are largely based on expert consensus or basic science studies looking at regulation of inflammatory cascades from cases of myocarditis [2, 3, 30, 47, 50].

The rationale for avoiding physical activity in pericarditis is to promote enhanced healing and reduce the risk of complications (progression to myocarditis, worsening pericardial effusion, cardiac tamponade, constrictive pericarditis) or recurrent/refractory symptoms. Several pathophysiologic mechanisms have been hypothesized on

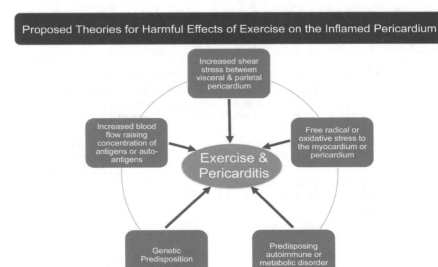

Fig. 9.3 Proposed theories for how exercise can be potentially harmful in cases of pericarditis. Mechanisms are postulated to be either immune-mediated, mechanical, or genetic. However, evidence is limited

how progression occurs (Fig. 9.3). The predominant theory to explain the development of complications associated with pericarditis is that a combination of immune mediation and mechanical and genetic factors are responsible, though these hypotheses are based on small animal and autopsy studies of myocarditis [10, 30, 50]. As noted with myocarditis, the period of immunosuppression after physical exertion can predispose the pericardium to infection or injury, which is then amplified by a subsequent surge of inflammation [10, 30, 51, 52]. Mouse models of myocarditis have shown that continued physical activity can further exaggerate this inflammatory response [24, 25, 53, 54]. Perhaps, the same is true for pericarditis.

It is also possible that exercise can further increase the inflammatory response through shear stress from increased friction between the two inflamed surfaces of the pericardium at higher heart rates. Oxidative stress from free radicals, due to increased blood flow related to both inflammation and exercise, may play a role as well. Lastly, genetic variations in the immune system may contribute, predisposing individuals to worsening inflammation from environmental triggers such as exercise [55]. Again, it is important to note that these mechanisms have not been extensively studied and further investigation is warranted.

Return to Play

Despite guideline recommendations to wait until resolution of inflammation prior to returning to play, the literature addressing the optimal time to return to sport or physical activity is limited. It is uncertain if one should gradually increase the intensity of the physical activity (low to moderate to high) or resume high-intensity activity right away after a period of physical restriction. One way to answer this question is to monitor the extent of LGE after other markers of active inflammation have resolved. In a retrospective analysis of 159 patients with recurrent pericarditis, quantitative assessment of pericardial LGE by CMR was associated with clinical outcomes and provided incremental prognostic value over baseline clinical and laboratory values [56]. Perhaps the quantitative assessment of pericardial LGE could guide return to activity. However, more research in this area is needed. Another area of investigation is the role of heart rate (HR) in the disease process. In a retrospective analysis of 73 patients with acute pericarditis, HR served as a prognostic marker and correlated with recurrence [57]. Further investigation is warranted to see if lower-average HR results in better outcomes in cases of pericarditis, especially in the era of mobile technologies and health applications that can monitor vitals continuously.

Conclusion

Inflammatory disorders of the heart such as myocarditis and pericarditis are associated with significant morbidity and mortality. In addition to medical treatment, exercise restriction is vital for healing and prevention of complications such as SCD. Both the AHA/ACC and EAPC sport participation guidelines for athletes are in agreement with physical activity restriction until there is evidence of resolution of inflammation. However, there are many unanswered questions regarding the role of CMR and LGE in later phases of myocarditis and the pathogenic mechanisms of exercise in pericarditis. Future research is warranted in these areas to help clinicians best manage athletes with inflammatory diseases of the heart.

References

1. Imazio M, Cooper LT. Management of myopericarditis. Expert Rev Cardiovasc Ther. 2013;11(2):193–201.
2. Maron BJ, Udelson JE, Bonow RO, et al. Eligibility and disqualification recommendations for competitive athletes with cardiovascular abnormalities: task force 3: hypertrophic cardiomyopathy, arrhythmogenic right ventricular cardiomyopathy and other cardiomyopathies, and myocarditis. Circulation. 2015;132:e273–80.
3. Pelliccia A, Solberg EE, Papadakis M, Adami PE, Biffi A, Caselli S, et al. Recommendations for participation in competitive and leisure time sport in athletes with cardiomyopathies, myocarditis, and pericarditis: position statement of the Sport Cardiology Section of the European Association of Preventive Cardiology (EAPC). Eur Heart J. 2019;40(1):19–33.
4. Basso C, Carturan E, Corrado D, Thiene G. Myocarditis and dilated cardiomyopathy in athletes: diagnosis, management, and recommendations for sport activity. Cardiol Clin. 2007;25(3):423–9.
5. Trachtenberg BH, Hare JM. Inflammatory cardiomyopathic syndromes. Circ Res. 2017;121(7):803–18.

6. Vikerfors T, Stjerna A, Olcén P, Malmcrona R, Magnius L. Acute myocarditis. Acta Med Scand. 2009;223(1):45–52.
7. Woodruff JF. Viral myocarditis. A review. Am J Pathol. 1980;101(2):425–84.
8. Caforio ALP, Marcolongo R, Basso C, Iliceto S. Clinical presentation and diagnosis of myocarditis. Heart. 2015;101(16):1332–44.
9. Shah NP, Phelan DM. Myocarditis in the athlete. Expert analysis. ACC.org. 2018.
10. Mazic S, Ilic V, Djelic M, Arandjelovic A. Sudden cardiac death in young athletes. Srp Arh Celok Lek. 2011;139(5–6):394–401.
11. Duraković Z, Misigoj Duraković M, Skavić J, Tomljenović A. Myopericarditis and sudden cardiac death due to physical exercise in male athletes. Coll Antropol. 2008;32(2):399–401.
12. Cooper LT, Keren A, Sliwa K, Matsumori A, Mensah GA. The global burden of myocarditis. Glob Heart. 2014;9(1):121–9.
13. Basso C. Postmortem diagnosis in sudden cardiac death victims: macroscopic, microscopic and molecular findings. Cardiovasc Res. 2001;50(2):290–300.
14. Kirschner RH. The cardiac pathology of sudden, unexplained nocturnal death in Southeast Asian Refugees. JAMA J Am Med Assoc. 1986;256(19):2700.
15. Corrado D. Sudden cardiac death in young people with apparently normal heart. Cardiovasc Res. 2001;50(2):399–408.
16. Phillips M. Sudden cardiac death in air force recruits. JAMA. 1986;256(19):2696.
17. Maron BJ. Sudden death in young athletes – lessons from the Hank Gathers affair. N Engl J Med. 1993;329(1):55–7.
18. Maron BJ, Haas TS, Murphy CJ, Ahluwalia A, Rutten-Ramos S. Incidence and causes of sudden death in U.S. college athletes. J Am Coll Cardiol. 2014;63(16):1636–43.
19. Larsson E, Wesslén L, Lindquist O, Baandrur U, Eriksson L, Olsen E, et al. Sudden unexpected cardiac deaths among young Swedish orienteers – morphological changes in hearts and other organs. APMIS. 1999;107(1–6):325–36.
20. Eckart RE, Scoville SL, Campbell CL, Shry EA, Stajduhar KC, Potter RN, et al. Sudden death in young adults: a 25-year review of autopsies in military recruits. Ann Intern Med. 2004;141(11):829.
21. Drory Y, Turetz Y, Hiss Y, Lev B, Fisman EZ, Pines A, et al. Sudden unexpected death in persons <40 years of age. Am J Cardiol. 1991;68(13):1388–92.
22. Wesslen L, Pahlso C, Lindquist O, Hjelm E, Gnarpe J, Larsson E, et al. An increase in sudden unexpected cardiac deaths among young Swedish orienteers during 1979–1992. Eur Heart J. 1996;17(6):902–10.
23. Corrado D, Basso C, Pavei A, Michieli P, Schiavon M, Thiene G. Trends in sudden cardiovascular death in young competitive athletes after implementation of a preparticipation screening program. JAMA. 2006;296(13):1593.
24. Gatmaitan BG. Augmentation of the virulence of murine coxsackie-virus B-3 myocardiopathy by exercise. J Exp Med. 1970;131(6):1121–36.
25. Ilbäck N-G, Fohlman J, Friman G. Exercise in coxsackie B3 myocarditis: effects on heart lymphocyte subpopulations and the inflammatory reaction. Am Heart J. 1989;117(6):1298–302.
26. Cabinian AE, Kiel RJ, Smith F, Ho KL, Khatib R, Reyes MP. Modification of exercise-aggravated coxsackievirus B3 murine myocarditis by T lymphocyte suppression in an inbred model. J Lab Clin Med. 1990;115(4):454–62.
27. Kiel RJ, Smith FE, Chason J, Khatib R, REYES MP. Coxsackievirus B3 myocarditis in C3H/HeJ mice: description of an inbred model and the effect of exercise on virulence. Eur J Epidemiol. 1989;5(3):348–50.
28. Hosenpud JD, Campbell SM, Niles NR, Lee J, Mendelson D, Hart MV. Exercise induced augmentation of cellular and humoral autoimmunity associated with increased cardiac dilatation in experimental autoimmune myocarditis. Cardiovasc Res. 1987;21(3):217–22.
29. Shephard RJ, Shek PN. Infectious diseases in athletes: new interest for an old problem. J Sports Med Phys Fitness. 1994;34(1):11–22.
30. MacKinnon LT. Overtraining effects on immunity and performance in athletes. Immunol Cell Biol. 2000;78(5):502–9.

31. Zorzi A, Perazzolo Marra M, Rigato I, De Lazzari M, Susana A, Niero A, et al. Nonischemic left ventricular scar as a substrate of life-threatening ventricular arrhythmias and sudden cardiac death in competitive athletes. Circ Arrhythm Electrophysiol. 2016;9(7):e004229.
32. Schnell F, Claessen G, La Gerche A, Bogaert J, Lentz P-A, Claus P, et al. Subepicardial delayed gadolinium enhancement in asymptomatic athletes: let sleeping dogs lie? Br J Sports Med. 2016;50(2):111–7.
33. Gräni C, Eichhorn C, Bière L, Murthy VL, Agarwal V, Kaneko K, et al. Prognostic value of cardiac magnetic resonance tissue characterization in risk stratifying patients with suspected myocarditis. J Am Coll Cardiol. 2017;70(16):1964–76.
34. Aquaro GD, Perfetti M, Camastra G, Monti L, Dellegrottaglie S, Moro C, et al. Cardiac MR with late gadolinium enhancement in acute myocarditis with preserved systolic function. J Am Coll Cardiol. 2017;70(16):1977–87.
35. Imazio M. Contemporary management of pericardial diseases. Curr Opin Cardiol. 2012;27(3):308–17.
36. Imazio M, Gaita F. Diagnosis and treatment of pericarditis. Heart. 2015;101(14):1159–68.
37. LeWinter MM. Clinical practice. Acute pericarditis. N Engl J Med. 2014;371(25):2410–6.
38. Imazio M, Bobbio M, Cecchi E, Demarie D, Demichelis B, Pomari F, et al. Colchicine in addition to conventional therapy for acute pericarditis. Circulation. 2005;112(13):2012–6.
39. Imazio M, Brucato A, Cemin R, Ferrua S, Maggiolini S, Beqaraj F, et al. A randomized trial of colchicine for acute pericarditis. N Engl J Med. 2013;369(16):1522–8.
40. Imazio M, Spodick DH, Brucato A, Trinchero R, Adler Y. Controversial issues in the management of pericardial diseases. Circulation. 2010;121(7):916–28.
41. Sliwa K, Mocumbi AO. Forgotten cardiovascular diseases in Africa. Clin Res Cardiol. 2010;99(2):65–74.
42. Cremer PC, Kumar A, Kontzias A, Tan CD, Rodriguez ER, Imazio M, et al. Complicated pericarditis. J Am Coll Cardiol. 2016;68(21):2311–28.
43. Adler Y, Charron P, Imazio M, Badano L, Barón-Esquivias G, Bogaert J, Brucato A, Gueret P, Klingel K, Lionis C, Maisch B, Mayosi B, Pavie A, Ristic AD, Sabaté Tenas M, Seferovic P, Swedberg K, Tomkowski W, ESC Scientific Document Group. 2015 ESC Guidelines for the diagnosis and management of pericardial diseases: the task force for the diagnosis and management of pericardial diseases of the European Society of Cardiology (ESC) Endorsed by: the European Association for Cardio-Thoracic Surgery (EACTS). Eur Heart J. 2015;36(42):2921–64.
44. Imazio M, Brucato A, Trinchero R, Spodick D, Adler Y. Individualized therapy for pericarditis. Expert Rev Cardiovasc Ther. 2009;7(8):965–75.
45. Imazio M, Brucato A, Trinchero R, Spodick D, Adler Y. Colchicine for pericarditis: hype or hope? Eur Heart J. 2009;30(5):532–9.
46. Imazio M, Brucato A, Belli R, Forno D, Ferro S, Trinchero R, et al. Colchicine for the prevention of pericarditis. J Cardiovasc Med. 2014;15(12):840–6.
47. Seidenberg PH, Haynes J. Pericarditis. Curr Sports Med Rep. 2006;5(2):74–9.
48. Shah NP, Phelan DM. Physical activity recommendations in patients with acute pericarditis. Expert analysis. ACC.org. 2017.
49. Shah N, Ala CK, Verma B, Bafadel A, Klein A. Exercise is good for the heart but not for the inflamed pericardium. J Am Coll Cardiol. 2018;71(11):A2339.
50. Pedersen BK, Hoffman-Goetz L. Exercise and the immune system: regulation, integration, and adaptation. Physiol Rev. 2000;80(3):1055–81.
51. Beisel KW, Srinivasappa J, Olsen MR, Stiff AC, Essani K, Prabhakar BS. A neutralizing monoclonal antibody against Coxsackievirus B4 cross-reacts with contractile muscle proteins. Microb Pathog. 1990;8(2):151–6.
52. Huber SA, Gauntt CJ, Sakkinen P. Enteroviruses and myocarditis: viral pathogenesis through replication, cytokine induction, and immunopathogenicity. Adv Virus Res. 1998;51:35–80.
53. Lerner A, Wilson FM, Reyes MP. Enteroviruses and the heart (with special emphasis on the probable role of coxsackieviruses, group B, types 1-5). II. Observations in humans. Mod Concepts Cardiovasc Dis. 1975;44(3):11–5.

54. Maisch B. Exercise and sports in cardiac patients and athletes at risk. Herz. 2015;40(3):395–401.
55. Lachmann HJ, Papa R, Gerhold K, Obici L, Touitou I, Cantarini L, et al. The phenotype of TNF receptor-associated autoinflammatory syndrome (TRAPS) at presentation: a series of 158 cases from the Eurofever/EUROTRAPS international registry. Ann Rheum Dis. 2014;73(12):2160–7.
56. Kumar A, Sato K, Yzeiraj E, Betancor J, Lin L, Tamarappoo BK, et al. Quantitative pericardial delayed hyperenhancement informs clinical course in recurrent pericarditis. JACC Cardiovasc Imaging. 2017;10(11):1337–46.
57. Khoueiry Z, Roubille C, Nagot N, Lattuca B, Piot C, Leclercq F, et al. Could heart rate play a role in pericardial inflammation? Med Hypotheses. 2012;79(4):512–5.

Chapter 10
Atrial Fibrillation

Kyle Mandsager and Dermot M. Phelan

Introduction

Atrial fibrillation (AF) is the most common cardiac arrhythmia, affecting between 2.7 and 6.1 million American adults and 8% of those over the age of 80. Risk factors for AF are well established and include advancing age as well as typical cardiac risk factors such as hypertension, obesity, diabetes, and obstructive sleep apnea. The relationship between exercise and AF is complex; regular exercise reduces the risk of AF compared to sedentary controls; however over the past several decades, AF has been increasingly recognized in highly trained athletes who otherwise lack traditional AF risk factors. Hypothesized mechanisms relate to changes in cardiac structure and autonomic function in response to chronic exposure to high-intensity exercise. This chapter will review the epidemiologic data and potential mechanisms underlying this clinical phenomenon, as well as focus on the unique aspects of managing atrial fibrillation in athletes.

K. Mandsager (✉)
Centennial Heart, TriStar Centennial Heart and Vascular Center, Nashville, TN, USA
e-mail: kyle.mandsager@hcahealthcare.com

D. M. Phelan
Sport Cardiology Center, Hypertrophic Cardiomyopathy Center, Atrium Health Sanger
Heart & Vascular Institute, Charlotte, NC, USA
e-mail: dermot.phelan@atriumhealth.org

© Springer Nature Switzerland AG 2021
D. J. Engel, D. M. Phelan (eds.), *Sports Cardiology*,
https://doi.org/10.1007/978-3-030-69384-8_10

Epidemiology

One of the earliest published reports of AF in athletes was from a study of veteran Finnish orienteers [1]. In a 10-year follow-up of 262 orienteers, 5.3% had been diagnosed with AF compared to 0.9% of controls ($p = 0.0012$). The age-specific prevalence of lone AF in this cohort was 4.2% for those aged 46–54 years, 5.6% for those aged 55–62 years, and 6.6% for those aged 63–70 years, compared to the general population prevalence of 0.5%, 1%, and 4% in the same respective age groups [2]. The increased prevalence of AF was present despite significantly lower mortality and fewer AF risk factors in the orienteers.

Similar findings have been subsequently published from a variety of highly trained athletic cohorts, including cyclists [3], runners [4], swimmers [5], and cross-country skiers [6–8]. While some studies of exercise habits and AF in the general population have been less conclusive [9, 10], overall there is compelling evidence that chronic, vigorous exercise increases the risk of developing AF. More recent evidence in support of this association includes large prospective cohort studies and several meta-analyses. In a large Scandinavian cohort of more than 20,000 adults followed for 20 years, the association between AF and exercise followed a J-shaped curve (Fig. 10.1a), in which the risk of those participating in "vigorous" exercise exceeded that of the sedentary group [11].

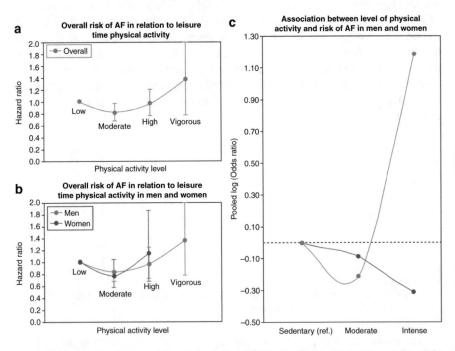

Fig. 10.1 Association between AF and physical activity in the Tromsø study (**a**) overall and (**b**) separated by gender, showing similar J-shaped relationship for males and females. (Reprinted with permission from Morseth et al. [11], Oxford University Press). (**c**) Gender-specific findings reported by Mohanty et al. [12], with divergent AF risk for men and women performing vigorous exercise. (Reprinted with permission from Mohanty et al. [12], John Wiley and Sons)

Table 10.1 Reported prevalence of atrial fibrillation (AF) among athlete cohorts

Study	Year	Cohort	AF prevalence
Karjalainen et al. [1]	1998	Orienteers ($n = 228$), mean age 47.5 ± 7, male 100%	5.30%
Baldesberger et al. [3]	2008	Former professional cyclists ($n = 134$), mean age 66 ± 6, male 100%	6%
Molina et al. [4]	2008	Marathon runners ($n = 252$), mean age 39 ± 9, male 100%	4.90%
Grimsmo et al. [7]	2010	Cross country skiers ($n = 78$), mean age 69.5 ± 10.2, male 100%	12.80%
Andersen et al. [8]	2013	Cross country skiers ($n = 52{,}755$), mean age not reported, male 90%	13.20%
Myrstad et al. [6]	2014	Cross country skiers ($n = 509$), mean age 68.9	Moderate PA 13% High PA 17.6%
Myrstad et al. [18]	2014	Cross country skiers ($n = 2366$), age ≥ 53, male 100%	12.50%
Schreiner et al. [5]	2016	Master's age competitive swimmers ($n = 40$), mean age 72.6 ± 4.9, male unreported	26.50%
Shapero et al. [48]	2016	Master's athletes ($n = 591$), mean age 50 ± 9, male 66%	4%
Boraita et al. [49]	2018	Spanish athletes ($n = 6813$), mean age 22 ± 7, male 65.0%	0.80%
Aagaard et al. [15]	2019	Former NFL players ($n = 460$), mean age 56 ± 12, male 100%	5%

PA physical activity

The true prevalence of AF in athletes is difficult to define but ranges from 0.8% to 26.5% in published studies (Table 10.1). This wide range is likely due to different cohort compositions, which differ by sport, age, gender, as well as definitions of "athletes" and/or quantification of exercise exposure. Larger studies and meta-analyses have found adjusted hazard ratios for AF between 1.4 and 5.3 for athletes compared to sedentary controls.

Whether gender plays a role in the risk of AF in athletes remains unclear, largely because few women were included in many of the initial cohort studies. Available studies of female athletes have offered discrepant findings than reported in male athletes. A recent meta-analysis by *Mohanty* et al. [12], which included several large population-based studies of physical activity in women, concluded that AF risk was lower in women who participated in exercise versus reference sedentary adults and lowest for women participating in vigorous exercise. Findings in men, in contrast, demonstrated the characteristic J-shaped relationship with increasing physical activity (Fig. 10.1c). Similar results were reported by *Everett* et al. [13], who showed progressive reduction in AF risk with increasing self-reported physical activity in a large cohort of nearly 35,000 women. The divergence of exercise-associated AF risk by gender is in contrast to the previously referenced study by *Morseth* et al., which showed a similar J-shaped relationship in both male and female athletes (Fig. 10.1b). Potential gender-specific findings may reflect a host of physiologic and clinical factors. Male athletes have been found to have more profound left atrial remodeling, higher resting and exertional systolic blood pressure, and more pronounced autonomic changes compared to female athletes, all of which may, in part, explain gender-related differences in AF risk [14]. Additionally there are social and behavioral factors, such as historical differences in sports participation, including specific differences in endurance sports participation, as well as gender-related training preferences which may lead to fewer female athletes exposing themselves to the cumulative training necessary to increase AF risk. These hypotheses remain speculative, and further study is needed to better define the influence of gender on the risk of AF in athletes.

Role of Training Intensity, Duration, and Sport

The increased prevalence of AF in athletes has largely been reported in those athletes participating in endurance exercise (e.g., cycling, running, cross-country skiing). The specific association with endurance exercise likely reflects the pronounced cardiovascular adaptations observed with prolonged endurance exercise exposure, many of which (e.g., left atrial enlargement, autonomic shifts, etc.) have been implicated in the pathophysiology of exercise-related AF. There is limited data to support an increased risk of AF in non-endurance athletes, though an increase in AF has been recently reported in a cohort of retired NFL athletes [15]. The mechanism of AF in this strength-style sport cohort is less well-defined although studies in active American Style Football players have reported high rates of obstructive sleep apnea and maladaptive ventricular remodeling which may be contributory [16, 17].

The duration and intensity of exercise or athletic exposure at which the risk of AF begins to increase remain ill-defined but likely requires >10 years of habitual (at least 3 hours/week), vigorous exercise. In a longitudinal cohort study of >52,000 cross-country skiers who participated in the *Vasaloppet* race in Sweden between 1989 and 1998, the risk of AF was higher in athletes who competed in multiple years, as well as in those with faster finishing times, suggesting that the risk of AF is related both to training duration and intensity [8]. In a similar study of 2300 male cross-country skiers who participated in the Birkebeiner ski race in 1999, a graded increase in AF and atrial flutter risk with cumulative years of exercise was observed in the skiers compared with a matched non-athletic cohort [18]. The risk of AF was higher after >20 cumulative years of exercise, whereas the risk of atrial flutter was increased with >10 years of exercise. In a small case-control study of 51 consecutive male patients with lone atrial fibrillation, >1500 lifetime hours of sport was found to be a threshold above which the risk of AF increased. A small, prospective study by *Opondo* et al. demonstrated that 10 months of high-intensity interval training in previously untrained adults were insufficient in producing the LA structural and electrical changes observed in masters athletes, suggesting that longer exposure to intense exercise is required to produce the cardiac adaptations implicated in AF development [19].

Pathophysiology

The mechanisms leading to the development in AF in athletes are thought to be related to cardiovascular adaptations to habitual, vigorous endurance exercise. These are broadly defined as structural changes of the left atrium (LA) and shifts in autonomic tone which lead to an arrhythmogenic LA substrate capable of triggering and maintaining AF (Fig. 10.2).

Animal Models

AF susceptibility was increased in rats following sustained exposure to intense exercise [20]. Key findings which appeared to contribute to AF susceptibility included LA dilation and fibrosis, as well as an increase in parasympathetic tone. A similar study in mice largely confirmed these findings, additionally implicating inflammatory pathways and the role of TNF-α in exercise-related AF [21]. The unique controlled nature of these studies and comprehensive physiologic and histologic assessment in these animals provides useful insight into the potential mechanisms behind AF development in human athletes.

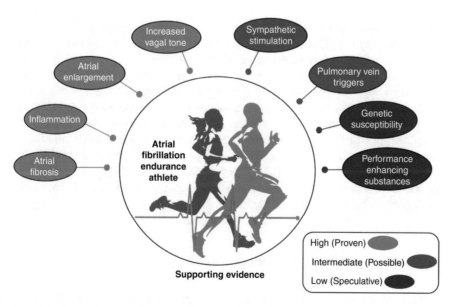

Fig. 10.2 Proposed mechanisms contributing to the development in AF in athletes. (Reprinted with permission from Estes et al. [47], Elsevier)

Left Atrial Enlargement

LA enlargement is recognized as a predictor of AF in the general population and is also a physiologic cardiac structural adaptation to endurance exercise. The degree of LA enlargement is proportional to cumulative lifetime hours of endurance training and can be profound in elite endurance athletes [22, 23]. While LA enlargement is seen after several months of athletic training, and generally returns to normal values with detraining, in former elite and professional athletes with prolonged exposure to high-level endurance training, these adaptive features appear to persist despite years of relative detraining [24, 25]. Permanent structural adaptations of the LA in athletes participating in years of intense endurance exercise may predispose to the development of AF. The clinical data to support this hypothesis is lacking, however. In a study by *Pelliccia* et al., there was no difference in AF development among athletes with or without LA enlargement, though the study was limited by the young age of the studied cohort (mean age at follow-up 33 ± 6 years) [26]. In a long-term echocardiographic follow-up study of the Birkebeiner cohort, LA size was associated with AF, though it is unclear if LA enlargement was a marker of exercise-related changes or simply a consequence of AF itself [7].

Vagal Tone

Another well-recognized adaptation to endurance exercise is heightened parasympathetic activity [27]. Cardioautonomic inputs have long been thought to contribute to both the initiation and maintenance of AF by affecting triggered activity in the pulmonary veins as well as altering the atrial refractory period [28, 29]. Cardiac ganglionic plexi are proposed extra-pulmonary vein targets for AF ablation, and vagal responses observed during AF ablation are associated with a reduction in arrhythmia recurrence [30]. The clinical syndrome of vagal-induced AF has been described, in which AF predominately occurs during periods of vagal stimulation (e.g., during sleep, after meals, or during post-exercise recovery), and has also been observed in athletes with AF [31]. Many of the electrocardiographic features of increased vagal tone, such as low heart rate and increased PR interval, have been associated with AF development in athletes [7].

Myocardial Inflammation and Fibrosis

There is significant evidence that inflammation plays a role in the development and maintenance of AF [32]. Intense endurance exercise has been shown to result in elevated levels of inflammatory cytokines, including IL-6 and TNF-α [33, 34]. A local inflammatory response in LA myocardium may theoretically be driven by intense bouts of exercise in the setting of acute rises in LA pressure. Over time, with repeated exposure and recurrent local myocardial inflammation, reactive atrial fibrosis and fibrotic atrial remodeling may lead to an arrhythmogenic substrate predisposed to AF development. In a small study of 16 endurance athletes, LA fibrosis, as detected by late gadolinium enhancement on cardiac MRI, was greater in endurance athletes compared to non-athlete controls [35]. Additionally, endurance exercise appeared to be a stronger predictor of LA fibrosis than more traditional clinical risk factors, such as obesity or hypertension. In the general AF population, atrial fibrosis is strongly associated with AF initiation and AF progression [36, 37], though it remains unclear whether LA fibrosis is involved in the development of AF or is the result of AF-induced fibrotic remodeling. More recent evidence suggests that LA fibrosis may precede AF onset and is predictive of AF development [38]. Whether LA fibrosis is predictive of AF occurrence in athletes remains unknown.

Other Factors

The acute effects of strenuous exercise may play a role in AF induction. Surges in sympathetic activity during exercise may trigger AF via autonomically responsive foci within the pulmonary veins or elsewhere within the atria. Electrolyte shifts, acid/base disturbances, and relative hypoxia, all of which may be encountered during extreme exercise, may additionally enhance focal AF triggers and/or increase the general arrhythmogenicity of the atrial substrate.

The use of performance enhancing substances is another potential mechanism for AF development in athletes. The use and potential arrhythmogenic effect of these substances is difficult to study, and any potential impact on AF risk remains speculative at best. Stimulant use provides a more logical mechanism to AF induction via the acute promotion of AF triggers. Both over-the-counter and prescribed stimulants have been associated with AF, but there is no specific data regarding their use and AF in athletes.

It is also important to recognize the potential role of traditional AF risk factors. While athletes tend to be healthier and without significant medical comorbidities, they are not immune to the development of traditional cardiac conditions (e.g., hypertension, obstructive sleep apnea), particularly in retired or former athletes. Other clinical contributors to AF, such as hyperthyroidism and structural heart disease, should also be considered.

Clinical Evaluation

All athletes with documented AF should undergo a basic clinical and cardiac evaluation to rule out contributing metabolic disorders and structural heart disease. This evaluation should include thyroid function testing, a resting ECG, and an echocardiogram. A careful history should be taken to evaluate for contributing substance use, family history, and other identifiable AF triggers. Screening for traditional AF risk factors as well as obstructive sleep apnea should be considered. Any concern for other cardiac pathologies should prompt further evaluation, which may include cardiac MRI and/or exercise stress testing. Coronary artery disease should be evaluated in the older athlete and should be excluded prior to the initiation of antiarrhythmic drug (AAD) therapy with 1C agents.

Management

The management of an athlete with AF can be challenging, as many available therapies may be undesirable, particularly in athletes who wish to continue to train and/or compete at a high level. Mainstay medical therapies, such as beta-blockers, are often poorly tolerated and may be prohibited in certain sports. Catheter ablation is often the most effective therapy, though it is an invasive procedure and carries some periprocedural risk. The appropriate treatment for an athlete with AF requires individualization of care, incorporation of athletic goals, and thoughtful discussion regarding the risks and benefits of different therapies, including their potential effects on athletic performance. A general approach to AF management in the athletes is presented in Fig. 10.3.

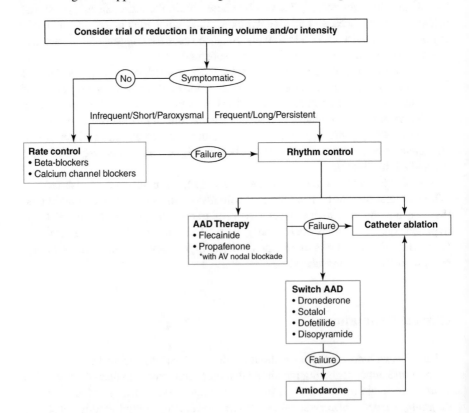

Fig. 10.3 Proposed management strategy for athletes with lone AF. AAD = antiarrhythmic drug

Ongoing Training and Competition

Rarely should AF alone require disqualification from competition. Current guidelines allow full sports participation for athletes with AF, so long as it is well tolerated and without associated hemodynamic compromise, rate-controlled, and self-terminating [39]. Athletes requiring anticoagulation should avoid sports that involve bodily collision. Given the implication that habitual exercise contributes to the development of AF, there is concern that ongoing exercise may further promote AF recurrence and/or decrease the success of other therapies. There are no prospective studies to guide clinicians in terms of exercise recommendations for athletes with AF, though observational data has suggested that detraining may be beneficial in some subsets of athletes [40, 41]. Depending on the goals of the individual athlete, a trial of detraining or a reduction in training may be worthwhile. In many cases, a reduction in training is not an acceptable approach, and other treatment strategies are warranted.

Medical Therapy

The initial decision regarding medical management of an athlete with AF is first deciding on a rate- or rhythm-control strategy. A rate-control strategy, typically using beta-blockers or calcium channel blockers, may be appropriate in athletes with infrequent AF episodes or in those with no or minimal symptoms. Unfortunately, rate-controlling medications are often poorly tolerated in athletes, owing to their resting bradycardia and the negative effect of these drugs on exercise capacity. The use of beta-blockers is also banned in certain sports.

For athletes with more frequent or prolonged AF episodes, AADs can be used to maintain sinus rhythm. The most commonly used AADs in athletes are 1C agents, such as flecainide and propafenone. These medications can be taken on a scheduled basis or as needed during AF episodes (the so-called "pill-in-the-pocket" approach). It is important to recognize that class 1C AADs can promote the organization of AF into atrial flutter with 1:1 conduction. This is a particular risk in athletes with robust AV nodal conduction and can be potentially life-threatening. These 1C drugs should always be given with an adequate dose of a beta-blocker or calcium channel blocker to reduce this risk. Alternative AAD options include sotalol, dofetilide, dronedarone, and amiodarone though the requirements for in-hospital drug loading (sotalol, dofetilide), inferior efficacy (dronedarone), or long-term side effect profiles (amiodarone) make them less desirable in younger athletes. Disopyramide is an additional option with specific efficacy in vagally mediated AF, though its anticholinergic and negative inotropic effects limit disopyramide to a second- or third-line option in athletes. While AADs are commonly used to treat AF in athletes, the potential pro-arrhythmic effect of these medications during intense exercise remains unknown.

Catheter Ablation

Catheter ablation, which principally involves the use of radiofrequency or cryoablation to isolate the pulmonary veins, has emerged as an effective therapy for patients with symptomatic AF. Current ACC/AHA guidelines support catheter ablation in athletes with AF, in part to obviate the need for long-term AAD therapy. Several small studies of AF ablation in athletes have demonstrated comparable efficacy to non-athletes [42, 43]. Overall, freedom from AF approaches 80–85% at 3 years following ablation, though approximately 20–40% of athletes require more than one procedure. Ablation is typically considered after failure of AAD therapy but can also be performed as first-line therapy in athletes who do not wish to take AADs. The consideration for early or first-line ablation is supported by observational data that early ablation, within 2 years of diagnosis, is associated with significantly lower AF recurrence in athletes [44]. The comparative efficacy of first-line ablation versus AAD therapy has not been studied in athletes, but has been shown to be superior in the general AF population [45].

The effect of catheter ablation on athletic performance is unknown. Theoretically, electrical isolation of the pulmonary veins and ablative scarring of the LA may disrupt the normal mechanical function of the LA and pulmonary veins, leading to a reduction in cardiorespiratory fitness. Catheter ablation can also affect cardioautonomic inputs, resulting in an increase in resting heart rate, with unknown impact on exercise capacity. The effect of AF ablation on athletic performance has only been studied in a small group of elite Italian athletes, all of which had severe AF-related symptoms precluding training and competition [46]. In this cohort, there was a significant improvement in maximal exercise capacity following ablation. In our own experience, athletes with AF often limit the frequency and intensity of training due to AF-related symptoms and/or the fear of exercise-induced AF episodes. Following successful ablation, the performance benefit from resumption of pre-AF training frequency and intensity likely far surpasses any potentially negative performance impact from ablation. However, further study is necessary to better understand the physiologic effects of AF ablation in athletes.

Anticoagulation

The risk of stroke and the indication for initiation of anticoagulation should be considered in any patient with AF. For most athletes, the underlying stroke risk is low and anticoagulation is not necessary, but athletes should be managed, as in non-athletes, based on their CHA_2DS_2VASc score. In athletes with risk factors for stroke, and in whom anticoagulation is initiated, continued sports participation and training should be limited to those with a low risk of impact and/or bodily injury. If continued sports participation is desired, the implantation of a left atrial appendage occlusion device, such as the WATCHMAN device (Boston Scientific; Natick, MA), could be considered, though this has not been studied in athletes.

Conclusion

AF in athletes is well-described, with an incidence that is approximately five times greater than in non-athletes, particularly among male endurance athletes. Cardiovascular and autonomic adaptations to habitual, vigorous exercise are thought to underlie this unique clinical risk. The treatment of AF in athletes can be challenging, but treatment options include consideration of detraining or reduction in training intensity and/or volume, rate-controlling agents, antiarrhythmic drug therapy, and catheter ablation. Anticoagulation is typically not indicated in the absence of additional established risk factors for stroke. In athletes with frequent, symptomatic AF, early catheter ablation should be considered and may obviate the need for long-term antiarrhythmic drug therapy.

References

1. Karjalainen J, Kujala UM, Kaprio J, Sarna S, Viitasalo M. Lone atrial fibrillation in vigorously exercising middle aged men: case-control study. BMJ [Internet]. 1998 June 13 [cited 2018 Jan 24];316(7147):1784–5. Available from: http://www.bmj.com/content/316/7147/1784.1.
2. Feinberg WM, Blackshear JL, Laupacis A, Kronmal R, Hart RG. Prevalence, age distribution, and gender of patients with atrial fibrillation. Analysis and implications. Arch Intern Med. 1995;155(5):469–73.
3. Baldesberger S, Bauersfeld U, Candinas R, Seifert B, Zuber M, Ritter M, et al. Sinus node disease and arrhythmias in the long-term follow-up of former professional cyclists. Eur Heart J. 2008;29(1):71–8.
4. Molina L, Mont L, Marrugat J, Berruezo A, Brugada J, Bruguera J, et al. Long-term endurance sport practice increases the incidence of lone atrial fibrillation in men: a follow-up study. Europace [Internet]. 2008 May 1 [cited 2019 May 28];10(5):618–23. Available from: http://academic.oup.com/europace/article/10/5/618/596326.
5. Schreiner AD, Keith BA, Abernathy KE, Zhang J, Brzezinski WA. Long-term, competitive swimming and the association with atrial fibrillation. Sports Med Open [Internet]. 2016 Oct 17 [cited 2019 May 28];2. Available from: https://www.ncbi.nlm.nih.gov/pmc/articles/PMC5067262/.
6. Myrstad M, Løchen M-L, Graff-Iversen S, Gulsvik AK, Thelle DS, Stigum H, et al. Increased risk of atrial fibrillation among elderly Norwegian men with a history of long-term endurance sport practice. Scand J Med Sci Sports [Internet]. 2014 Aug [cited 2019 May 28];24(4):e238–44. Available from: https://www.ncbi.nlm.nih.gov/pmc/articles/PMC4282367/.
7. Grimsmo J, Grundvold I, Maehlum S, Arnesen H. High prevalence of atrial fibrillation in long-term endurance cross-country skiers: echocardiographic findings and possible predictors — a 28–30 years follow-up study. Eur J Cardiovasc Prev Rehabil [Internet]. 2010 Feb 1 [cited 2018 Jan 24];17(1):100–5. Available from: https://doi.org/10.1097/HJR.0b013e32833226be.
8. Andersen K, Farahmand B, Ahlbom A, Held C, Ljunghall S, Michaëlsson K, et al. Risk of arrhythmias in 52 755 long-distance cross-country skiers: a cohort study. Eur Heart J [Internet]. 2013 Dec 14 [cited 2019 May 28];34(47):3624–31. Available from: https://academic.oup.com/eurheartj/article/34/47/3624/619893.
9. Aizer A, Gaziano JM, Cook NR, Manson JE, Buring JE, Albert CM. Relation of vigorous exercise to risk of atrial fibrillation. Am J Cardiol [Internet]. 2009 June 1 [cited 2019 May 28];103(11):1572–7. Available from: http://www.sciencedirect.com/science/article/pii/S0002914909005499.

10. Drca N, Wolk A, Jensen-Urstad M, Larsson SC. Atrial fibrillation is associated with different levels of physical activity levels at different ages in men. Heart [Internet]. 2014 July 1 [cited 2019 May 28];100(13):1037–42. Available from: https://heart.bmj.com/content/100/13/1037.
11. Morseth B, Graff-Iversen S, Jacobsen BK, Jørgensen L, Nyrnes A, Thelle DS, et al. Physical activity, resting heart rate, and atrial fibrillation: the Tromsø Study. Eur Heart J [Internet]. 2016 Aug 1 [cited 2018 Jan 24];37(29):2307–13. Available from: https://academic.oup.com/eurheartj/article/37/29/2307/2237632.
12. Mohanty S, Mohanty P, Tamaki M, Natale V, Gianni C, Trivedi C, et al. Differential association of exercise intensity with risk of atrial fibrillation in men and women: evidence from a meta-analysis. J Cardiovasc Electrophysiol. 2016;27(9):1021–9.
13. Everett BM, Conen D, Buring JE, Moorthy MV, Lee IM, Albert CM. Physical activity and the risk of incident atrial fibrillation in women. Circ Cardiovasc Qual Outcomes [Internet]. 2011 May 1 [cited 2019 June 1];4(3):321–7. Available from: https://www.ahajournals.org/doi/10.1161/CIRCOUTCOMES.110.951442.
14. Wilhelm M, Roten L, Tanner H, Wilhelm I, Schmid J-P, Saner H. Gender differences of atrial and ventricular remodeling and autonomic tone in nonelite athletes. Am J Cardiol [Internet]. 2011 Nov 15 [cited 2019 June 1];108(10):1489–95. Available from: http://www.sciencedirect.com/science/article/pii/S0002914911022806.
15. Aagaard P, Sharma S, McNamara DA, Joshi P, Ayers CR, de Lemos JA, et al. Arrhythmias and adaptations of the cardiac conduction system in former National Football League players. J Am Heart Assoc. 2019;8(15):e010401.
16. Kim JH, Hollowed C, Irwin-Weyant M, Patel K, Hosny K, Aida H, et al. Sleep-disordered breathing and cardiovascular correlates in college football players. Am J Cardiol. 2017;120(8):1410–5.
17. Lin J, Wang F, Weiner RB, DeLuca JR, Wasfy MM, Berkstresser B, et al. Blood pressure and LV remodeling among American-style football players. JACC Cardiovasc Imaging. 2016;9(12):1367–76.
18. Myrstad M, Nystad W, Graff-Iversen S, Thelle DS, Stigum H, Aarønæs M, et al. Effect of years of endurance exercise on risk of atrial fibrillation and atrial flutter. Am J Cardiol [Internet]. 2014 Oct 15 [cited 2019 June 1];114(8):1229–33. Available from: http://www.sciencedirect.com/science/article/pii/S0002914914015082.
19. Opondo MA, Aiad N, Cain MA, Sarma S, Howden E, Stoller DA, et al. Does high-intensity endurance training increase the risk of atrial fibrillation? A longitudinal study of left atrial structure and function. Circ Arrhythm Electrophysiol. 2018;11(5):e005598.
20. Guasch E, Benito B, Qi X, Cifelli C, Naud P, Shi Y, et al. Atrial fibrillation promotion by endurance exercise: demonstration and mechanistic exploration in an animal model. J Am Coll Cardiol [Internet]. 2013 July 2 [cited 2018 Feb 23];62(1):68–77. Available from: http://www.onlinejacc.org/content/62/1/68.
21. Aschar-Sobbi R, Izaddoustdar F, Korogyi AS, Wang Q, Farman GP, Yang F, et al. Increased atrial arrhythmia susceptibility induced by intense endurance exercise in mice requires TNFα. Nat Commun [Internet]. 2015 Jan 19 [cited 2019 June 2];6:6018. Available from: https://www.nature.com/articles/ncomms7018.
22. Wilhelm M, Roten L, Tanner H, Wilhelm I, Schmid J-P, Saner H. Atrial remodeling, autonomic tone, and lifetime training hours in nonelite athletes. Am J Cardiol. 2011;108(4):580–5.
23. Iskandar A, Mujtaba MT, Thompson PD. Left atrium size in elite athletes. JACC Cardiovasc Imaging. 2015;8(7):753–62.
24. Pelliccia A, Maron BJ, De Luca R, Di Paolo FM, Spataro A, Culasso F. Remodeling of left ventricular hypertrophy in elite athletes after long-term deconditioning. Circulation [Internet]. 2002 Feb 26 [cited 2019 June 2];105(8):944–9. Available from: http://www.ahajournals.org/doi/full/10.1161/hc0802.104534.
25. Luthi P, Zuber M, Ritter M, Oechslin EN, Jenni R, Seifert B, et al. Echocardiographic findings in former professional cyclists after long-term deconditioning of more than 30 years. Eur J Echocardiogr. 2008;9(2):261–7.

26. Pelliccia A, Maron BJ, Di Paolo FM, Biffi A, Quattrini FM, Pisicchio C, et al. Prevalence and clinical significance of left atrial remodeling in competitive athletes. J Am Coll Cardiol [Internet]. 2005 Aug 16 [cited 2019 June 2];46(4):690–6. Available from: http://www.science-direct.com/science/article/pii/S0735109705011733.
27. Dorey TW, O'Brien MW, Kimmerly DS. The influence of aerobic fitness on electrocardiographic and heart rate variability parameters in young and older adults. Auton Neurosci [Internet]. 2019 Mar 1 [cited 2019 Apr 5];217:66–70. Available from: http://www.sciencedirect.com/science/article/pii/S1566070218302455.
28. Liu L, Nattel S. Differing sympathetic and vagal effects on atrial fibrillation in dogs: role of refractoriness heterogeneity. Am J Phys. 1997;273(2 Pt 2):H805–16.
29. Po SS, Li Y, Tang D, Liu H, Geng N, Jackman WM, et al. Rapid and stable re-entry within the pulmonary vein as a mechanism initiating paroxysmal atrial fibrillation. J Am Coll Cardiol [Internet]. 2005 June 7 [cited 2019 June 2];45(11):1871–7. Available from: http://www.sciencedirect.com/science/article/pii/S0735109705006285.
30. Yorgun H, Aytemir K, Canpolat U, Şahiner L, Kaya EB, Oto A. Additional benefit of cryoballoon-based atrial fibrillation ablation beyond pulmonary vein isolation: modification of ganglionated plexi. Europace [Internet]. 2014 May 1 [cited 2019 June 2];16(5):645–51. Available from: https://academic.oup.com/europace/article-lookup/doi/10.1093/europace/eut240.
31. Coumel P, Attuel P, Lavallée J, Flammang D, Leclercq JF, Slama R. The atrial arrhythmia syndrome of vagal origin. Arch Mal Coeur Vaiss [Internet]. 1978 June [cited 2019 June 2];71(6):645–56. Available from: http://europepmc.org/abstract/med/28709.
32. Engelmann MDM, Svendsen JH. Inflammation in the genesis and perpetuation of atrial fibrillation. Eur Heart J [Internet]. 2005 Oct 1 [cited 2019 June 2];26(20):2083–92. Available from: https://academic.oup.com/eurheartj/article/26/20/2083/446740.
33. La Gerche A, Inder WJ, Roberts TJ, Brosnan MJ, Heidbuchel H, Prior DL. Relationship between inflammatory cytokines and indices of cardiac dysfunction following intense endurance exercise. PLoS One. 2015;10(6):e0130031.
34. Bernecker C, Scherr J, Schinner S, Braun S, Scherbaum WA, Halle M. Evidence for an exercise induced increase of TNF-α and IL-6 in marathon runners. Scand J Med Sci Sports. 2013;23(2):207–14.
35. Peritz D, Kaur G, Wasmund S, Kheirkhahan M, Loveless B, Marrouche NF, et al. P4692Endurance training is associated with increased left atrial fibrosis. Eur Heart J [Internet]. 2018 Aug 1 [cited 2019 June 2];39(Suppl_1). Available from: http://academic.oup.com/eurheartj/article/39/suppl_1/ehy563.P4692/5082161.
36. Platonov PG, Mitrofanova LB, Orshanskaya V, Ho SY. Structural abnormalities in atrial walls are associated with presence and persistency of atrial fibrillation but not with age. J Am Coll Cardiol. 2011;58(21):2225–32.
37. Oakes RS, Badger TJ, Kholmovski EG, Akoum N, Burgon NS, Fish EN, et al. Detection and quantification of left atrial structural remodeling with delayed-enhancement magnetic resonance imaging in patients with atrial fibrillation. Circulation [Internet]. 2009 Apr 7 [cited 2019 June 2];119(13):1758–67. Available from: http://www.ahajournals.org/doi/10.1161/CIRCULATIONAHA.108.811877.
38. Siebermair J, Suksaranjit P, McGann CJ, Peterson KA, Kheirkhahan M, Baher AA, et al. Atrial fibrosis in non-atrial fibrillation individuals and prediction of atrial fibrillation by use of late gadolinium enhancement magnetic resonance imaging. J Cardiovasc Electrophysiol. 2019;30(4):550–6.
39. Zipes DP, Link MS, Ackerman MJ, Kovacs RJ, Myerburg RJ, Estes NAM. Eligibility and disqualification recommendations for competitive athletes with cardiovascular abnormalities: task force 9: arrhythmias and conduction defects: a scientific statement from the American Heart Association and American College of Cardiology. J Am Coll Cardiol [Internet]. 2015 Dec 1 [cited 2019 June 2];66(21):2412–23. Available from: http://www.onlinejacc.org/content/66/21/2412.

40. Hoogsteen J, Schep G, Van Hemel NM, Van Der Wall EE. Paroxysmal atrial fibrillation in male endurance athletes. A 9-year follow up. Europace. 2004;6(3):222–8.
41. Furlanello F, Bertoldi A, Dallago M, Galassi A, Fernando F, Biffi A, et al. Atrial fibrillation in elite athletes. J Cardiovasc Electrophysiol. 1998;9(8 Suppl):S63–8.
42. Calvo N, Mont L, Tamborero D, Berruezo A, Viola G, Guasch E, et al. Efficacy of circumferential pulmonary vein ablation of atrial fibrillation in endurance athletes. Europace. 2010;12(1):30–6.
43. Koopman P, Nuyens D, Garweg C, La Gerche A, De Buck S, Van Casteren L, et al. Efficacy of radiofrequency catheter ablation in athletes with atrial fibrillation. Europace. 2011;13(10):1386–93.
44. Mandsager KT, Phelan DM, Diab M, Baranowski B, Saliba WI, Tarakji KG, et al. Outcomes of pulmonary vein isolation in athletes. JACC Clin Electrophysiol. 2020;6(10):1265–74.
45. Morillo CA, Verma A, Connolly SJ, Kuck KH, Nair GM, Champagne J, et al. Radiofrequency ablation vs antiarrhythmic drugs as first-line treatment of paroxysmal atrial fibrillation (RAAFT-2): a randomized trial. JAMA. 2014;311(7):692–700.
46. Furlanello F, Lupo P, Pittalis M, Foresti S, Vitali-Serdoz L, Francia P, et al. Radiofrequency catheter ablation of atrial fibrillation in athletes referred for disabling symptoms preventing usual training schedule and sport competition. J Cardiovasc Electrophysiol. 2008;19(5):457–62.
47. Estes NAM, Madias C. Atrial fibrillation in athletes: a lesson in the virtue of moderation. JACC Clin Electrophysiol [Internet]. 2017 Sep 18 [cited 2018 Feb 23];3(9):921–8. Available from: http://electrophysiology.onlinejacc.org/content/3/9/921.
48. Shapero K, Deluca J, Contursi M, Wasfy M, Weiner RB, Lewis GD, et al. Cardiovascular risk and disease among masters endurance athletes: insights from the Boston MASTER (Masters Athletes Survey To Evaluate Risk) Initiative. Sports Med Open [Internet]. 2016 Aug 9 [cited 2019 Aug 18];2. Available from: https://www.ncbi.nlm.nih.gov/pmc/articles/PMC4978752/.
49. Boraita A, Santos-Lozano A, Heras ME, González-Amigo F, López-Ortiz S, Villacastín JP, et al. Incidence of atrial fibrillation in elite athletes. JAMA Cardiol [Internet]. 2018 Dec 1 [cited 2019 May 14];3(12):1200–5. Available from: https://jamanetwork.com/journals/jamacardiology/fullarticle/2711895.

Chapter 11
Sports Participation in Patients with Congenital Long QT Syndrome

Salima Bhimani, Jared Klein, and Peter F. Aziz

Introduction

Congenital long QT syndrome (LQTS) is an inherited ion channelopathy that can manifest as syncope, seizures, and most importantly sudden cardiac death in the absence of morphologic heart disease [1]. It is the most common cardiac channelopathy and is characterized by prolongation of the corrected QT interval (QTc) on electrocardiogram (ECG) [2]. It has an estimated prevalence of 1 in 2500 live births and accounts for approximately 5000 deaths per year in the United States of America [2, 3]. However, this may be an underestimation when accounting for the subpopulation of "concealed LQTS" (genotype positive, phenotype negative) [4]. LQTS was first reported in 1957 when Jervell and Lange-Neilsen reported a disease cluster with an autosomal recessive inheritance in a family where several children experienced recurrent syncope and sudden death in the context of a prolonged QT interval and profound sensorineural hearing loss [5]. Since then, it has been identified that individuals with LQTS have an increased susceptibility to fatal ventricular arrhythmias with an annual rate of sudden death in untreated individuals between 0.33% and 0.9% [6, 7].

Before the advent of the genetic era, LQTS was viewed in a different paradigm with the first diagnostic criteria proposed in 1985 [8]. Although clinically useful, these criteria were relatively qualitative; hence, Schwartz et al. published a revised version in 1993, incorporating objective parameters by assigning points to patient's symptoms, medical and family history, and ECG findings [9]. With progressive understanding of genetic interplay in this disease, realization arose that these criteria did not include those with "concealed LQTS" or silent variants [8]. The criteria, thus, had a limited use in those with a normal or borderline QT interval. In 2011,

S. Bhimani · J. Klein · P. F. Aziz (✉)
Cleveland Clinic Children's, Cleveland, OH, USA
e-mail: BHIMANS@ccf.org; Kleinj4@ccf.org; Azizp@ccf.org

© Springer Nature Switzerland AG 2021
D. J. Engel, D. M. Phelan (eds.), *Sports Cardiology*,
https://doi.org/10.1007/978-3-030-69384-8_11

Table 11.1 1993–2011 LQTS Diagnostic Criteria. (Adapted from: Schwartz and Crotti [8])

	Points
Electrocardiographic findings[a]	
A QTc[b]	
≥480 ms	3
460–479 ms	2
450–459 ms (in males)	1
B QTc[b] 4th minute of recovery from exercise stress test ≥480 ms	1
C Torsade de pointes[c]	2
D T wave alternans	1
E Notched T wave in 3 leads	1
F Low heart rate for age[d]	0.5
Clinical history	
A Syncope[e]	
With stress	2
Without stress	1
B Congenital deafness	0.5
Family history	
A Family members with definite LQTS[f]	1
B Unexplained sudden cardiac death below age 30 among immediate family members[f]	0.5

[a]In the absence of medications or disorders known to affect these electrocardiographic features
[b]QTc calculated by Bazett's formula where $QTc=QT/\sqrt{RR}$
[c]Mutually exclusive
[d]Resting heart rate below the 2nd percentile for age
[e]The same family member cannot be counted in A and B
SCORE: ≤1 point: low probability of LQTS
1.5 to 3 points: intermediate probability of LQTS
≥3.5 points high probability

multiple studies demonstrated that QTc prolongation during the recovery phase of postexercise testing could unmask LQTS in those with a concealed subtype [8–10]. The current Schwartz diagnostic criteria have therefore evolved with time to accommodate these additional objective parameters as summarized in Table 11.1.

Today, about 75–80% of patients with LQTS have identifiable genetic variants [11]. Variants in 17 genes have been associated with LQTS, each resulting in dysfunction of sodium, potassium, or calcium ion channels [6, 12]. Each variant leads to distinct clinical features with the majority inherited in an autosomal-dominant pattern (historically described as Romano Ward Syndrome) [13, 14]. Medical management of LQTS includes therapy with beta blockade and avoidance of QTc-prolonging medications. Beta blockade has shown to reduce the risk of a first time event in all patients with LQTS but is particularly beneficial in the LQT1 subset [2].

The phenomenon of variable penetrance in genotype positive LQTS may result in clinically diverse presentations within members of the same family making individual risk prediction of fatal arrhythmias particularly challenging [15]. This becomes even more relevant when reviewing the transition in sports restriction

Table 11.2 Evolution of sports participation guidelines with respect to LQTS

	European Society of Cardiology (2005)	Bethesda 36th Conference (2005)	Task Force 10 (2015)
Upper limits for QTc for guideline applications	>440 Males >460 Females	>470 Males >480 Females	>470 Males >480 Females
Concealed LQTS (genotype +, phenotype −)	All sports restricted	No restrictions	No restrictions
Symptomatic	All sports restricted	Class 1A	No restrictions (except for LQT1 swimmers). Must be asymptomatic for 3 months on therapy.
ICD	All sports restricted	Class 1A	Class 1A (consult an expert otherwise)

Adapted from Furst and Aziz [53]

guidelines in those with manifest LQTS and those with concealed LQTS. Historically, all individuals with concealed LQTS were restricted from all sports participation. Over the years, the necessity of this restriction has been questioned. With the advent of cascade screening, many genotype positive, phenotype negative patients are being identified who remain asymptomatic [16]. Successive studies demonstrating risk reduction in cardiac events with the introduction of beta blockers as a standard of care have also hastened this transition. This evolution is pictorially depicted in Table 11.2.

LQTS is a clinical diagnosis encompassing clinical presentation, family history, and ECG characteristics, as summarized in Table 11.1 [8, 17]. It is also important to emphasize that expert consensus states that individuals suspected of having a cardiac channelopathy should undergo a comprehensive evaluation by an experienced heart rhythm specialist or genetic cardiologist with sufficient expertize prior to sports participation [18]. Due to intricacies of genotype-phenotype interplay and importance of sports participation in this era of shared decision making (SDM), it is crucial to review risk stratification, particularly in athletes with LQTS.

Challenges of QTc Measurement in Athletes

The accuracy of computer generated QT is estimated to be 90–95% [15]. It is ideally measured manually from the earliest onset of QRS to the offset of T-wave in order to yield the most accurate results. This is ideally done using the lead with the most prominent T-wave amplitude (lead II or V5) [19, 20].

The QT interval may fluctuate with variation in heart rate; several formulae exist to correct the QT interval for heart rate. Bazett's formula is recommended for QTc calculation in athletes, since the majority of existing LQTS data has utilized this approach [21]. It entails using the RR interval immediately preceding the measured QT interval and incorporating it into the following equation:

$$QTc = QT / \sqrt{RR}$$

Figure 11.1 displays the accurate method of QTc measurement on a standard ECG. Defining the end of T-wave can often be challenging, but is better achieved by drawing a tangent to the steepest portion of the descending part of the T-wave and marking its intercept with the isoelectric line as the end of the T-wave [19, 20, 22]. The accuracy of this approach is suboptimal at the extremes of heart rate specifically rates that are less than 40 bpm and greater than 120 bpm [21, 23, 24]. This is important to note in athletes who typically have lower resting sympathetic stimulation and a relatively higher resting vagal tone. It has been previously demonstrated that vagal stimulation and acetylcholine prolong the QT interval independent of their bradycardia inducing ability [23, 24]. Hence, at lower heart rates, the QTc may be underestimated in athletes using the Bazett's formula.

Factors that may affect the QTc interval include certain medications, electrolyte disturbances, changes in cardiac after load (sympathetic and parasympathetic autonomic interplay), metabolic, and neurologic diseases [18].

Fig. 11.1 Pictorial representation of QTc measurement. The red line constitutes the tangent drawn from the maximum T-wave slope to the iso-electric line. (Figure obtained from the "Life in the Fast Lane" website by Ed Burns MD. https://litfl.com/qt-interval-ecg-library/)

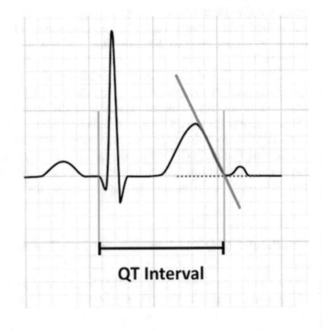

Pathophysiology of Malignant Arrhythmia in LQTS

LQTS-related ion channelopathy results in prolonged action potentials and increased dispersion of myocardial repolarization, predisposing these individuals to torsades de pointes (TdP) with potential to degenerate into ventricular fibrillation (VF) [25]. This risk increases with progressive QT prolongation with the highest risk incurred in those with a QTc greater than 500 ms [26]. Adrenergic stress states have been implicated as a substrate for syncopal events in patients with congenital LQTS [27]. Interplay between sympathetic and vagal stimulation has also been suggested in literature to play an important role in dynamic change in the QT interval prior to initiation of TdP [28]. Age and gender variation serve as risk modifiers amongst different subtypes making the understanding of this entity even more intricate. For instance, males with LQT1 have a higher risk of first cardiac events in adolescence (<16 years of age) when compared to their female cohort. After adolescence, the overall risk decreases in males with LQT1 but remains higher in females [29].

The early molecular studies suggested that all genes associated with LQTS phenotype encode for proteins forming the subunits of transmembrane ion channel, however more recent studies have brought to light variants in genes coding for regulatory proteins acting as modulators of these ion channels [30]. Although now 17 genetic variants have been implicated to date in LQTS, the majority of the disease is caused by variants in *KCNQ1* and *KCNH2* (coding for cardiac potassium channels in LQT1 and LQT2, respectively) and *SCN5A* (coding for cardiac sodium channels in LQT3) [26].

Diagnosis of LQTS

As stated previously, the diagnosis of LQTS is clinical [17]. Normal QTc values are dependent on age and gender. The first step in the diagnostic evaluation is a resting ECG. The typical "prolonged" interval is greater than 470 milliseconds in males and 480 milliseconds in females, though various "cutoffs" have been employed [31]. Regardless, up to 50% of patients with LQTS display a nondiagnostic resting QTc [14]. Various clinical criteria scores exist including the Schwartz and Keating criteria, though these scales are hindered by low sensitivity [14].

The most common subtype is LQT1, constituting about 35% of the population of patients with LQTS. The mechanism behind this disorder is loss of function in the *KCNQ1* gene [16]. *KCNQ1* encodes the alpha subunit of the K+ channel, which is essential for QT adaption with an increase in heart rate during exercise [17]. When this channel is defective, the QT interval does not shorten during tachycardia,

Table 11.3 LQTS as summarized through genotype

Genotype	LQT1	LQT2	LQT3
Gene mutation frequency	35%	30%	10%
Affected gene	*KCNQ1*	*KCNH2*	*SCN5A*
Affect on current	↓ I_{Ks}	↓ I_{Kr}	↑ I_{Na}
Effect on myocyte action potential	Phases 3 > 2	Phase 2 > 3	Phase 0
Most common triggers for a cardiac event	Exercise and sympathetic tone	Auditory stimuli and emotion	Sleep, rest without arousal
Percentage of events triggered by exercise*	62%	13%	13%
Patient characteristics for higher risk	Males prior to adolescence	Females after adolescence	Males after adolescence
Response to beta-blockade	+++	++	+

*Schwartz et al. [31].

Adapted from Schwartz et al. [32]
[a]Schwartz et al. [31]

resulting in dysrhythmias [14]. The main trigger for syncopal events in this subtype is exercise, particularly swimming. LQT2 is the second most common subtype and is caused by loss-of-function in the *KCNH2* gene. The most common triggers of significant cardiac events in this subgroup are through auditory stimuli, emotional events, or startle. In LQT3, arrhythmias most often occur during sleep, making this subtype particularly difficult to prevent.

Exercise testing can be used for differentiating LQT1, LQT2, and unaffected individuals. A QTc that remains prolonged at 7 minutes is predictive for LQT1 and LQT2 compared to normal control subjects [18]. Provocative testing with epinephrine administered in graded infusions can also be diagnostic of LQTS as a positive result will demonstrate paradoxical prolonging of the QTc [14]. This is comprehensively summarized in Table 11.3 [32].

Utility of Beta Blockade and Other Treatments in LQTS

The mainstay of treatment for LQTS is beta blockade as this has been shown to decrease the number of significant cardiac events and degeneration into TdP [30, 31]. One study showed a greater than 90% reduction in risk with full compliance and avoidance of QT-prolonging medications in LQT1 patients [33]. While there are multiple treatment options, nadolol has been demonstrated as the treatment with the most efficacy as compared to metoprolol, which should be avoided in the treatment of LQTS patients due to a higher number of breakthrough cardiac events [34]. Propranolol has demonstrated to be similar in efficacy as nadolol and is used in infants and younger children due to its availability in a liquid form.

Beta blockers are most effective among LQT1 patients but there is significant benefit in LQT2 and LQT3 [35]. Noncompliance with medications and use of QT-prolonging drugs are the most common cause of treatment failures. With the increasing evidence that beta blockade is effective at preventing cardiac events, practitioners have become more comfortable with sports eligibility liberalization.

Role of ICD in the Management of LQTS

While implanted cardiac defibrillators (ICD) are rarely used in the treatment of LQTS, some patients deemed at high risk for sudden death independent of sports participation may be advised to undergo ICD placement. Theoretically, this device should provide protection during sports, but concerns about inappropriate shocks or lead fracture have made experts reluctant to make different recommendations for sports participation for athletes with an ICD [31]. The 2012 ACCF/AHA/HRS guidelines state as a class III recommendation (may cause harm), that an ICD should NOT be implanted for the sole purpose of permitting sporting participation [36, 37]. Indications for ICD placement vary but can include previous history of cardiac arrest, syncope despite beta blocker therapy, ventricular arrhythmias despite beta blocker therapy, and those with atrioventricular heart block [37]. The risks of inappropriate shocks, lead fractures, and the high likelihood of device re-intervention need to be considered against the likelihood of requiring defibrillation to treat a cardiac event in a discussion between the clinician and the patient before an ICD is placed [38]. A recent study exploring long-term outcomes of the multinational ICD registry prospectively evaluated 129 young athletes participating in competitive sports. These individuals were followed for 42 months with the observation that 35 athletes received 38 shocks without any occurrences of death, arrest, or injury related to arrhythmia during sports, implying relative safety of sports participation in this cohort. These results however are limited by the small sample size and may not be generalizable [38].

Surgical Management in LQTS

One potential surgical option for LQTS is left cardiac sympathetic denervation. This procedure entails removal of the first 3–4 ganglia of the sympathetic chain [39]. This modality is reserved for those in which medical therapy has been ineffective, not tolerated, or with a severely prolonged QTc (>500 ms). The effectiveness of this procedure has been variable. One large cohort found a significant reduction in the QTc duration as well as the incidence of aborted cardiac arrest and syncopal episodes [40]. However, this procedure has also been found to be ineffective at shortening the QTc with limited literature [41]. Side effects of this procedure include left sided dryness, flushing, transient ptosis, thermoregulation difficulties, and left arm paresthesia.

History of LQTS and Sports Participation

Sports eligibility has largely been based on clinical interpretation of risk that has evolved with our understanding of genotype–phenotype correlations along with the physiologic response to exercise testing. In 1998, when only 4 genes linked to LQTS had been identified, Zareba et al. were the first group to demonstrate that distinct LQTS genotypes were associated with variable overall risk for significant cardiac events [42]. This study marked the beginning of risk stratification based upon genotype–phenotype correlation for sudden cardiac death. QTc prolongation was found to be an independent risk factor for cardiac events. Although those in the study population with LQT1 had the lowest mean QTc, those who did have a QTc greater than 500 ms were found to have the highest risk for cardiac events including syncope, aborted cardiac arrest, or sudden death [42].

Early guidelines regarding sports participation were based upon the evidence that exercise is a general trigger for cardiac events in patients with LQTS. According to the Bethesda consensus guidelines published in 2005, suspicion for a diagnosis of LQTS in athletes should be based upon a QTc exceeding 470 ms in males and 480 ms in females. The recommendations stated that any patient with LQTS who met the QTc criteria, had a history of LQTS-related symptoms, or had an ICD implanted should be restricted from all athletic participation aside from the Class IA category of sports that includes billiards, bowling, cricket, curling, golf, and riflery. These sports had been broadly categorized as involving the lowest possible dynamic and static components. The authors of this classification, however, conceded that the matrix of sports they created should not be used rigidly as several sports are heterogeneous depending on differences in roles within each sport (such as athletes who play as a forward versus those who play as the goalkeeper in soccer) and differences in how intensely individuals perform in any given sport [43].

While the Bethesda guidelines were based upon the best evidence at that time, the counsel admitted that in the absence of empiric data from large, well-designed studies, their recommendations were more based upon the "art of medicine" [43, 44]. Nevertheless, these guidelines did include the recommendation that genotype-positive, phenotype-negative patients who do not fulfill one of the aforementioned criteria should not be restricted from athletic activity, which was based upon strong evidence of a very low incidence of cardiac events in these patients [45]. The one exception to this allowance was swimming in genetically confirmed LQT1 patients. Research at that point had clearly demonstrated this particular vulnerability, and this was the first recognition within published guidelines that LQTS genotype confers differential risk [46]. These guidelines were broad in order to maximize the prevention of cardiac events from sports participation in LQTS patients; however, and did not allow for individualized approach to patient care nor was patient autonomy recognized.

In the same year, the European Society of Cardiology (ESC) also published consensus recommendations for athletic participation for patients with LQTS. These guidelines were even more rigid than the Bethesda consensus guidelines in that all patients with a diagnosis of LQTS, including those who are phenotypically negative, should be restricted from all forms of athletic participation. Furthermore, they endorsed a more conservative QTc threshold for recommending genetic testing for LQTS of 440 ms in males and 460 ms in females. There were no additional recommendations for patients who were genotype negative with borderline QTc [16]. Both the Bethesda and ESC guidelines did exclude all those with ICD placement from participation in all but Class IA activities. Pellicia et al. later discussed the reasoning behind the more conservative guidelines of the ESC, suggesting that it is likely due to differences in the liability within the medical systems of Europe, in particular [44].

Current Risk Stratification in Athletes

Considering that arrhythmias, particularly in LQT1, are often the consequence of catecholaminergic surges which are typical in competitive sports, expert consensus was particularly conservative regarding sports participation [47]. This was specifically evident in the 36th Bethesda Conference guidelines where these individuals were restricted to low static/low dynamic competitive participation, disqualifying even those asymptomatic from partaking in commonly played competitive sports [44]. Ensuing literature brought forth new evidence that sports liberalization is a possibility in these patients and may be safer than previously believed. This was highlighted by a single center study retrospectively examining a cohort of 212 genotype positive patients with LQTS on beta blockade therapy. Of these 212 patients, 103 participated in either competitive or recreational sports. None of these patients had LQTS symptoms during sports participation. Five appropriate ICD shocks were delivered in 2 patients none of which were related to sports participation. Thus, this study concluded that there were no serious cardiac events or deaths during sports participation in LQTS patients who were treatment compliant [47]. Another study evaluated 353 patients with LQTS followed over a period of approximately 5 years. This study mirrored similar results with only one patient of their cohort receiving an appropriate shock from ICD for ventricular fibrillation on two separate occasions in the setting of admitted nonadherence to beta blockade therapy [48]. This study also concluded a low rate of LQTS-triggered cardiac events during sports participation.

Providing impetus that participation may in fact be "safer" in the treated LQTS patient, the above studies provided support for the evolution of prior consensus. The most recent guideline is the report of the AHA/ACC scientific statement "Eligibility and Disqualification Recommendations for Competitive Athletes with Cardiovascular Abnormalities: Task Force 10: The Cardiac Channelopathies" [49]. The previous recommendations were deemed too restrictive as disqualification carries its own set of health and psychological consequences [31]. These guidelines recommend asymptomatic athletes who are genotype-positive/phenotype-negative for LQTS be allowed to participate in all sports with appropriate precautionary measures such as avoidance of dehydration and having an automatic external defibrillator on-site at all practice and games. As for those who have been symptomatic in the past, sports participation can be considered if one has been asymptomatic on medical treatment for at least 3 months. In the circumstance of athletes with ICDs, Task Force 9: Eligibility and Disqualification Recommendations for Competitive Athletes with Cardiovascular Abnormalities: Arrhythmias and Conduction Defects, states that these athletes can participate in 1A sports if episode free for 3 months on device interrogation [18]. Contact sports should still be avoided for risk of ICD damage. Participation in other sports with higher static and dynamic aspects can be considered if the athlete is free from cardiac events for more than 3 months with appropriate counseling of the higher likelihood of appropriate and inappropriate shocks.

Beyond Medical Therapy- Counseling and Preparedness on the Field

The presence of effective pharmacologic therapy should not undermine the importance of general measures of prudence in an athlete with a channelopathy. This was comprehensively summarized by Task Force 10 as universal precautions that athletes and organized teams should adhere to. These include: avoiding QT-prolonging drugs for athletes with LQTS (http://www.crediblemeds.org), electrolyte replenishment and avoidance of dehydration for all athletes, avoiding hyperthermia and treating hyperthermia from febrile illnesses or training-related heat exhaustion/heat stroke for athletes with LQTS, procurement of a personal automatic external defibrillator (AED) as part of the athlete's personal sports safety gear, and establishing an emergency action plan with the appropriate school/team officials [18]. In addition, coaching staff should also be made aware of their athletes' cardiac conditions and undergo AHA-approved CPR training [18].

Role of Shared Decision Making in Athletes with LQTS

In the modern era, shared decision making (SDM) has come to the forefront as a way to improve clinical care for patients by encouraging the production and dissemination of accurate, balanced, understandable health information while increasing patient participation in care [50–52]. The physician's responsibility in SDM is to give accurate medical information, elicit and acknowledge patients' preferences for sports participation, give the patients choices about how the decision making process will proceed and respect patients' choices. In this setting, patients have the responsibility to communicate their values, goals, and preferences to the physician. Finally when a treatment decision is made, both parties agree to the decision. The approach to the pediatric athlete provides additional complexity. Not only should the SDM be contractual between the physician and patient, but also it is our institutional practice to have all caregivers agree and support the child's decision to participate. This process may have to involve the school or team officials as they may have the final say on return to play [15]. Using this paradigm, it is hopeful that a joint decision will be made that will be safe and beneficial for the patient.

Future Directions

Current treatment methods for LQTS have been effective and will continue to be improved upon. There has been decades-worth of studies involving the link between specific genotypes and the natural history of patients with LQTS; however, several of these studies have limitations with regard to selection bias. Though LQTS and channelopathy research have experienced an explosion in genotype–phenotype correlation, many of these associations are observational, nonrandomized, and retrospective. Another aspect challenging our interpretation of genotype is the complexity of variable penetrance and modifier genes that are still poorly understood and may account for the variance between different families with the same variant. Until we are able to elucidate this complexity, sports participation guidelines will often be too restrictive in some patients and not restrictive enough in others.

The studied efficacy of beta blockade in treatment of patients, particularly those with LQT1, has largely led to the recognition that the psychological and health benefits of sports participation may outweigh the potential risks of a sudden cardiac event. In the future, we hope to stratify risk based on each individual's specific gene variant (or combination) and the electrophysiological characteristics of their repolarization to determine their specific therapy and their ability to participate in all types of competitive sports. The development of such tools, however, will be dependent upon more rigorous studies to better define the link between exercise and cardiac events in LQTS. Consistent with that aim, there is an on-going study designed to prospectively assess safety in sports participation (NIH RO1 HL125918-01). This will yield invaluable data in terms of understanding the long-term prognosis and outcome of sports participation in these individuals. Keeping patient safety in mind, a more personalized approach may be taken in diagnosis and treatment of LQTS while incorporating a comprehensive evaluation and assessment of these individuals by an expert heart rhythm specialist.

References

1. Li K, Yang J, Guo W, Lv T, Guo J, Li J, Zhang P. GW29-e0961 video-assisted thoracoscopic left cardiac sympathetic denervation in Chinese patients with long QT syndrome. J Am Coll Cardiol. 2018. https://doi.org/10.1016/j.jacc.2018.08.768.
2. Aziz PF, Saarel EV. Sports participation in long QT syndrome. Cardiol Young. 2017;27:S43–8.
3. Gibbs C, Thalamus J, Tveten K, Busk ØL, Hysing J, Haugaa KH, Holla ØL. Genetic and phenotypic characterization of community hospital patients with QT prolongation. J Am Heart Assoc. 2018. https://doi.org/10.1161/JAHA.118.009706.
4. Schwartz PJ, Stramba-Badiale M, Crotti L, et al. Prevalence of the congenital long-qt syndrome. 2009. Circulation https://doi.org/10.1161/CIRCULATIONAHA.109.863209.
5. Jervell A, Lange-Nielsen F. Congenital deaf-mutism, functional heart disease with prolongation of the Q-T interval, and sudden death. Am Heart J. 1957. https://doi.org/10.1016/0002-8703(57)90079-0.
6. Priori SG, Schwartz PJ, Napolitano C, et al. Risk stratification in the long-QT syndrome. 2003;348:1866–74.
7. Moss AJ, Schwartz PJ, Crampton RS, Tzivoni D, Locati EH, MacCluer J, Hall WJ, Weitkamp L, Vincent GM, Garson A Jr, et al. The long QT syndrome. Prospective longitudinal study of 328 families. Circulation. 1991;84(3):1136–44. https://doi.org/10.1161/01.cir.84.3.1136. PMID: 1884444.
8. Schwartz PJ, Crotti L. QTc behavior during exercise and genetic testing for the long-qt syndrome. Circulation. 2011. 124:2181–2184. https://doi.org/10.1161/CIRCULATIONAHA.111.062182.
9. Hayashi K, Konno T, Fujino N, et al. Impact of updated diagnostic criteria for long QT syndrome on clinical detection of diseased patients. JACC Clin Electrophysiol. 2016;2:279–87.
10. Aziz PF, Wieand TS, Ganley J, Henderson J, Patel AR, Iyer VR, Vogel RL, McBride M, Vetter VL, Shah MJ. Genotype- and mutation site-specific QT adaptation during exercise, recovery, and postural changes in children with long-QT syndrome. Circ Arrhythm Electrophysiol. 2011;4:867–73.
11. Kwok S, Liu AP, Chan CY, Lun K, Fung JL, Mak CC, Chung BH, Yung T. Clinical and genetic profile of congenital long QT syndrome in Hong Kong: a 20-year experience in paediatrics. Hong Kong Med J. 2018. https://doi.org/10.12809/hkmj187487.
12. Giudicessi JR, Ackerman MJ. Calcium revisited. Circ Arrhythm Electrophysiol. 2016;9:1–11.
13. Kaufman ES. Mechanisms and clinical management of inherited channelopathies: long QT syndrome, Brugada syndrome, catecholaminergic polymorphic ventricular tachycardia, and short QT syndrome. Heart Rhythm. 2009. https://doi.org/10.1016/j.hrthm.2009.02.009.
14. Skinner JR, Winbo A, Abrams D, Vohra J, Wilde AA. Channelopathies that lead to sudden cardiac death: clinical and genetic aspects. Heart Lung Circ. 2018. https://doi.org/10.1016/j.hlc.2018.09.007.
15. Schnell F, Behar N, Carré F. Long-QT Syndrome and Competitive Sports. Arrhythm Electrophysiol Rev. 2018;7(3):187–92. https://doi.org/10.15420/aer.2018.39.3. PMID: 30416732; PMCID: PMC6141947.
16. Ackerman MJ. Long QT syndrome and sports participation. JACC Clin Electrophysiol. 2015;1:71–3.
17. Shah SR, Park K, Alweis R. Long QT syndrome: a comprehensive review of the literature and current evidence. Curr Probl Cardiol. 2019;44:92–106.
18. Ackerman MJ, Link MS, Estes NAM, Myerburg RJ, Kovacs RJ, Zipes DP. Eligibility and disqualification recommendations for competitive athletes with cardiovascular abnormalities: task force 9: arrhythmias and conduction defects. J Am Coll Cardiol. 2015;66:2412–23.
19. Funck-Brentano C, Jaillon P. Rate-corrected QT interval: techniques and limitations. Am J Cardiol. 1993. https://doi.org/10.1016/0002-9149(93)90035-B.
20. Garson A. How to measure the QT interval-what is normal? Am J Cardiol. 1993. https://doi.org/10.1016/0002-9149(93)90034-A.
21. Sharma S, Drezner JA, Baggish A, et al. International recommendations for electrocardiographic interpretation in athletes. J Am Coll Cardiol. 2017;69:1057–75.

22. Cadogan M, Burns E. How to measure QTc interval. In: Life fast lane-QT interval. 2019. https://litfl.com/qt-interval-ecg-library/. Accessed 6 Jan 2020.
23. Davidowski TA. Pathophysiology and natural history the QT interval during reflex cardiovascular adaptation. Circulation. 1983:22–5.
24. Litovsky SH, Antzelevitch C. Differences in the electrophysiological response to canine ventricular subendocardium and subepicardium to acetylcholine and isoproterenol. A direct effect of acetylcholine in ventricular myocardium. Circ Res. 1990;67:615–27.
25. Charisopoulou D, Koulaouzidis G, Rydberg A, Henein MY. Exercise worsening of electromechanical disturbances: A predictor of arrhythmia in long QT syndrome. Clin Cardiol. 2019;42(7):701. https://doi.org/10.1002/clc.23216. Epub 2019 Jun 18. Erratum for: Clin Cardiol. 2019;42(2):235–40. PMID: 31265760; PMCID: PMC6605001.
26. Etheridge SP, Asaki SY, Niu MC-I. A personalized approach to long QT syndrome. Curr Opin Cardiol. 2018;34:46–56.
27. Viskin S, Alla SR, Barron HV, Heller K, Saxon L, Kitzis I, Van Hare GF, Wong MJ, Lesh MD, Scheinman MM. Mode of onset of torsade de pointes in congenital long QT syndrome. J Am Coll Cardiol. 1996;28:1262–8.
28. Fujiki A, Nishida K, Mizumaki K. Spontaneous onset of torsade de pointes in long-QT. Jpn Circ J. 2001;65:1087–90.
29. Zareba W, Moss AJ, Locati EH, et al. Modulating effects of age and gender on the clinical course of long QT syndrome by genotype. J Am Coll Cardiol. 2003;42:103–9.
30. Ruan Y, Liu N, Napolitano C, Priori SG. Therapeutic strategies for long-QT syndrome. Circ Arrhythm Electrophysiol. 2008;1:290–7.
31. Ackerman MJ, Zipes DP, Kovacs RJ, Maron BJ. Eligibility and disqualification recommendations for competitive athletes with cardiovascular abnormalities: task force 10: the cardiac channelopathies. J Am Coll Cardiol. 2015;66:2424–8.
32. Schwartz PJ, Priori SG, Spazzolini C, et al. Genotype-phenotype correlation in the long-QT syndrome gene-specific triggers for life-threatening arrhythmias. Circulation. 2001;103:89–95.
33. Vincent GM, Schwartz PJ, Denjoy I, et al. High efficacy of β-blockers in long-QT syndrome type 1: contribution of noncompliance and QT-prolonging drugs to the occurrence of β-blocker treatment "failures". Circulation. 2009;119:215–21.
34. Chockalingam P, Crotti L, Girardengo G, et al. Not all beta-blockers are equal in the management of long QT syndrome types 1 and 2: higher recurrence of events under metoprolol. J Am Coll Cardiol. 2012. https://doi.org/10.1016/j.jacc.2012.07.046.
35. Barsheshet A, Dotsenko O, Goldenberg I. Congenital long QT syndromes: prevalence, pathophysiology and management. Pediatr Drugs. 2014. https://doi.org/10.1007/s40272-014-0090-4.
36. Tracy CM, Epstein AE, Darbar D, et al. 2012 ACCF/AHA/HRS focused update incorporated into the ACCF/AHA/HRS 2008 guidelines for device-based therapy of cardiac rhythm abnormalities. J Am Coll Cardiol. 2013;61:e6–e75.
37. Etheridge SP, Sanatani S, Cohen MI, Albaro CA, Saarel EV, Bradley DJ. Long QT syndrome in children in the era of implantable defibrillators. J Am Coll Cardiol. 2007;50:1335–40.
38. Saarel EV, Law I, Berul CI, et al. Safety of sports for young patients with implantable cardioverter-defibrillators. Circ Arrhythm Electrophysiol. 2018;11:e006305.
39. Schwartz PJ, Crotti L, Insolia R. Long-QT syndrome from genetics to management. Circ Arrhythm Electrophysiol. 2012;5:868–77.
40. Schwartz PJ, Priori SG, Cerrone M, et al. Left cardiac sympathetic denervation in the management of high-risk patients affected by the long-QT syndrome. Circulation. 2004;109:1826–33.
41. Waddell-Smith KE, Ertresvaag KN, Li J, Chaudhuri K, Crawford JR, Hamill JK, Haydock D, Skinner JR. Physical and psychological consequences of left cardiac sympathetic denervation in long-QT syndrome and catecholaminergic polymorphic ventricular tachycardia. Circ Arrhythm Electrophysiol. 2015;8:1151–8.
42. Mag O, Matteo S, Cardiology M, Maugeri FS, Hospital BC, Lake S, Hospital S, Program F. The New England Journal of Medicine influence of the genotype on the clinical course. N Engl J Med. 1998;339:960–5.
43. Mitchell JH, Haskell W, Snell P, Van Camp SP. Task force 8: classification of sports. J Am Coll Cardiol. 2005;45:1364–7.

44. Pelliccia A, Zipes DP, Maron BJ. Bethesda conference #36 and the European Society of Cardiology consensus recommendations revisited. J Am Coll Cardiol. 2008;52:1990–6.
45. Liu JF, Jons C, Moss AJ, et al. Risk factors for recurrent syncope and subsequent fatal or near-fatal events in children and adolescents with long QT syndrome. J Am Coll Cardiol. 2011;57:941–50.
46. Albertella L, Crawford J, Skinner JR. Presentation and outcome of water-related events in children with long QT syndrome. Arch Dis Child. 2011;96:704–7.
47. Aziz PF, Sweeten T, Vogel RL, Bonney WJ, Henderson J, Patel AR, Shah MJ. Sports participation in genotype positive children with long QT syndrome. JACC Clin Electrophysiol. 2015;1:62–70.
48. Johnson JN, Ackerman MJ. Competitive sports participation in athletes with congenital long QT syndrome. JAMA J Am Med Assoc. 2012. https://doi.org/10.1001/jama.2012.9334.
49. Maron BJ, Zipes DP, Kovacs RJ. Eligibility and disqualification recommendations for competitive athletes with cardiovascular abnormalities: preamble, principles, and general considerations. Circulation. 2015; https://doi.org/10.1161/CIR.0000000000000236.
50. Lin GA, Fagerlin A. Shared decision making state of the science. Circ Cardiovasc Qual Outcomes. 2014;7:328–34.
51. Baggish AL, Ackerman MJ, Lampert R. Competitive sport participation among athletes with heart disease. Circulation. 2017;136:1569–71.
52. Etheridge SP, Saarel EV, Martinez MW. Exercise participation and shared decision-making in patients with inherited channelopathies and cardiomyopathies. Heart Rhythm. 2018;15:915–20.
53. Furst ML, Aziz PF. The evolution of sports participation guidelines and the influence of genotype-phenotype correlation in long QT syndrome. Trends Cardiovasc Med. 2016;26:690–7.

Chapter 12
Other Arrhythmic Disorders: WPW, CPVT, Brugada and Idiopathic VF/VT

Jeffrey J. Hsu and Eugene H. Chung

Introduction

Sudden cardiac death (SCD) occurs in approximately 1 in 40,000 to 200,000 athletes every year [1–5]. In addition to the arrhythmias presented in the preceding chapters, there are several categories of arrhythmic disorders that raise particular concerns in athletes, as strenuous physical activity may precipitate life-threatening manifestations of these disorders. The focus of this chapter is to discuss these arrhythmic disorders in the context of the athletic patient and to review how management needs to be specially tailored to the physically active lifestyle of this patient population. Diagnostic work-up, advanced treatment options and guidance recommendations will also be reviewed.

Wolff-Parkinson-White Syndrome

First described by Drs. Louis Wolff, John Parkinson, and Paul D. White in 1930 in a case series of young and otherwise healthy adults [6], the Wolff-Parkinson-White (WPW) ECG identifies one or more accessory conduction pathway between the atria and ventricles. While these accessory pathways may be present in asymptomatic individuals, symptoms along with the WPW pattern on ECG (i.e., WPW syndrome) may first manifest as palpitations, near syncope, syncope, or sudden cardiac death (SCD).

J. J. Hsu
Department of Medicine (Cardiology), University of California, Los Angeles, CA, USA
e-mail: JJHsu@mednet.ucla.edu

E. H. Chung (✉)
Department of Medicine, University of Michigan, Ann Arbor, MI, USA
e-mail: chungeug@umich.edu

© Springer Nature Switzerland AG 2021
D. J. Engel, D. M. Phelan (eds.), *Sports Cardiology*,
https://doi.org/10.1007/978-3-030-69384-8_12

Background & Epidemiology

Patients who present with the ECG findings alone, without any obvious symptoms such as presyncope, syncope, or palpitations, are considered to have a **WPW ECG pattern**. Symptomatic patients who have the ECG findings are diagnosed with **WPW syndrome**.

The prevalence of WPW syndrome (hereafter referred to as WPW) ranges from 1 to 4.5 per 1000 people in pediatric and adult studies, though this may underestimate the true prevalence as the WPW pattern may present intermittently on ECG. WPW syndrome is thought to account for at least 1% of sudden cardiac death (SCD) in athletes [2]. The true number may be higher due to the difficulty of determining WPW pathology in autopsy studies.

Risk factors for WPW include: male sex, young age (<30 years), a history of atrial fibrillation, a family history of WPW, and a history of congenital heart disease (i.e., Ebstein's anomaly, hypertrophic cardiomyopathy) [7].

Pathophysiology

Normal conduction between the atria and ventricles occurs through the atrioventricular (AV) node and bundle of His. In conditions such as atrial fibrillation, in which the atria may conduct at rapid rates, the AV node acts as a "toll bridge," limiting conduction (i.e., decremental conduction) to the ventricles.

WPW describes a condition in which rapid conduction between the atria and ventricles can occur via one or more accessory pathways. The presence of an accessory pathway presents another route whereby depolarization can be conducted, without decrement, to the ventricles. If this conduction occurs before the signal is propagated through the AV node, then there is ventricular "pre-excitation" via the accessory pathway. A supraventricular tachycardia such as atrial fibrillation could thus result in rapid atrial rates directly conducted via the accessory pathway(s) to the ventricles and induce ventricular fibrillation. That said, an accessory pathway may not be able to "keep up" with rapid atrial rates, at which point conduction would block in the accessory pathway and conduction would preferentially follow the normal path down the AV node and His-Purkinje system.

Diagnosis

If the pathway conducts antegrade down the accessory pathway and preexcites the ventricle ahead of the normal conduction path, a delta wave will be observed on ECG. Of note, *concealed* accessory pathways may conduct slowly (relative to the AV node, such as with some left lateral accessory pathways) or not at all but are able

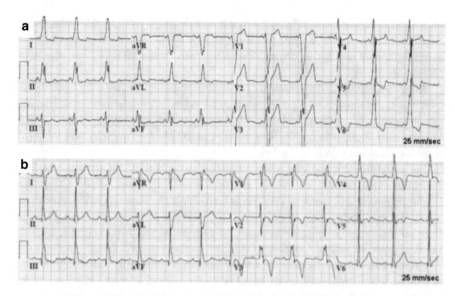

Fig. 12.1 Wolff-Parkinson-White (WPW) ECG pattern. (**a**) 12-lead ECG of a young patient diagnosed with WPW. Accessory pathways are suggested by the presence of a short PR interval and delta-waves in most leads, best seen in leads I, II, aVF. (**b**) Shortly post-ablation of the accessory pathway, normalization of the PR-interval and loss of the delta-waves are seen on follow-up ECG. The deep T-wave inversions seen steadily improved after recovery from ablation

to conduct retrograde (ventricle to atria). In this case, a delta wave will not be seen on the ECG, but ventricular to atria conduction could be provoked during an electrophysiology study. Retrograde conduction via an accessory pathway can form the substrate for a supraventricular tachycardia called orthodromic atrioventricular reentrant tachycardia (i.e., down the AVN, up the accessory pathway).

WPW ECG pattern can be diagnosed on a 12-lead ECG (Fig. 12.1) by the following pathognomonic criteria:

- Shortened PR interval (<120 ms), and
- Slurring of the initial component of the QRS complex (termed the "delta wave").

Observation of a delta wave may vary depending on the location of the accessory pathway and its conduction velocity relative to the AVN. A subtle or intermittently appearing delta wave can make the diagnosis more challenging.

Management

For athletes who are found to have either WPW pattern or WPW syndrome, non-invasive imaging (transthoracic echocardiography) should be performed. This imaging assessment should place focus on evaluating for congenital heart disease, particularly Ebstein's anomaly, as this has been associated with WPW. Additionally, careful attention should be placed on evaluating for phenocopies of hypertrophic cardiomyopathy (HCM), as disorders such as Danon's and PRKAG2 are also associated with WPW.

After evaluating for the presence of structural heart disease, then the major bifurcation in the management algorithm hinges on whether the athlete is symptomatic. For symptomatic athletes, ablation of the accessory pathway is recommended. Success rate of ablation for WPW according in the MAP-IT registry was 95% [8], with complication rate of about 1%.

For asymptomatic athletes who are found to have a WPW pattern, the 36th Bethesda Conference as well as the latest Pediatric and Congenital Electrophysiological Society (PACES)/Heart Rhythm Society (HRS) consensus statement recommend risk stratification with invasive electrophysiological studies (EPS) if the athlete is engaged in moderate-to-high intensity sports [7, 9], whereas the European Society of Cardiology (ESC) recommends EPS for all athletes [10]. The American Heart Association (AHA)/American College of Cardiology (ACC) Scientific Statement recommends initial risk stratification by exercise stress testing, and if an athlete is deemed not to be at low risk, EPS is recommended (Class IIa, Level B) [11].

Previously, a patient with an intermittent WPW pattern on ECG, in which the presence of a delta intermittently appears, was considered low risk for ventricular arrhythmia [7]. Recent studies have found that an intermittent pattern on resting ECG is not necessarily indicative of a low risk substrate [12, 13], and an intermittent pattern does not preclude patients from developing a supraventricular tachycardia (SVT). In one study, 8.3% of patients with an intermittent pattern of WPW developed a reentrant SVT over long-term follow-up [14]. The most recent PACES/HRS consensus statement recommends that patients with an intermittent WPW pattern can proceed with competitive sport participation without additional workup [7]. However, if there remains concern, exercise stress testing can be performed, with particular attention paid to whether there is a clear and abrupt termination of preexcitation at physiologic heart rates during exercise. Yet this assessment is highly observer-dependent, and its accuracy in detecting low-risk WPW (as assessed by electrophysiological testing parameters) was found to be low in a pediatric population [15].

If the patient undergoes electrophysiological testing, risk stratification can be performed by measuring the shortest pre-excited RR interval (SPERRI). A short SPERRI, defined as ≤ 250 ms, suggests an increased risk of SCD, while a longer SPERRI (>250 ms) is suggestive of a lower risk phenotype. However, the utility of SPERRI in risk stratification is still up for debate: in one study, up to 37% of children with a life-threatening event had a SPERRI >250 ms [16].

If an athlete with atrial fibrillation is found to have a bypass tract capable of anterograde conduction on EPS with a short refractory period, then ablation of the accessory pathway should be performed prior to being allowed to return to athletic competition (Class I, Level B) [11]. If the athlete is asymptomatic but is deemed to have a high risk pathway on EPS, then ablation of the accessory pathway is reasonable (Class IIa, Level B) [11].

If the athlete is deemed to be at low risk and ablation is not performed, the athlete can return to play and should be advised to maintain close follow-up with a physician to monitor for any new symptoms. If an athlete undergoes an ablation of the accessory pathway, the athlete may be advised to return to competition as long as there is documentation of successful ablation and loss of the accessory pathway on follow-up ECGs.

Catecholaminergic Polymorphic Ventricular Tachycardia (CPVT)

Catecholaminergic polymorphic ventricular tachycardia (CPVT) is an uncommon yet life-threatening genetic channelopathy that is a potential cause of SCD in athletes. In CPVT, situations that precipitate elevated levels of catecholamines, such as exercise or stress, can precipitate polymorphic ventricular arrhythmias in people with normal resting ECGs and otherwise structurally normal hearts. There has been progress in identifying genetic mutations that are associated with the CPVT disease process, allowing for genetic testing evaluation of this heritable condition.

Background & Epidemiology

After the first published description of a child with bidirectional ventricular tachycardia precipitated by effort and emotional stress in 1975 [17], Leenhardt and colleagues described a case series of 21 children with normal resting ECG and no evidence of structural heart disease who presented with stress- or emotion-induced syncope with associated polymorphic ventricular arrhythmias [18]. The first clinical manifestation of disease typically is either syncope or seizure, which upon further evaluation is found to be triggered by physical or emotional stress and associated with polymorphic ventricular tachycardia. CPVT most commonly presents in the first or second decade of life.

The true prevalence of CPVT is difficult to assess, but some estimates list it to be as common as 1 in every 10,000 people [19]. The prognosis of CPVT is rather poor, with some studies demonstrating a 13% fatal or near-fatal event rate within 8 years of follow-up [20].

Pathophysiology

CPVT is a genetically diverse disease process, with several associated mutations identified, and the clinical presentations can be diverse with variable penetrance. However, the underlying mechanism in CPVT is deregulated calcium handling in cardiac myocytes that leads to leakage of Ca^{2+} ions from the sarcoplasmic reticulum into the cytoplasm during diastole. This Ca^{2+} overload state increases the transient inward current and promotes delayed after depolarizations (DADs), which can precipitate ventricular arrhythmias.

The genetic mutations associated with CPVT center around proteins involved in intracellular calcium handling. The most commonly observed mutations in CPVT affect the cardiac ryanodine receptor 2 (*Ryr2*) gene, which is transmitted in an autosomal dominant fashion, and the calsequestrin 2 (*Casq2*) gene, which is autosomal recessive. Other mutations that have been associated with CPVT are *KCNJ2* (cardiac inward rectifier K channel), *Ank2, TRDN,* and calmodulin (*CALM1*).

CPVT Subtypes

There are several CPVT subtypes that have been described. The most common of the subtypes is CPVT1, which accounts for more than 50% of CPVT cases and is caused by a mutation in the *Ryr2* gene. The inheritance of CPVT1 is autosomal dominant.

CPVT2 is the second most common subtype and is a result of a mutation in the *Casq2* gene. It is generally inherited in an autosomal recessive fashion [21], though there have been autosomal dominant mutations reported [22]. The other CPVT subtypes, as well as their general characteristics, are summarized in Table 12.1.

Table 12.1 CPVT Subtypes. (Reprinted with permission from Ref. [23])

Subtypes	Juvenile type					CPVT related diseases		Adult type
	CPVT1	CPVT2	CPVT3	CPVT4	CPVT5	ATS	LQT4	
Incidence (%)	50–60	1	<< 1	<< 1	<< 1	<< 1	<< 1	≈ 30
Inheritance	AD	AR	AR	AD	Sporadic	AD	AD	Sporadic
Onset of symptoms	10 years	7 years	10 years	4 years	2, 26 years	14, 9, 17 years	?	> 20 years (40 years)
Sex	Ml:F = 1:1	M:F = 1:1	M:F = 1:1	M:F = 1:1	M = 3	F > M?	?	F >> M
Chromosome locus	1q43	1p13.1	7p22– p14	I4q32.11	6q22.31	17q24.3	4q25-26	
Gene	*RyR2*	*CASQ2*	?	*CALM1*	*TRD*	*KCNJ2*	*ANK2*	*RYR2* ≈30%
Protein				CaM		$K_{ir}2.1\alpha$	Ankyrin-B	
Sudden death (%)	≈ 10	≈ 42	≈ 75	≈ 18	≈ 25	?	?	0

Diagnosis

At rest, patients with CPVT have a normal 12-lead ECG, with the exception of possibly a sinus bradycardia. Traditional imaging modalities such as transthoracic echocardiography reveal normal structural anatomy of the heart. A history of exercise-or emotional stress-induced syncope and/or seizure should prompt the evaluation for CPVT.

In order to make the diagnosis of CPVT, patients can undergo an exercise stress test or EPS with epinephrine challenge. In patients with CPVT, exercise will precipitate the steady onset of monomorphic PVCs, which are followed by polymorphic PVCs or bidirectional PVC bigeminy, followed by bidirectional or polymorphic VT. This rhythm can then degenerate further into ventricular fibrillation if untreated.

If exercise testing produces these findings, then genetic testing of the patient should be considered given the known heritability of the CPVT-associated mutations. If any of these positive variants are identified, then testing of family members may help identify those who are at risk of CPVT (concealed mutation-positive patients) and who may benefit from initiating medical therapy [19].

An expert consensus statement by the Heart Rhythm Society, European Heart Rhythm Association, and Asia Pacific Heart Rhythm Society [19] states CPVT can be diagnosed in:

1. Patients <40 years old who have a structurally normal heart and normal ECG, and unexplained exercise- or catecholamine-induced bidirectional VT, PVCs, or VT,
2. Patients who are found to have a pathogenic mutation,
3. Family members of a CPVT index patient who also have a structurally normal heart who manifest exercise-induced PVCs or bidirectional/polymorphic VT, or
4. Patients >40 years old who have a structurally normal heart and coronary arteries, normal ECG, and unexplained exercise- or catecholamine-induced bidirectional VT, PVCs, or VT [19].

Electrophysiological study (EPS) is not indicated in CPVT. There have been studies evaluating the use of catecholamine infusion (i.e., epinephrine) to assist with the diagnosis, but the sensitivity was found to be low (28%). As such, there are currently no recommendations regarding catecholamine infusions from the professional societies [24].

Notably, CPVT is also associated with atrial arrhythmias, including atrial fibrillation [25]. Thus, the presence of atrial fibrillation in a child or young adult should prompt evaluation for CPVT. Another possibility is Brugada syndrome (also associated with atrial fibrillation [26]) as well as paroxysmal atrial fibrillation.

Management

When CPVT is diagnosed in an athlete, the first step of management is counseling the athlete with recommendations on physical activity and competition, as well as medications to help prevent ventricular arrhythmias. Given that the catecholamine surge during exercise and especially competitive sports can elicit life-threatening arrhythmias in CPVT, the recommendations from multiple societies are conservative. While the AHA/ACC do not explicitly give recommendations for activity restrictions in CPVT [11], the ESC recommends avoidance of competitive sports, strenuous exercise, and stressful environments in patients diagnosed with CPVT (Class I, Level C).

The first line of medical therapy in CPVT is a beta-blocker for all symptomatic patients. Nadolol, a long-acting beta-blocker, is the preferred agent for prophylactic therapy, but it may not be available in all countries. Propranolol has also been found to be similarly effective. It is crucial to emphasize to the patient the importance of adherence to the prescribed regimen and the potential consequences of non-adherence. Notably, arrhythmic events have been reported to occur despite beta-blocker therapy, with an annual event rate ranging between 3–11% per year [20]. Guidelines list beta-blocker therapy as a Class I recommendation for all symptomatic patients with CPVT, and as a Class IIa recommendation for patients with a known pathogenic mutation for CPVT without clinical manifestations [19].

Another potential medication is the non-dihydropyridine calcium channel blocker, verapamil [27], with some evidence for the use of combination therapy alongside beta-blockers [28]. The class IC anti-arrhythmic medication, flecainide, has been demonstrated to be effective as well [29–31]. In genotype-positive patients, flecainide was found to be effective in 74% of cases [29], while in genotype-negative, it was effective in 92% of cases [31]. Flecainide use as an adjunctive therapy with beta-blockers is a Class IIa recommendation in symptomatic patients with CPVT [19].

Left cardiac sympathetic denervation (LCSD) is a surgical intervention that can be considered in drug-refractory patients with CPVT. Small trials have demonstrated promise [32, 33], but larger studies are needed to demonstrate long-term efficacy and safety. LCSD is a Class IIb recommendation for symptomatic patients with CPVT.

ICD implantation in patients with CPVT is recommended for patients who have experienced cardiac arrest, recurrent syncope or polymorphic/bidirectional VT despite optimal medical therapy. However, studies that have shown that ICD shocks may promote catecholaminergic surges that can trigger more arrhythmia and more shocks [34]. Thus, the decision for ICD implantation should be taken carefully via a shared-decision making process with the symptomatic patient. For asymptomatic patients with CPVT, there are no recommendations for ICD implantation for primary prevention. However, in a meta-analysis of 1429 patients with CPVT, 35.2% of patients had received an ICD (47.3% of whom received an ICD for primary prevention) [35]. Only 12.8% of patients were on optimal antiarrhythmic therapy, and there was a high burden of shocks and complications (e.g., lead failure, endocarditis, need for surgical revision). Thus, every attempt should be made to optimize patients on medical therapy prior to considering ICD implantation for primary prevention.

For athletes diagnosed with CPVT, the AHA, ACC, and ESC recommendations state that competitive sports participation and strenuous activity should be avoided, given the concern that the catecholaminergic surge that occurs with competition or exercise may precipitate life-threatening ventricular arrhythmias [11, 36]. However, the AHA and ACC statement does leave room for possible return to competition if there is evidence of adequate suppression of ventricular arrhythmias with medical therapy. There is limited data on continued athletic competition in patients diagnosed with CPVT. In one retrospective study performed on patients >6 years of age at the time of CPVT diagnosis, 21 of 24 patients (88%) who were classified as athletes continued to compete after their diagnosis [37]. Of these 21 patients, 3 (14%) experienced CPVT-triggered events, with none resulting in death. Interestingly, in patients who were not considered athletes and did not compete in sports after their diagnosis, 6 of 42 patients (14%) experienced CPVT-triggered events. This single-center experience suggests that with appropriate therapy, the risk of exercise-associated events can be mitigated, but still exist. Thus, a shared-decision making approach is of the utmost importance in counseling athletes with the diagnosis of CPVT.

Brugada Syndrome

Background

First described in 1989 by a group from the University of Padua in Italy [38] and first characterized in 1992 by Drs. Pedro Brugada and Josep Brugada [39], Brugada syndrome is an inherited disorder that predisposes individuals with presumably structurally normal hearts to sudden cardiac death (SCD). It is considered a primary electrical cardiac disease, as there are no known associated structural abnormalities, and it is associated with characteristic ECG patterns, called the Brugada pattern, with the classic pattern being an atypical right bundle branch block (RBBB) pattern in the right precordial leads, with associated ST-segment elevation and T-wave inversions. Since its first description, there have been advances in identifying the inheritance patterns and associated gene mutations, which predominantly affect the cardiac sodium channel. The diagnosis of Brugada syndrome poses a particular challenge in athletes, as there exists some overlap between athletic ECG findings and Brugada ECG findings. Yet as the diagnosis of Brugada syndrome can significantly impact the management of an athlete, it is crucial to meticulously complete the evaluation for the disorder when suspected.

Epidemiology

The prevalence of Brugada syndrome is estimated to be in the range of 1 in every 1000 to 10,000 people. It is more commonly seen in patients of southeast Asian descent and is more common in men than women. The typical age for symptoms to present is in the 4th decade however, symptoms may manifest at any age, including childhood. Approximately 4% of SCD worldwide is attributed to Brugada syndrome; up to 20% of SCD in cases with structurally normal hearts are attributed to the disorder [40, 41].

Clinically, patients with Brugada syndrome may present with a syncopal event, atrial and/or ventricular arrhythmias, and SCD. The Brugada pattern may incidentally be found in asymptomatic patients on a screening ECG, but the pattern can also be intermittent. Factors that are known to elicit or accentuate the Brugada ECG pattern include increased vagal tone (such as occurs during sleep), fever, electrolyte abnormalities, and sodium channel inhibitors (such as Class I antiarrhythmic drugs).

Pathophysiology

There are multiple hypotheses for the pathophysiology governing the characteristic ECG changes in Brugada syndrome [42]. One hypothesis is that abnormal repolarization occurs due to mutations in the sodium channel SCN5A, which results in the loss of Na^+ current and unopposed outward K^+ current through the I_{to} channel [43]. A voltage gradient is created between the epicardium and endocardium in the right ventricle (RV) and right ventricular outflow tract (RVOT), explaining the location of the ECG changes in the right precordial leads. Another hypothesis is that the ECG changes are due to delayed depolarization in the RV and RVOT. It is possible that both repolarization and depolarization abnormalities are present, and this could generate the substrate for initiation of arrhythmias, including polymorphic ventricular tachycardia or ventricular fibrillation. Using a non-invasive ECG imaging modality (ECGI) developed by Dr. Yoram Rudy at Washington University in St. Louis, patients with Brugada syndrome were found to have abnormal conduction and depolarization in electrophysiological substrate confined to the RVOT [44]. Epicardial ablation of this substrate is a possible treatment option [44, 45].

Further, while there are numerous gene mutations (>8) that have been associated with Brugada syndrome, mutations in SCN5A account for >75% of genotype-positive patients [46]. However, the majority of cases are genetically elusive.

Diagnosis

The diagnosis of Brugada syndrome should consist of the presence of symptoms as well as meeting the criteria for the Brugada ECG pattern. However, more recent recommendations consider meeting the Brugada Type 1 ECG pattern alone, with or without the presence of symptoms, diagnostic of Brugada syndrome [43].

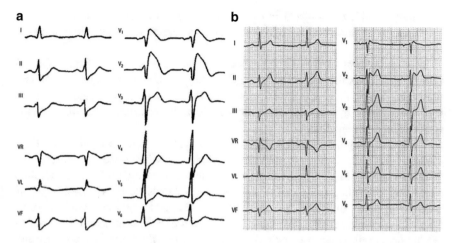

Fig. 12.2 Brugada ECG patterns. (**a**) The Type 1 pattern, with its associated atypical RBBB morphology and ST-segment elevations in leads V1-V2, is the classic Brugada pattern considered to be diagnostic of the disorder. (**b**) The Type 2 "saddle-back" pattern. (Figure used with permission from Ref. [43])

There are now two recognized categories of ECG patterns in potential patients with Brugada syndrome (Fig. 12.2). Type 1 is the classic Brugada pattern, in which there is a coved ST-segment elevation ≥2 mm, negative T wave, and no isoelectric separation of the T wave (no clear r') in the right precordial leads (V1–V2). The Type 2 pattern consists of a saddle-back appearance in the ST-T segment of leads V1–V2, with a positive or biphasic T wave.

The diagnosis can be made if the Type 1 Brugada ECG pattern is seen spontaneously or during intravenous administration of a sodium channel inhibitor (e.g., procainamide, flecainide, ajmaline, pilsicainide) in either V1 or V2. Appropriate lead placement of V1 or V2 is critical in the standard position when performing any ECG. Placing V1 and V2 leads in a superior position (up to the 2nd intercostal space) can potentially increase the diagnostic yield of the ECG. However, superior positioning should only be considered if highly suspicious for Brugada syndrome, as high lead placement on routine screening ECGs may lead to overdiagnosis of Brugada ECG patterns, especially in taller and heavier male athletes [47]. Superior positioning can accentuate a Type 1 Brugada ECG pattern in a patient with known Brugada syndrome, but can cause an rSr' pattern in a patient without Brugada syndrome [48].

Differentiation from the Athlete's ECG

While the Type 1 Brugada ECG pattern has a characteristic pattern, the Type 2 Brugada ECG pattern shares similarities to normal variants, including those often seen in athletes [49]. The term "Brugada phenocopy" has been proposed to describe situations in which a Brugada ECG can be elicited in a person without Brugada syndrome by conditions such as hyperkalemia, hypothyroidism, and alcohol intoxication [42].

In addition to athletic ECG changes considered to be a normal variant, the differential diagnosis for "Brugada-like" ECG changes includes incomplete right bundle branch block (also a normal variant), as well as pathological causes, such as right ventricular hypertrophy, arrhythmogenic right ventricular cardiomyopathy (ARVC), and hyperkalemia.

To help distinguish between Brugada ECG patterns and "Brugada-like" ECG variants that can be seen in athletes, multiple tools have been proposed. The "Corrado index" (Fig. 12.3a, b) compares the ratio of the heights of the ST elevation in lead V1 at the beginning of the ST segment (ST_J) and 80 ms afterwards (ST_{80}), whereby a value of $ST_J:ST_{80} > 1$ is seen in Brugada syndrome while a value $ST_J:ST_{80} < 1$ is present in repolarization abnormalities seen in athletes [50]. Another distinguishing finding is the angle (β) formed between the ascending and descending limbs of r' (Fig. 12.3c) [51, 52]. Patients with Type 2 Brugada ECG pattern typically have a larger β, and a cutoff of 58° has been shown to have discriminative value, with a positive predictive value of 73% and negative predictive value of 87% [51]. In addition, if a triangle is drawn using the up- and downslope of the r', the length of the triangle 5 mm below the peak of the r' can be measured (d; Fig. 12.3d). A value $d \geq 4$ mm (or 160 msec) was found to have a specificity of 95.6%, sensitivity of 85%, positive predictive value of 94.4%, and negative predictive value of 87.9% [53].

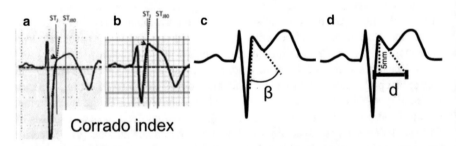

Fig. 12.3 Distinguishing parameters between Brugada ECG pattern and normal variants. (**a, b**) "Corrado index" compares the heights of the ST_J and ST_{80} segments. An $ST_J:ST_{80} < 1$ is seen in normal variants, such as early repolarization seen in athletes (**a**), while $ST_J:ST_{80} > 1$ is seen in Brugada ECG pattern (**b**). (**c**) The angle β describes the angle between the upslope and downslope of r', and a larger value is seen in Brugada ECG pattern. (**d**) A triangle can be drawn using the upsloping and downsloping segments of r'. If the third wall of the triangle consists of a line drawn 5 mm below the r' peak, the length of the line, d, can be measured, with a larger d seen in Brugada ECG pattern. (Figures **a, b** adapted with permission from Ref. [54])

Management

While asymptomatic patients with the Type 2 Brugada ECG pattern (and no concerning family history) do not warrant further workup [55], cardiology consultation to discuss ECG findings is reasonable. The management of asymptomatic patients with the Type 1 Brugada ECG pattern (and thus a diagnosis of Brugada syndrome) remains controversial [36, 56]. The mainstay of management in asymptomatic Brugada patients is avoidance of drugs that are known to elicit the Brugada pattern (which can be found at http://www.brugadadrugs.org), avoidance of excessive alcohol intake and large meals, and prompt treatment of any fever. (Class I, Level C) [36].

For patients with a diagnosis of Brugada syndrome who have experienced cardiac arrest or have documented spontaneous sustained VT, ICD implantation is recommended (Class I, Level C) [11, 19, 36]. In patients with a spontaneous Type 1 Brugada ECG pattern who have a history of syncope, ICD implantation is also recommended (Class IIa, Level C) [19, 36].

With regards to whether athletes with a diagnosis of Brugada syndrome should refrain from competitive sports, the recommendations have evolved over the last few decades [57]. While the Bethesda guidelines from 2005 previously advised restriction to Class IA sports for athletes diagnosed with Brugada syndrome, regardless of the presence of symptoms [9], the most recent task force recommendations provide a more nuanced approach. For symptomatic athletes with suspected or diagnosed Brugada syndrome, restriction from all competitive sports is recommended while the athlete and family are informed of the diagnosis and implications, and a treatment program (i.e., ICD placement) is initiated (Class I, Level C). If after ICD placement, the athlete is asymptomatic for 3 months and there is no evidence of ventricular arrhythmias that require device therapy, participation in sports with higher demands that Class IA sports may be considered after a thorough shared decision-making discussion (Class IIb, Level C) [11]. Participation of athletes with implanted ICDs in sports has been evaluated in a prospective ICD Sports Registry, and no patients with Brugada syndrome with an ICD experienced an arrhythmic storm during competition [58, 59]. For asymptomatic athletes with a diagnosis of Brugada syndrome, there are no specific activity restrictions recommended, but an emergency action plan (EAP) must be in place [11].

Idiopathic Ventricular Tachycardia/Ventricular Fibrillation

Ventricular tachycardia (VT) most commonly occurs in the setting of an underlying cardiomyopathy, but VT can also occur in patients who have no known structural heart abnormalities or ischemic heart disease. VT that occurs in the absence of clinically apparent structural heart disease is classified as idiopathic VT. Similarly, idiopathic ventricular fibrillation (VF) is the occurrence of VF in the setting of a structurally normal heart. Both idiopathic VT and VF can lead to SCD and establishing the diagnosis in the athlete is crucial as there are effective treatment strategies to present SCD while potentially still allowing the athlete to return to competition.

Background & Epidemiology

The true prevalence of idiopathic VT and idiopathic VF in SCD is difficult to measure, since autopsy studies are unrevealing in the setting of structurally normal hearts seen in idiopathic VT/VF. Yet SCD occurs in the setting of structurally normal hearts in roughly 5–14% of SCD cases [60–62]. In a study performed on SCD in collegiate athletes in the United States, the most common finding at death was a structurally normal heart (31%) [4]. In a study of premature deaths attributed to sudden arrhythmic death syndrome (SADS) of people ages 4–64 years old in the United Kingdom, 52.8% of the presumed arrhythmic deaths were found to not have any identifiable structural abnormality or familial syndrome [63].

Haïssaguerre and colleagues identified an association between idiopathic VF and early repolarization on baseline ECG [64]. In their initial study, they found that 31% of patients who experienced cardiac arrest due to idiopathic VF had early repolarization on ECG, while only 5% of control patients had early repolarization. This finding has been confirmed on repeat studies by their group and others [65–67]. Now termed Haïssaguerre syndrome, the pathophysiology of the association between early repolarization with idiopathic VF is still unclear. The degree of J-point elevation is important as patients who experienced idiopathic VF were more likely to have a J-point elevation >1.0 mm compared to young athletes with early repolarization [67]. Additionally, J-point elevation was more commonly seen in the inferior leads and in leads I and aVL in patients with idiopathic VF, whereas the presence of J-point elevation in leads V4–V6 was similar between groups [67].

Further research is needed to better characterize high risk features of early repolarization patterns. The ST-segment morphology after the J-point in early repolarization has been found to have discriminatory value (Fig. 12.4) [68]. In a study comparing early repolarization patterns in Finnish and American athletes, and a middle-aged Finnish population, the early repolarization patterns seen in young and healthy athletes were more likely to have an ascending/upsloping ST-segment after the J-point (Fig. 12.4a, b). In the middle-aged Finnish population, subjects who had a horizontal/descending ST-segment after the J-point (Fig. 12.4c, d) had an increased hazard ratio of arrhythmic death. An ascending/upsloping ST-segment in this population was not associated with an increased risk of arrhythmic death [68]. Other features such as T-wave amplitude, T/R ratio, J-wave duration, and J-wave slope have been studied as well and may also have discriminatory value [69, 70].

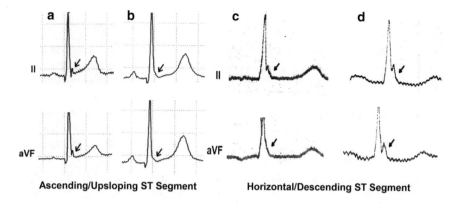

Fig. 12.4 Early repolarization patterns. (**a, b**) Inferior leads from two young Finnish athletes, demonstrating (**a**) notching and (**b**) slurring of the terminal QRS portion (arrows), followed by an ascending/upsloping ST segment. (**c, d**) Inferior leads from two middle-aged subjects from the general Finnish population. After the notching or slurring in the terminal QRS portion (arrows), the ST-segment has a horizontal/descending pattern, which was found to be more likely to be present in subjects with arrhythmic death. (Figures adapted with permission from Ref. [68])

Pathophysiology

Idiopathic VT can originate from a variety of locations within the heart; most commonly, idiopathic VTs originate from the ventricular outflow tracts, particularly the right ventricular outflow tract (RVOT; ~70% of outflow tract VTs) [71]. Other sites of outflow tract origin include the aortic sinuses of Valsalva, left ventricular outflow tract (LVOT), great cardiac veins, epicardial myocardium, aorto-mitral curtain, and the pulmonary artery. The mechanisms of these outflow tract VTs are thought to be focal secondary to automaticity, micro-re-entry, or triggered activity. RVOT VT is mediated by cyclic AMP-mediated intracellular calcium overload [72–74].

Idiopathic VT can also originate from the left ventricle, including fascicular VT (also known as Belhassen Tachycardia, which is the most common idiopathic VT from the left ventricle) and papillary muscle VT. Fascicular VT is a result of reentry involving a portion of the left ventricular Purkinje fiber system and is often verapamil-sensitive.

In endurance athletes, idiopathic VTs most frequently originate from the right ventricle, and there is evidence to suggest that, at least in a portion of athletes in this group, this predisposition to right-sided VTs may be a result of the endurance exercise itself [75]. In what has been termed "exercise-induced right ventricular arrhythmogenic cardiomyopathy," the hypothesis is that the chronic right-sided pressure overload that can occur with years of extreme endurance training can lead to deleterious effects on the right ventricle, including fibrosis and functional abnormalities, which can in effect predispose to arrhythmia susceptibility. Thought to be on a similar spectrum as ARVC, it is possible that this phenomenon may instead be capturing a genetic defect not yet identified, in what has been termed "gene-elusive ARVC" [76].

Diagnosis

The first step of managing an athlete with suspected idiopathic VT is ruling out structural heart disease, which can be done with routine imaging modalities such as transthoracic echocardiography or cardiac magnetic resonance imaging (cMRI).

Once structural heart disease has been excluded, attempts should be made to obtain ECG tracings (ideally 12-lead) of the VT, if possible. Analysis of a multi-lead ECG tracing of the VT can assist with determining its potential origin, and this information can help to inform management options, particularly planning for radiofrequency catheter ablation.

Idiopathic VF, unless otherwise captured on ambulatory or telemetry monitoring, is typically a diagnosis of exclusion in a patient who has suffered a sudden cardiac arrest. If VF is documented and the patient survives, then a thorough workup for secondary causes of VF should be performed to evaluate for cardiac, respiratory, metabolic, or toxicological etiologies [19].

Management

In general, the risk of syncope and sudden cardiac death from idiopathic VT is very low. Medical therapy with beta blockers or calcium channel blockers is typically the first line therapy considered in symptomatic patients with idiopathic outflow tract VT (Class I, Level B) [62]. Some patients, particularly those with interfascicular VT, oral verapamil may be useful (Class IIa, Level C), but intravenous verapamil can be used for acute termination of VT (Class I, Level B).

While medical therapy is typically the first line of therapy in idiopathic VT, medications can be difficult to use in athletes given their potential effects on athletic performance. Medical therapy may be considered if radiofrequency catheter ablation (RFA) is not possible or not desired [77, 78], or the location of VT origin is deemed high risk. For instance, fascicular VT is usually responsive to the non-dihidropyridine calcium channel blocker, verapamil, as well as beta-blockers. For outflow tract VT, class IC and class III anti-arrhythmic medications are more effective than beta-blockers or calcium channel blockers and can be considered as long as there is no evidence of structural heart disease [77]. However, the side effect profiles of anti-arrhythmic medications need to be strongly considered prior to initiation in any athlete and beta blockers are usually the first choice given the safety profile.

In addition to medical therapy, radiofrequency catheter ablation (RFA) is being increasingly performed successfully to treat VT, including idiopathic VT [79]. For athletes with idiopathic VT, RFA may be considered if the arrhythmia does not respond to medical therapy or if the athlete is unable or unwilling to take medications [11]. Notably, in contrast to medications, RFA can be curative of idiopathic VT. For ectopy with an RVOT origin, RFA was found to be more effective than antiarrhythmic drug therapy in preventing recurrence [80], and acute success rates as high as 84% have been achieved with a low complication rate (2–3%) [81].

In athletes with idiopathic VT who have undergone successful catheter ablation and who remain free of VT (spontaneous or induced) at least 3 months post-procedure can resume full competition with no restrictions (Class I, Level C) [11]. If catheter ablation is not performed and medical therapy is prescribed, the recommendation is to allow for 3 months of medical therapy optimization; if there is no evidence of recurrence or inducibility by exercise testing or electrophysiological study (EPS), then full competition can be resumed with no restriction (Class I, Level C) [11].

In any athlete with idiopathic VT or VF who has survived from sudden cardiac arrest, ICD implantation is recommended (Class I, Level B) [62].

Conclusion

- Management of arrhythmic conditions such as Wolff Parkinson White (WPW), Brugada syndrome, catecholaminergic polymorphic ventricular tachycardia (CPVT), and idiopathic ventricular fibrillation (VF) or ventricular tachycardia (VT) in the athlete is challenging.
- Risk stratification for WPW continues to evolve, and new studies suggest that characteristics such as an intermittent pattern or SPERRI >250 ms may not be as low risk as previously thought.
- While the general recommendation is to recommend restriction of athletic participation in patients with CPVT, recent studies suggest that return to athletic activity can be considered on an individual basis for patients who demonstrate adequate suppression of ventricular arrhythmias on optimal medical therapy. However, the risk of exercise-associated SCD still exists.
- Differentiating between a Brugada ECG pattern and the athlete's ECG pattern can be challenging, and new tools (i.e., Corrado index) are proving valuable to assist with the diagnosis.
- Further research is needed to better characterize high risk features of early repolarization patterns that are associated with idiopathic VT and VF.
- Guidelines and recommendations for management of these conditions in athletes are evolving as therapies such as radiofrequency ablation improve.
- A shared decision-making approach is essential when counseling athletes on their management and providing treatment options.

References

1. Maron BJ, Shirani J, Poliac LC, Mathenge R, Roberts WC, Mueller FO. Sudden death in young competitive athletes. Clinical, demographic, and pathological profiles. JAMA. 1996;276:199–204.
2. Maron BJ, Doerer JJ, Haas TS, Tierney DM, Mueller FO. Sudden deaths in young competitive athletes: analysis of 1866 deaths in the United States, 1980–2006. Circulation. 2009;119:1085–92.

3. Maron BJ. Sudden death in young athletes. N Engl J Med. 2003;349:1064–75.
4. Harmon KG, Asif IM, Maleszewski JJ, Owens DS, Prutkin JM, Salerno JC, Zigman ML, Ellenbogen R, Rao AL, Ackerman MJ, Drezner JA. Incidence, cause, and comparative frequency of sudden cardiac death in National Collegiate Athletic Association Athletes: a decade in review. Circulation. 2015;132:10–9.
5. Toresdahl BG, Rao AL, Harmon KG, Drezner JA. Incidence of sudden cardiac arrest in high school student athletes on school campus. Heart Rhythm. 2014;11:1190–4.
6. Wolff L, Parkinson J, White PD. Bundle-branch block with short PR interval in healthy young people to paroxysmal tachycardia. Am Heart J. 1930;5:685–704.
7. Pediatric and Congenital Electrophysiology Society (PACES), Heart Rhythm Society (HRS), American College of Cardiology Foundation (ACCF), American Heart Association (AHA), American Academy of Pediatrics (AAP), Canadian Heart Rhythm Society (CHRS), Cohen MI, Triedman JK, Cannon BC, Davis AM, Drago F, Janousek J, Klein GJ, Law IH, Morady FJ, Paul T, Perry JC, Sanatani S, Tanel RE. PACES/HRS expert consensus statement on the management of the asymptomatic young patient with a Wolff-Parkinson-White (WPW, ventricular preexcitation) electrocardiographic pattern: developed in partnership between the Pediatric and Congenital Electrophysiology Society (PACES) and the Heart Rhythm Society (HRS). Endorsed by the governing bodies of PACES, HRS, the American College of Cardiology Foundation (ACCF), the American Heart Association (AHA), the American Academy of Pediatrics (AAP), and the Canadian Heart Rhythm Society (CHRS). Heart Rhythm. 2012;9:1006–24.
8. Dubin AM, Jorgensen NW, Radbill AE, Bradley DJ, Silva JN, Tsao S, Kanter RJ, Tanel RE, Trivedi B, Young M-L, Pflaumer A, McCormack J, Seslar SP. What have we learned in the last 20 years? A comparison of a modern era pediatric and congenital catheter ablation registry to previous pediatric ablation registries. Heart Rhythm. 2019;16:57–63.
9. Maron BJ, Zipes DP. Introduction: eligibility recommendations for competitive athletes with cardiovascular abnormalities-general considerations. J Am Coll Cardiol. 2005;45:1318–21.
10. Corrado D, Pelliccia A, Bjørnstad HH, Vanhees L, Biffi A, Borjesson M, Panhuyzen-Goedkoop N, Deligiannis A, Solberg E, Dugmore D, Mellwig KP, Assanelli D, Delise P, van-Buuren F, Anastasakis A, Heidbuchel H, Hoffmann E, Fagard R, Priori SG, Basso C, Arbustini E, Blomstrom-Lundqvist C, McKenna WJ, Thiene G, Study Group of Sport Cardiology of the Working Group of Cardiac Rehabilitation and Exercise Physiology and the Working Group of Myocardial and Pericardial Diseases of the European Society of Cardiology. Cardiovascular pre-participation screening of young competitive athletes for prevention of sudden death: proposal for a common European protocol. Consensus Statement of the Study Group of Sport Cardiology of the Working Group of Cardiac Rehabilitation and Exercise Physiology and the Working Group of Myocardial and Pericardial Diseases of the European Society of Cardiology. Eur Heart J. 2005;26:516–24.
11. Zipes DP, Link MS, Ackerman MJ, Kovacs RJ, Myerburg RJ, Estes NAM. Eligibility and disqualification recommendations for competitive athletes with cardiovascular abnormalities: task force 9: arrhythmias and conduction defects: a scientific statement from the American Heart Association and American College of Cardiology. J Am Coll Cardiol. 2015;66:2412–23.
12. Kiger ME, McCanta AC, Tong S, Schaffer M, Runciman M, Collins KK. Intermittent versus persistent Wolff-Parkinson-White syndrome in children: electrophysiologic properties and clinical outcomes. Pacing Clin Electrophysiol. 2016;39:14–20.
13. Mah DY, Sherwin ED, Alexander ME, Cecchin F, Abrams DJ, Walsh EP, Triedman JK. The electrophysiological characteristics of accessory pathways in pediatric patients with intermittent preexcitation. Pacing Clin Electrophysiol. 2013;36:1117–22.
14. Fitzsimmons PJ, McWhirter PD, Peterson DW, Kruyer WB. The natural history of Wolff-Parkinson-White syndrome in 228 military aviators: a long-term follow-up of 22 years. Am Heart J. 2001;142:530–6.
15. Dalili M, Vahidshahi K, Aarabi-Moghaddam MY, Rao JY, Brugada P. Exercise testing in children with Wolff-Parkinson-White syndrome: what is its value? Pediatr Cardiol. 2014;35:1142–6.

16. Etheridge SP, Escudero CA, Blaufox AD, Law IH, Dechert-Crooks BE, Stephenson EA, Dubin AM, Ceresnak SR, Motonaga KS, Skinner JR, Marcondes LD, Perry JC, Collins KK, Seslar SP, Cabrera M, Uzun O, Cannon BC, Aziz PF, Kubuš P, Tanel RE, Valdes SO, Sami S, Kertesz NJ, Maldonado J, Erickson C, Moore JP, Asakai H, Mill L, Abcede M, Spector ZZ, Menon S, Shwayder M, Bradley DJ, Cohen MI, Sanatani S. Life-threatening event risk in children with wolff-parkinson-white syndrome: a multicenter international study. JACC Clin Electrophysiol. 2018;4:433–44.
17. Reid DS, Tynan M, Braidwood L, Fitzgerald GR. Bidirectional tachycardia in a child. A study using His bundle electrography. Br Heart J. 1975;37:339–44.
18. Leenhardt A, Lucet V, Denjoy I, Grau F, Ngoc DD, Coumel P. Catecholaminergic polymorphic ventricular tachycardia in children. A 7-year follow-up of 21 patients. Circulation. 1995;91:1512–9.
19. Priori SG, Wilde AA, Horie M, Cho Y, Behr ER, Berul C, Blom N, Brugada J, Chiang C-E, Huikuri H, Kannankeril P, Krahn A, Leenhardt A, Moss A, Schwartz PJ, Shimizu W, Tomaselli G, Tracy C. Executive summary: HRS/EHRA/APHRS expert consensus statement on the diagnosis and management of patients with inherited primary arrhythmia syndromes. Heart Rhythm. 2013;10:e85–108.
20. Hayashi M, Denjoy I, Extramiana F, Maltret A, Buisson NR, Lupoglazoff J-M, Klug D, Hayashi M, Takatsuki S, Villain E, Kamblock J, Messali A, Guicheney P, Lunardi J, Leenhardt A. Incidence and risk factors of arrhythmic events in catecholaminergic polymorphic ventricular tachycardia. Circulation. 2009;119:2426–34.
21. Lahat H, Eldar M, Levy-Nissenbaum E, Bahan T, Friedman E, Khoury A, Lorber A, Kastner DL, Goldman B, Pras E. Autosomal recessive catecholamine- or exercise-induced polymorphic ventricular tachycardia: clinical features and assignment of the disease gene to chromosome 1p13-21. Circulation. 2001;103:2822–7.
22. Postma AV, Denjoy I, Hoorntje TM, Lupoglazoff J-M, Da Costa A, Sebillon P, Mannens MMAM, Wilde AAM, Guicheney P. Absence of calsequestrin 2 causes severe forms of catecholaminergic polymorphic ventricular tachycardia. Circ Res. 2002;91:e21–6.
23. Sumitomo N. Current topics in catecholaminergic polymorphic ventricular tachycardia. J Arrhythm. 2016;32:344–51.
24. Marjamaa A, Hiippala A, Arrhenius B, Lahtinen AM, Kontula K, Toivonen L, Happonen J-M, Swan H. Intravenous epinephrine infusion test in diagnosis of catecholaminergic polymorphic ventricular tachycardia. J Cardiovasc Electrophysiol. 2012;23:194–9.
25. Sumitomo N, Sakurada H, Taniguchi K, Matsumura M, Abe O, Miyashita M, Kanamaru H, Karasawa K, Ayusawa M, Fukamizu S, Nagaoka I, Horie M, Harada K, Hiraoka M. Association of atrial arrhythmia and sinus node dysfunction in patients with catecholaminergic polymorphic ventricular tachycardia. Circ J. 2007;71:1606–9.
26. Morita H, Kusano-Fukushima K, Nagase S, Fujimoto Y, Hisamatsu K, Fujio H, Haraoka K, Kobayashi M, Morita ST, Nakamura K, Emori T, Matsubara H, Hina K, Kita T, Fukatani M, Ohe T. Atrial fibrillation and atrial vulnerability in patients with Brugada syndrome. J Am Coll Cardiol. 2002;40:1437–44.
27. Swan H, Laitinen P, Kontula K, Toivonen L. Calcium channel antagonism reduces exercise-induced ventricular arrhythmias in catecholaminergic polymorphic ventricular tachycardia patients with RyR2 mutations. J Cardiovasc Electrophysiol. 2005;16:162–6.
28. Rosso R, Kalman JM, Rogowski O, Diamant S, Birger A, Biner S, Belhassen B, Viskin S. Calcium channel blockers and beta-blockers versus beta-blockers alone for preventing exercise-induced arrhythmias in catecholaminergic polymorphic ventricular tachycardia. Heart Rhythm. 2007;4:1149–54.
29. Watanabe H, Chopra N, Laver D, Hwang HS, Davies SS, Roach DE, Duff HJ, Roden DM, Wilde AAM, Knollmann BC. Flecainide prevents catecholaminergic polymorphic ventricular tachycardia in mice and humans. Nat Med. 2009;15:380–3.
30. van der Werf C, Kannankeril PJ, Sacher F, Krahn AD, Viskin S, Leenhardt A, Shimizu W, Sumitomo N, Fish FA, Bhuiyan ZA, Willems AR, van der Veen MJ, Watanabe H, Laborderie J, Haïssaguerre M, Knollmann BC, Wilde AAM. Flecainide therapy reduces exercise-induced

ventricular arrhythmias in patients with catecholaminergic polymorphic ventricular tachycardia. J Am Coll Cardiol. 2011;57:2244–54.

31. Watanabe H, van der Werf C, Roses-Noguer F, Adler A, Sumitomo N, Veltmann C, Rosso R, Bhuiyan ZA, Bikker H, Kannankeril PJ, Horie M, Minamino T, Viskin S, Knollmann BC, Till J, Wilde AAM. Effects of flecainide on exercise-induced ventricular arrhythmias and recurrences in genotype-negative patients with catecholaminergic polymorphic ventricular tachycardia. Heart Rhythm. 2013;10:542–7.

32. Wilde AAM, Bhuiyan ZA, Crotti L, Facchini M, De Ferrari GM, Paul T, Ferrandi C, Koolbergen DR, Odero A, Schwartz PJ. Left cardiac sympathetic denervation for catecholaminergic polymorphic ventricular tachycardia. N Engl J Med. 2008;358:2024–9.

33. Collura CA, Johnson JN, Moir C, Ackerman MJ. Left cardiac sympathetic denervation for the treatment of long QT syndrome and catecholaminergic polymorphic ventricular tachycardia using video-assisted thoracic surgery. Heart Rhythm. 2009;6:752–9.

34. Roses-Noguer F, Jarman JWE, Clague JR, Till J. Outcomes of defibrillator therapy in catecholaminergic polymorphic ventricular tachycardia. Heart Rhythm. 2014;11:58–66.

35. Roston TM, Jones K, Hawkins NM, Bos JM, Schwartz PJ, Perry F, Ackerman MJ, Laksman ZWM, Kaul P, Lieve KVV, Atallah J, Krahn AD, Sanatani S. Implantable cardioverter-defibrillator use in catecholaminergic polymorphic ventricular tachycardia: a systematic review. Heart Rhythm. 2018;15:1791–9.

36. Priori SG, Blomström-Lundqvist C, Mazzanti A, Blom N, Borggrefe M, Camm J, Elliott PM, Fitzsimons D, Hatala R, Hindricks G, Kirchhof P, Kjeldsen K, Kuck K-H, Hernandez-Madrid A, Nikolaou N, Norekvål TM, Spaulding C, Van Veldhuisen DJ, ESC Scientific Document Group. 2015 ESC guidelines for the management of patients with ventricular arrhythmias and the prevention of sudden cardiac death: the task force for the management of patients with ventricular arrhythmias and the prevention of sudden cardiac death of the European Society of Cardiology (ESC). Endorsed by: Association for European Paediatric and Congenital Cardiology (AEPC). Eur Heart J. 2015;36:2793–867.

37. Ostby SA, Bos JM, Owen HJ, Wackel PL, Cannon BC, Ackerman MJ. Competitive sports participation in patients with catecholaminergic polymorphic ventricular tachycardia: a single center's early experience. JACC Clin Electrophysiol. 2016;2:253–62.

38. Martini B, Nava A, Thiene G, Buja GF, Canciani B, Scognamiglio R, Daliento L, Dalla VS. Ventricular fibrillation without apparent heart disease: description of six cases. Am Heart J. 1989;118:1203–9.

39. Brugada P, Brugada J. Right bundle branch block, persistent ST segment elevation and sudden cardiac death: a distinct clinical and electrocardiographic syndrome. A multicenter report. J Am Coll Cardiol. 1992;20:1391–6.

40. Derval N, Simpson CS, Birnie DH, Healey JS, Chauhan V, Champagne J, Gardner M, Sanatani S, Yee R, Skanes AC, Gula LJ, Leong-Sit P, Ahmad K, Gollob MH, Haïssaguerre M, Klein GJ, Krahn AD. Prevalence and characteristics of early repolarization in the CASPER registry: cardiac arrest survivors with preserved ejection fraction registry. J Am Coll Cardiol. 2011;58:722–8.

41. Hiraoka M. Brugada syndrome in Japan. Circ J. 2007;71 Suppl A:A61–8.

42. Baranchuk A, Nguyen T, Ryu MH, Femenía F, Zareba W, Wilde AAM, Shimizu W, Brugada P, Pérez-Riera AR. Brugada phenocopy: new terminology and proposed classification. Ann Noninvasive Electrocardiol. 2012;17:299–314.

43. Bayés de Luna A, Brugada J, Baranchuk A, Borggrefe M, Breithardt G, Goldwasser D, Lambiase P, Riera AP, Garcia-Niebla J, Pastore C, Oreto G, McKenna W, Zareba W, Brugada R, Brugada P. Current electrocardiographic criteria for diagnosis of Brugada pattern: a consensus report. J Electrocardiol. 2012;45:433–42.

44. Zhang J, Sacher F, Hoffmayer K, O'Hara T, Strom M, Cuculich P, Silva J, Cooper D, Faddis M, Hocini M, Haïssaguerre M, Scheinman M, Rudy Y. Cardiac electrophysiological substrate underlying the ECG phenotype and electrogram abnormalities in Brugada syndrome patients. Circulation. 2015;131:1950–9.

45. Nademanee K, Hocini M, Haïssaguerre M. Epicardial substrate ablation for Brugada syndrome. Heart Rhythm. 2017;14:457–61.
46. Ackerman MJ, Priori SG, Willems S, Berul C, Brugada R, Calkins H, Camm AJ, Ellinor PT, Gollob M, Hamilton R, Hershberger RE, Judge DP, Le Marec H, McKenna WJ, Schulze-Bahr E, Semsarian C, Towbin JA, Watkins H, Wilde A, Wolpert C, Zipes DP, Heart Rhythm Society (HRS), European Heart Rhythm Association (EHRA). HRS/EHRA expert consensus statement on the state of genetic testing for the channelopathies and cardiomyopathies: this document was developed as a partnership between the Heart Rhythm Society (HRS) and the European Heart Rhythm Association (EHRA). Europace. 2011;13:1077–109.
47. Chung EH, McNeely DE, Gehi AK, Brickner T, Evans S, Pryski E, Waicus K, Stafford H, Mounsey JP, Schwartz JD, Huang S, Pursell I, Ciocca M. Brugada-type patterns are easily observed in high precordial lead ECGs in collegiate athletes. J Electrocardiol. 2014;47:1–6.
48. Shimizu W, Matsuo K, Takagi M, Tanabe Y, Aiba T, Taguchi A, Suyama K, Kurita T, Aihara N, Kamakura S. Body surface distribution and response to drugs of ST segment elevation in Brugada syndrome: clinical implication of eighty-seven-lead body surface potential mapping and its application to twelve-lead electrocardiograms. J Cardiovasc Electrophysiol. 2000;11:396–404.
49. Chung EH. Brugada ECG patterns in athletes. J Electrocardiol. 2015;48:539–43.
50. Corrado D, Pelliccia A, Heidbuchel H, Sharma S, Link M, Basso C, Biffi A, Buja G, Delise P, Gussac I, Anastasakis A, Borjesson M, Bjørnstad HH, Carrè F, Deligiannis A, Dugmore D, Fagard R, Hoogsteen J, Mellwig KP, Panhuyzen-Goedkoop N, Solberg E, Vanhees L, Drezner J, Estes NAM, Iliceto S, Maron BJ, Peidro R, Schwartz PJ, Stein R, Thiene G, Zeppilli P, McKenna WJ, Section of Sports Cardiology, European Association of Cardiovascular Prevention and Rehabilitation. Recommendations for interpretation of 12-lead electrocardiogram in the athlete. Eur Heart J. 2010;31:243–59.
51. Chevallier S, Forclaz A, Tenkorang J, Ahmad Y, Faouzi M, Graf D, Schlaepfer J, Pruvot E. New electrocardiographic criteria for discriminating between Brugada types 2 and 3 patterns and incomplete right bundle branch block. J Am Coll Cardiol. 2011;58:2290–8.
52. Ohkubo K, Watanabe I, Okumura Y, Ashino S, Kofune M, Nagashima K, Nakai T, Kunimoto S, Kasamaki Y, Hirayama A. A new criteria differentiating type 2 and 3 Brugada patterns from ordinary incomplete right bundle branch block. Int Heart J. 2011;52:159–63.
53. Serra G, Baranchuk A, Bayés-De-Luna A, Brugada J, Goldwasser D, Capulzini L, Arazo D, Boraita A, Heras M-E, Garcia-Niebla J, Elosua R, Brugada R, Brugada P. New electrocardiographic criteria to differentiate the Type-2 Brugada pattern from electrocardiogram of healthy athletes with r'-wave in leads V1/V2. Europace. 2014;16:1639–45.
54. Zorzi A, Leoni L, Di Paolo FM, Rigato I, Migliore F, Bauce B, Pelliccia A, Corrado D. Differential diagnosis between early repolarization of athlete's heart and coved-type Brugada electrocardiogram. Am J Cardiol. 2015;115:529–32.
55. Zorzi A, Migliore F, Marras E, Marinelli A, Baritussio A, Allocca G, Leoni L, Perazzolo Marra M, Basso C, Buja G, Thiene G, Iliceto S, Delise P, Corrado D. Should all individuals with a nondiagnostic Brugada-electrocardiogram undergo sodium-channel blocker test? Heart Rhythm. 2012;9:909–16.
56. Nunn L, Bhar-Amato J, Lambiase P. Brugada syndrome: controversies in risk stratification and management. Indian Pacing Electrophysiol J. 2010;10:400–9.
57. Mascia G, Arbelo E, Hernandez-Ojeda J, Solimene F, Brugada R, Brugada J. Brugada syndrome and exercise practice: current knowledge, shortcomings and open questions. Int J Sports Med. 2017;38:573–81.
58. Lampert R, Olshansky B, Heidbuchel H, Lawless C, Saarel E, Ackerman M, Calkins H, Estes NAM, Link MS, Maron BJ, Marcus F, Scheinman M, Wilkoff BL, Zipes DP, Berul CI, Cheng A, Jordaens L, Law I, Loomis M, Willems R, Barth C, Broos K, Brandt C, Dziura J, Li F, Simone L, Vandenberghe K, Cannom D. Safety of sports for athletes with implantable cardioverter-defibrillators: long-term results of a prospective multinational registry. Circulation. 2017;135:2310–2.

59. Lampert R, Olshansky B, Heidbuchel H, Lawless C, Saarel E, Ackerman M, Calkins H, Estes NAM, Link MS, Maron BJ, Marcus F, Scheinman M, Wilkoff BL, Zipes DP, Berul CI, Cheng A, Law I, Loomis M, Barth C, Brandt C, Dziura J, Li F, Cannom D. Safety of sports for athletes with implantable cardioverter-defibrillators: results of a prospective, multinational registry. Circulation. 2013;127:2021–30.
60. Corrado D, Basso C, Thiene G. Sudden cardiac death in young people with apparently normal heart. Cardiovasc Res. 2001;50:399–408.
61. Chugh SS, Kelly KL, Titus JL. Sudden cardiac death with apparently normal heart. Circulation. 2000;102:649–54.
62. Al-Khatib SM, Stevenson WG, Ackerman MJ, Bryant WJ, Callans DJ, Curtis AB, Deal BJ, Dickfeld T, Field ME, Fonarow GC, Gillis AM, Granger CB, Hammill SC, Hlatky MA, Joglar JA, Kay GN, Matlock DD, Myerburg RJ, Page RL. 2017 AHA/ACC/HRS guideline for management of patients with ventricular arrhythmias and the prevention of sudden cardiac death: a report of the American College of Cardiology/American Heart Association task force on clinical practice guidelines and the Heart Rhythm Society. J Am Coll Cardiol. 2018;72:e91–e220.
63. Papadakis M, Raju H, Behr ER, De Noronha SV, Spath N, Kouloubinis A, Sheppard MN, Sharma S. Sudden cardiac death with autopsy findings of uncertain significance: potential for erroneous interpretation. Circ Arrhythm Electrophysiol. 2013;6:588–96.
64. Haïssaguerre M, Derval N, Sacher F, Jesel L, Deisenhofer I, de Roy L, Pasquié J-L, Nogami A, Babuty D, Yli-Mayry S, De Chillou C, Scanu P, Mabo P, Matsuo S, Probst V, Le Scouarnec S, Defaye P, Schlaepfer J, Rostock T, Lacroix D, Lamaison D, Lavergne T, Aizawa Y, Englund A, Anselme F, O'Neill M, Hocini M, Lim KT, Knecht S, Veenhuyzen GD, Bordachar P, Chauvin M, Jais P, Coureau G, Chene G, Klein GJ, Clémenty J. Sudden cardiac arrest associated with early repolarization. N Engl J Med. 2008;358:2016–23.
65. Haïssaguerre M, Sacher F, Nogami A, Komiya N, Bernard A, Probst V, Yli-Mayry S, Defaye P, Aizawa Y, Frank R, Mantovan R, Cappato R, Wolpert C, Leenhardt A, de Roy L, Heidbuchel H, Deisenhofer I, Arentz T, Pasquié J-L, Weerasooriya R, Hocini M, Jais P, Derval N, Bordachar P, Clémenty J. Characteristics of recurrent ventricular fibrillation associated with inferolateral early repolarization role of drug therapy. J Am Coll Cardiol. 2009;53:612–9.
66. Nam G-B, Kim Y-H, Antzelevitch C. Augmentation of J waves and electrical storms in patients with early repolarization. N Engl J Med. 2008;358:2078–9.
67. Rosso R, Kogan E, Belhassen B, Rozovski U, Scheinman MM, Zeltser D, Halkin A, Steinvil A, Heller K, Glikson M, Katz A, Viskin S. J-point elevation in survivors of primary ventricular fibrillation and matched control subjects: incidence and clinical significance. J Am Coll Cardiol. 2008;52:1231–8.
68. Tikkanen JT, Junttila MJ, Anttonen O, Aro AL, Luttinen S, Kerola T, Sager SJ, Rissanen HA, Myerburg RJ, Reunanen A, Huikuri HV. Early repolarization: electrocardiographic phenotypes associated with favorable long-term outcome. Circulation. 2011;123:2666–73.
69. Cristoforetti Y, Biasco L, Giustetto C, De Backer O, Castagno D, Astegiano P, Ganzit G, Gribaudo CG, Moccetti M, Gaita F. J-wave duration and slope as potential tools to discriminate between benign and malignant early repolarization. Heart Rhythm. 2016;13:806–11.
70. Roten L, Derval N, Maury P, Mahida S, Pascale P, Leenhardt A, Jesel L, Deisenhofer I, Kautzner J, Probst V, Rollin A, Ruidavets J-B, Ferrières J, Sacher F, Heg D, Scherr D, Komatsu Y, Daly M, Denis A, Shah A, Hocini M, Jaïs P, Haïssaguerre M. Benign vs. malignant inferolateral early repolarization: focus on the T wave. Heart Rhythm. 2016;13:894–902.
71. Yamada T, McElderry HT, Doppalapudi H, Murakami Y, Yoshida Y, Yoshida N, Okada T, Tsuboi N, Inden Y, Murohara T, Epstein AE, Plumb VJ, Singh SP, Kay GN. Idiopathic ventricular arrhythmias originating from the aortic root prevalence, electrocardiographic and electrophysiologic characteristics, and results of radiofrequency catheter ablation. J Am Coll Cardiol. 2008;52:139–47.
72. Lerman BB, Belardinelli L, West GA, Berne RM, DiMarco JP. Adenosine-sensitive ventricular tachycardia: evidence suggesting cyclic AMP-mediated triggered activity. Circulation. 1986;74:270–80.

73. Lerman BB. Response of nonreentrant catecholamine-mediated ventricular tachycardia to endogenous adenosine and acetylcholine. Evidence for myocardial receptor-mediated effects. Circulation. 1993;87:382–90.
74. Lerman BB, Stein K, Engelstein ED, Battleman DS, Lippman N, Bei D, Catanzaro D. Mechanism of repetitive monomorphic ventricular tachycardia. Circulation. 1995;92:421–9.
75. Heidbuchel H, Prior DL, La Gerche A. Ventricular arrhythmias associated with long-term endurance sports: what is the evidence? Br J Sports Med. 2012;46(Suppl 1):i44–50.
76. Sawant AC, Bhonsale A, te Riele ASJM, Tichnell C, Murray B, Russell SD, Tandri H, Tedford RJ, Judge DP, Calkins H, James CA. Exercise has a disproportionate role in the pathogenesis of arrhythmogenic right ventricular dysplasia/cardiomyopathy in patients without desmosomal mutations. J Am Heart Assoc. 2014;3:e001471.
77. Saeid AK, Klein GJ, Leong-Sit P. Sustained ventricular tachycardia in apparently normal hearts: medical therapy should be the first step in management. Card Electrophysiol Clin. 2016;8:631–9.
78. Lai E, Chung EH. Management of arrhythmias in athletes: atrial fibrillation, premature ventricular contractions, and ventricular tachycardia. Curr Treat Options Cardiovasc Med. 2017;19:86.
79. Bradfield JS, Shivkumar K. Anatomy for ventricular tachycardia ablation in structural heart disease. Card Electrophysiol Clin. 2017;9:11–24.
80. Ling Z, Liu Z, Su L, Zipunnikov V, Wu J, Du H, Woo K, Chen S, Zhong B, Lan X, Fan J, Xu Y, Chen W, Yin Y, Nazarian S, Zrenner B. Radiofrequency ablation versus antiarrhythmic medication for treatment of ventricular premature beats from the right ventricular outflow tract: prospective randomized study. Circ Arrhythm Electrophysiol. 2014;7:237–43.
81. Latchamsetty R, Yokokawa M, Morady F, Kim HM, Mathew S, Tilz R, Kuck K-H, Nagashima K, Tedrow U, Stevenson WG, Yu R, Tung R, Shivkumar K, Sarrazin J-F, Arya A, Hindricks G, Vunnam R, Dickfeld T, Daoud EG, Oza NM, Bogun F. Multicenter outcomes for catheter ablation of idiopathic premature ventricular complexes. JACC Clin Electrophysiol. 2015;1:116–23.

Chapter 13
Cardiovascular Implantable Electronic Devices in Athletes

Benjamin H. Hammond and Elizabeth V. Saarel

Introduction

Cardiovascular implantable electronic devices (CIEDs) were invented in the 1950s at which time the first permanent pacemakers were implanted in patients with acquired complete heart block. Implantable cardioverter-defibrillator (ICD) technology developed many years later and the first ICD devices were placed in humans in the mid 1980s. These early CIEDS required large pulse generators with surgical lead placement on the epicardium. It was not until transvenous leads and compact pulse generators were developed in the early 1990s that sports participation became possible for patients with CIEDs.

In 1994, an elite high school senior basketball player, Nicholas Knapp, collapsed playing recreational basketball and required resuscitation with defibrillation. Within 10 days of his cardiac arrest, he underwent placement of an ICD. He had been offered a full athletic scholarship at Northwestern University, which he retained, but he was informed that he could not be medically cleared to play pursuant to the guideline recommendations for sports eligibility from the 26th American College of Cardiology Bethesda Conference [1]. This disqualification led to his filing of a discrimination suit against the university that was initially upheld, but later struck down by a higher court that determined playing basketball at the collegiate level was not a basic function of life, and therefore this activity did not qualify for protection under section 504(a) of the Rehabilitation Act of 1973 [2]. After enrolling in a different collegiate basketball program and being cleared to play by that college's team physician, he had an appropriate shock during a basketball practice due to a cardiac dysrhythmia and did not return to complete that season [3]. In the years since the Knapp case, the safety of competitive sports for patients with ICDs has been questioned and studied.

B. H. Hammond · E. V. Saarel (✉)
Division of Pediatric Cardiology, St. Luke's Health System, Boise, ID, USA
e-mail: hammonb4@ccf.org; saarele@slhs.org

© Springer Nature Switzerland AG 2021
D. J. Engel, D. M. Phelan (eds.), *Sports Cardiology*,
https://doi.org/10.1007/978-3-030-69384-8_13

Some athletes who have had a pacemaker or ICD placed continue vigorous and competitive sports participation after implantation. More than 40% of electrophysiologists surveyed in a study published in 2006 had at least one patient who continued to participate in sports more vigorous than golf after ICD implantation [4]. This finding was surprisingly inconsistent with the contemporary 2005 36th Bethesda Conference eligibility recommendations which, similar to prior recommendations, suggested that only Class IA sports such as bowling, billiards, and golf were safe for patients with ICDs [5]. Subsequent studies have demonstrated a low incidence of adverse sequelae associated with competitive sports participation in patients with ICDs, despite the fact that sports can be arrhythmogenic in some athletes [6, 7]. This chapter will review the current recommendations for athletic participation in athletes with CIEDs, present data demonstrating the safety of CIEDs while highlighting potential adverse outcomes associated with competitive sports participation, and review quality of life factors for athletes with CIEDs.

Pacemakers

Indications for pacemakers include heart failure, refractory arrhythmias, atrioventricular block, and sinus node dysfunction [8]. In contrast with those patients with ICDs, patients with pacemakers have not been restricted from participation in competitive sports in consensus guidelines, though there is little published data regarding the degree of participation or the safety of sports in this population. A study from the Netherlands in 2004 looked at nine long distance runners with pacemakers. These athletes were followed through a 9-month training program with cardiac monitoring and intermittent device interrogation. The runners with underlying complete heart block required adjustment of the upper rate parameter to 170–180 beats per minute to ensure atrioventricular synchrony with high atrial rates. Otherwise, pacemaker dysfunction was not observed in any of these athletes during the training program or when athletes were surveyed 2 years after completing the training program [9].

In 1992, Schuger et al. described significant damage to two right-sided transvenous leads in a 23-year-old softball player with a pacemaker. He was right-hand-dominant and was participating in daily softball games with intense throwing practices. He presented to the hospital with bradycardia leading to syncope and was found to have pacemaker dysfunction. There was complete transection of his ventricular lead and damage to the atrial lead believed to have resulted from frequent, repetitive arm movements causing the leads to be being crushed between the clavicle and the first rib [10]. While implant techniques and lead design have improved over the years, there is still potential risk for damage to pacemaker or ICD leads with repetitive and forceful arm movements especially for hardware located between the clavicle and the first rib.

The risks to the athlete with a pacemaker, most of whom have structurally normal hearts without cardiomyopathy or a primary inherited arrhythmia syndrome, center on the potential for damage to the device including the pulse generator and leads. In those with underlying congenital, acquired or arrhythmogenic heart disease, it is important to risk-stratify the patient according to their underlying cardiac diagnosis. With regards to the potential for device damage, participation in contact/collision sports for these athletes has been discouraged by serial task force recommendations due to perceived risk [1, 5, 11]. A list of these contact sports from the most recent 2015 American Heart Association (AHA)/American College of Cardiology (ACC) Task Force guidelines is shown in Table 13.1.

Athletes with heart block are recommended to have dual chamber pacemaker devices placed which allow for more physiologic pacing and chronotropic competence including atrial sensing and ventricular pacing, or sensing/pacing of both chambers

Table 13.1   AHA/ACC classification of sports according to risk of impact

	Junior high school	High school/college
Impact expected	American football Ice hockey Lacrosse Wrestling Karate/judo Fencing Boxing	American football Soccer Ice hockey Lacrosse Basketball Wrestling Karate/judo Downhill skiing Squash Fencing Boxing
Impact may occur	Soccer Basketball Field hockey Downhill skiing Equestrian Squash Cycling	Field hockey Equestrian Cycling Baseball/softball Gymnastics Figure skating
Impact not expected	Baseball/softball Cricket Golf Riflery Gymnastics Volleyball Swimming Track and field Tennis Figure skating Cross-country skiing Rowing Sailing Archery Weightlifting Badminton	Cricket Golf Riflery Volleyball Swimming Track and field Tennis Cross-country skiing Rowing Sailing Archery Weightlifting Badminton

Reprinted with permission from: Levine et al. [12], Elsevier

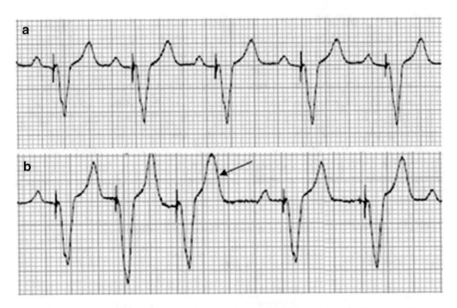

Fig. 13.1 Upper Rate Behavior. (**a**) Atrial-sensed, ventricular-paced rhythm. (**b**) Sensed P-wave followed by a paced QRS. The following two-paced QRS complexes are preceded by an enhanced T-wave suggestive of a P-wave falling within the T-wave that is sensed, and ventricular pacing occurs. The fourth P-wave falling within the T-wave (indicated by arrow) occurs within the post-ventricular atrial refractory period (PVARP) and is not sensed and ventricular pacing is not triggered, resulting in heart rate slowing. (Reprinted with permission from [14], Elsevier)

[13]. High upper heart rate parameters are important for athletic participation in order to avoid pacemaker upper rate behavior, as previously referenced in the Netherlands pacemaker study [9]. Upper rate behavior occurs when a sensed atrial systole (P-wave) falls within the programmed postventricular atrial refractory period (PVARP), and is therefore un-sensed, causing a Wenckebach pattern with sudden slowing of the ventricular rate when the athlete is potentially at peak exercise. An example of this phenomenon is shown in Fig. 13.1. Exercise testing can aid in determining appropriate pacemaker parameters for athletes and should be utilized for all athletes with pacemakers before allowing return to sports participation after implantation.

Implantable Cardioverter-Defibrillator (ICD) Devices

Class I indications for ICD implantation include:

- Secondary prevention for survivors of cardiac arrest.
- Structural heart disease plus spontaneous sustained ventricular tachycardia (VT).
- Syncope of undetermined origin plus sustained VT induced by electrophysiology (EP) study.

- Left ventricular ejection fraction (LVEF) ≤35%, ≥40 days postmyocardial infarction (MI) with New York Heart Association (NYHA) II or III symptoms.
- Nonischemic cardiomyopathy with LVEF ≤35% and NYHA II or III symptoms.
- LVEF ≤30%, ≥40 days post-MI, with NYHA I symptoms.
- Nonsustained VT due to prior MI, LVEF ≤40%.
- Inducible ventricular fibrillation (VF) or sustained VT in an EP study.

Class IIa and IIb indications include additional patients with significant risk factors for sudden cardiac death [8]. One important point of emphasis in serial AHA/ACC athletic recommendations is that an ICD should never be placed for the sole or primary reason of allowing athletes to compete in high-intensity sports (class III indication) [8].

An ICD system can be placed in a variety of configurations. Most commonly the ICD system includes transvenous pacing/sensing leads in the right ventricular endomyocardium with one or two high-voltage coils in the right ventricle (RV) and/or superior vena cava (SVC), but ICDs systems may also include epicardial leads and coils on the RV or LV surfaces, or a subcutaneous parasternal sensing lead and coil. An ICD pulse generator is usually placed subcutaneously in the right or left chest in transvenous lead systems, but generators may also be placed in a subpectoral position, in the abdomen, or in the axilla. Modern endocardial ICD leads typically consist of pacing and sensing electrodes and high-voltage coils surrounded by silicone insulation with an outer polyurethane insulation. Recalled high-voltage ICD leads, most common in thin leads, have demonstrated early fracture when flexing with the heart during the cardiac cycle, if there is a constrained portion of the cable to create a hinge point [15]. Additionally, there can be insulation breaches due to deformation of the silicone insulation and damage due to friction. Initial damage to an ICD lead, either by fracture or insulation breach, is most likely to cause over-sensing with normal pacing impedance [15]. In this case, over-sensing of noise may lead to inappropriate ICD shocks. In rare circumstances, perforation of the myocardium can occur (particularly at the RV apex), but this is less likely related to sports participation and more likely caused by high-forward lead pressure at the tip at the time of implant causing local migration through the myocardium.

While ICD shocks have traditionally been referred to as "appropriate" and "inappropriate", recent literature has suggested that more accurate terminology would be "necessary" and "unnecessary" shocks [16]. Necessary shocks appropriately terminate ventricular tachyarrhythmias that could not be terminated by antitachycardia pacing (ATP) or resolve spontaneously. Patients receiving a necessary shock would typically be symptomatic and potentially unconscious, needing resuscitation. Unnecessary shocks include shocks delivered for supraventricular tachycardia (SVT) or monomorphic VT with a heart rate that exceeds the programmed rate threshold, but these shocks would likely occur in a hemodynamically stable, conscious patient. Over-sensing can lead to false detection of a ventricular tachyarrhythmia. Unnecessary shocks have been documented in up to 50% of device discharges [16].

In 2006, an ICD Sports Safety Registry was established and initiated as a multinational, prospective, and observational registry, to identify and quantify risks associated with sports participation for patients with ICDs. Findings from this registry that included 372 athletes who competed in organized sports of greater than class IA intensity, ranging in age from 10 to 60 years old, were first published by Lampert et al. in 2013 [17]. The most common underlying cardiac diagnoses for these athletes in the registry were:

1. Long QT syndrome (20%)
2. Hypertrophic cardiomyopathy (17%)
3. Arrhythmogenic right ventricular dysplasia (14%)
4. Coronary artery disease (11%)
5. Idiopathic VT/VF (structurally normal heart – 11%)
6. Dilated cardiomyopathy (8%)
7. Congenital heart disease (8%)
8. Catecholaminergic polymorphic VT (3%)
9. Brugada syndrome (2%)

Twenty-seven percent of the patients with these underlying conditions in the cohort underwent ICD implantation after ventricular fibrillation/cardiac arrest, 14% had a prior incidence of sustained VT, and 27% had syncope [17]. With these data in mind, it is justified that there exists a certain amount of fear for cardiologists and patients alike in considering further sports participation after placement of such a device is deemed clinically necessary. At the same time, some individuals may erroneously view ICD placement to be a "safety net" that will protect and save them regardless of their level of sport participation. Proper assessment of an athlete's underlying cardiac disease is necessary to provide appropriate recommendations regarding sport participation to an athlete with an ICD. Defibrillatory shocks are not benign and have been shown in older patients to increase mortality risk secondary to progressive heart failure [18]. The risk inherent in necessary and unnecessary shocks is an additional important consideration, particularly in those with significant underlying heart disease.

Recommendations for Athletes with CIEDs for Competitive Sports Participation

Pacemakers were first mentioned in the 1985 report of the 16th Bethesda Conference providing recommendations regarding eligibility for competition in sports for patients with cardiovascular disease. The recommendation by this expert panel for individuals with pacemakers was to "not engage in competitive sports with a danger of body collision" [19]. Twenty years later, the 36th Bethesda Conference addressed the increased use of ICDs [5], stating:

> Although differences of opinion exist and little direct evidence is available, the panel asserts that the presence of an ICD (whether for primary or secondary prevention of sudden death) should disqualify athletes from most competitive sports (with the exception of low-intensity, class IA), including those that potentially involve bodily trauma. The presence of an

implantable device in high-risk patients with cardiovascular disease should not be regarded as protective therapy and therefore a justification for permitting participation in competitive sports that would otherwise be restricted.

The panel additionally raised concern that there was uncertainty of device performance at peak exercise, raising the potential for necessary and unnecessary discharges and associated risk of injury to the athlete [5].

Subsequent to the publication of these recommendations, the aforementioned ICD Sports Safety Registry was established to address these concerns expressed at the 36th Bethesda Conference. The first results of the registry were published in 2013. In the registry, 13% of athletes had a necessary ICD shock, and 11% of athletes had an unnecessary shock over a median follow-up of 31 months. In those athletes receiving either a necessary or an unnecessary shock, there was no difference in the timing of shocks between competition/practice and other physical activity. Regarding injury to the device, there were some lead malfunctions with an estimated lead survival without definite or possible malfunction of 97% at 5 years and 90% at 10 years. The registry data suggested that many athletes with ICDs can engage in competitive sports without physical injury or failure to terminate arrhythmias despite the occurrence of both necessary and unnecessary shocks [17]. The registry data were re-evaluated 4 years later, showing similar results in a cohort of 440 patients [20].

The 2015 AHA/ACC eligibility and disqualification recommendations for competitive athletes with cardiovascular disease incorporated the early data studying ICDs in athletes, recognizing the potential for safe participation in some competitive sports. The authors stated that it was reasonable to allow athletes with ICDs to participate in class IA sports, but they supplemented their recommendations by stating that it was possible for athletes to engage in more intensive sports through a shared decision making construct whereby the athlete assumes a portion of the potential risk for adverse events. Shared decision making in this context was summarized: [11]

> Participation in sports with higher peak static and dynamic components than class IA may be considered if the athlete is free of episodes of ventricular flutter or ventricular fibrillation requiring device therapy for 3 months. The decision regarding athletic participation should be made with consideration of, and counseling of, the athlete regarding the higher likelihood of appropriate and inappropriate shocks and the potential for device-related trauma in high-impact sports.

The guidelines also re-affirmed that eligibility and safety for athletic participation should never be the indication for placement of an ICD device [11]. Physicians were advised to prioritize the patient's underlying cardiovascular disease and clinical context instead of making sports participation recommendations based solely on the presence of an ICD. Decision-trees incorporating the most recent competitive sports guidelines for athletes with pacemakers and ICDs are shown in Figs. 13.2 and 13.3.

Athletes with Permanent
Pacemakers (PPM)

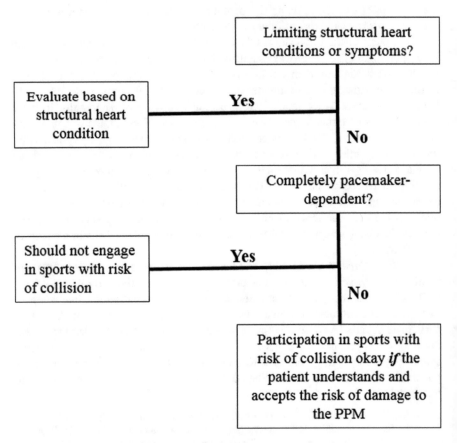

Fig. 13.2 Decision-tree for athletes with permanent pacemakers

Pediatric Athletes

Saarel et al. separately examined patients enrolled in the ICD registry who were ≤21 years of age (age range 10–21 years) [21]. The majority of patients had normal underlying ventricular function; the most common diagnoses were long QT syndrome (38%), hypertrophic cardiomyopathy (23%), congenital heart disease (12%); other less prevalent diagnoses included arrhythmogenic right ventricular cardiomyopathy, idiopathic VT/VF, catecholaminergic polymorphic VT (CPVT), dilated cardiomyopathy, and Brugada Syndrome. There were 117 patients who participated in competitive sports and 12 who participated in dangerous sports as classified by ACC/AHA guidelines (Table 13.2) [11]; 79 athletes participated in sports at the high school or college level. In this subgroup of the larger of athlete ICD registry,

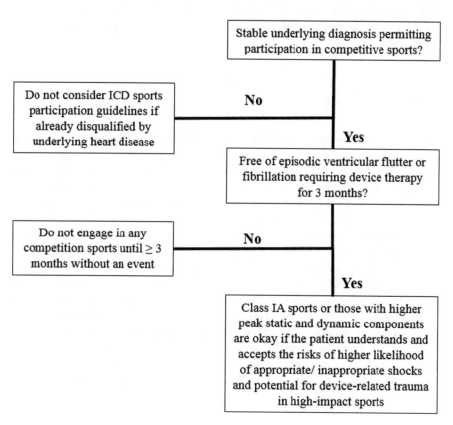

Fig. 13.3 Decision-tree for athletes with ICDs

Table 13.2 Dangerous sports as classified by AHA/ACC guidelines with respect to risk if syncope occurs

Dangerous sports (increased risk if syncope occurs)		
Auto racing	Gymnastics	Synchronized swimming
Body building	Motorcycling	Triathlon
Cycling	Rodeoing	Water skiing
Diving	Skateboarding	Weight lifting
Equestrian	Snowboarding	Windsurfing

similar findings to the larger cohort were observed with no tachyarrhythmic deaths, externally resuscitated tachyarrhythmias, or severe injury. There were low rates of device malfunction. Six necessary shocks were delivered in four individuals that occurred during competition or practice, giving a rate of 1.5 necessary shocks during sports per one hundred person-years. Overall, 27% of athletes received at least one shock, and there were a significant number of unnecessary shocks (35% of all shocks were unnecessary) due to noise, SVT, and over-sensing. These findings regarding shocks were also similar to the larger registry findings. Importantly, 105/117 athletes in this study stopped participation in all or some sports during the follow-up period: the majority for nonmedical reasons and 7 of them because of an ICD shock [21].

Sideline Management

Several problems can occur in athletes with ICDs during active athletic activity and competition. The most serious of these would be a ventricular tachyarrhythmia with shock failure leading to death. For this reason, it is essential to be prepared with an automated external defibrillator (AED) on the sideline during competitive sports participation (including practices). There is a risk of postshock pulseless electrical activity (PEA), such that sideline preparation should include CPR-trained bystanders. Knowledge of the underlying cardiac diagnosis and associated mechanism of sudden cardiac death are essential in anticipating outcomes. Rarely, patients with CPVT can have proarrhythmic ICD discharges due to the release of catecholamines leading to a clustering of recurrent episodes of VT or VF in a brief period. This sequence of events has been referred to as an "electrical storm" [22]. Unnecessary shocks can cause discomfort and can induce further ventricular arrhythmia. Other consequences to anticipate on the sideline are injuries from syncopal arrhythmias and potential injury to the patient's ICD leads or generator. It is important when there is suspicion of damage to the device components that all vigorous activity is suspended and the athlete is evaluated promptly by an electophysiologist.

External Defibrillation in Shock Failure

First responders to a symptomatic athlete should be made aware of the presence of an ICD and allow 30–60 seconds for the device to cycle prior to attaching an automated external defibrillator (AED) device. Rarely, the shock from an AED can conflict with the shock cycle of the ICD. Placement of the AED pads should be at least 1 inch (2.5 cm) away from the device generator [23]. First responders should be reminded that shocks delivered by the ICD to the patient during resuscitation will not pose a danger to those performing CPR, though responders may experience a tingling sensation when a shock is delivered [24]. When external defibrillation is required, it is important to subsequently have the ICD device checked by an electrophysiologist to assess for any damage to the device.

Unnecessary ICD Shocks

An unnecessary shock was reported in 40 patients in the ICD Sports Safety Registry (11% of cohort) [17]. Table 13.3 shows the underlying rhythms responsible for unnecessary shocks, including sinus tachycardia exceeding programmed thresholds, atrial fibrillation being read as a ventricular arrhythmia, noise, T-wave oversensing, and other causes including SVT [17]. Lead fracture can cause noise on the high-voltage lead, as demonstrated in Fig. 13.4, and cause an unnecessary shock. In rare and extreme cases, patients can have an unnecessary shock that degenerates into a ventricular arrhythmia. Shocks that occur in a conscious patient can be uncomfortable and can even lead to post-traumatic stress disorder or severe anxiety as the patient lives in fear of an unnecessary shock. Assessment by an electrophysiologist is important if an unnecessary shock occurs to understand the reason for the shock and to check for device damage or malfunction.

Damage to Pacemakers/ICDs

The potential of damage to a patient's implanted electrical device is not confined to direct traumatic impact during sports participation. Dislodgement and fracture of the leads can occur due to repetitive muscular movements. There can be gross electrode dislodgement or partial electrode dislodgement with the latter being the more

Table 13.3 Number of shock events and underlying rhythms leading to necessary and unnecessary shocks in the ICD sports safety registry

Rhythm	Competition related, n^a	Physical activity related, n^b	Other, n	Total, n (%)
Ventricular tachycardia	22/16	14/11	11/8	47/35 (9)
Ventricular fibrillation	8/6	3/3	10/5	21/14 (4)
Sinus tachycardia	7/6	6/3	1/1	14/10 (3)
Atrial fibrillation	5/3	10/6	3/3	18/12 (3)
Other supraventricular tachycardia	2/2	2/2	0/0	4/4 (1)
Noise	0/0	2/2	6/5	8/7 (2)
T-wave oversensing	2/2	1/1	1/1	4/4 (1)
Other	3/2	1/1	1/1	5/4 (1)
Total, n (%)	49/36 (10)	39/29 (8)	33/23 (6)	121/77 (21)

Values refer to number of events/number of unique individuals. Percents refer to percent of the study population. Eighteen shocks did not have available implantable cardioverter-defibrillator–stored data, so the diagnosis is based on that of the treating physician. Of these, 4 were ventricular arrhythmia, 2 were supraventricular, 7 were noise, and 5 were other
[a]Includes competition, postcompetition, or practice for competition
[b]Includes physical activity and post-physical activity
Reprinted with permission from [17], Wolters Kluwer Health, Inc.

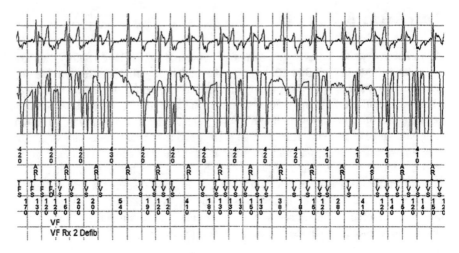

Fig. 13.4 ICD over-sensing. Device interrogation in a 14-year-old female with an ICD demonstrating inappropriate ventricular lead sensing due to noise artifact from lead fracture. Note the increased ventricular-sensed (VS) intracardiac electrogram signals in comparison with actual QRS complexes

common. Lead fracture can also occur at points of significant pressure and stress on the lead. The points on the lead that experiences consistent mechanical stress and high pressure include the portions inside the suture sleeve, adjacent to the tricuspid valve, and in proximity to the first rib and clavicle [25]. Direct impact trauma, as inherent in full contact sports, can also cause fracture or dislodgement of the leads and damage to the generator. The ICD Sports Safety Registry reported outcomes in the patients participating in "moderate" and "aggressive" contact sports. Examples of moderate contact sports included basketball and soccer; examples of aggressive contact sports included tackle football and ice hockey. Despite a significant number of athletes participating in moderate contact sports, the number of athletes with possible or definite device damage was low, with 93% and 84% malfunction-free survival at 5 and 10 years, respectively [17]. Impact/collision sports have been classified as high-risk by the 2015 AHA/ACC guidelines (Table 13.1) for patients on chronic anticoagulation therapy, and this classification can reasonably also be applied for those athletes with CIEDs. Wearable shields and padded shirts currently on the market claim to be engineered to protect pacemakers, ICDs, and subcutaneous ICDs from direct impact though they are untested. It is important to note that these devices may provide false reassurance and place the athlete at risk of damage to their device.

Syncope During Sports Participation

As discussed previously, a significant portion of athletes have ICDs implanted for secondary prevention of further cardiac arrest. The presence of an ICD is not preventative for syncopal events during sports participation. An athlete can also lose control when a shock (necessary or unnecessary) is delivered. Certain sports have therefore been considered dangerous or high-risk, where "a brief loss of control could result in injury" [17] (Table 13.2). Of the 372 patients in the ICD Sports Safety Registry, there were no serious injuries or moderate injuries despite having some patients who participated in dangerous or high-risk sports.

Quality of Life in Athletes with CIEDs

In the general population, several studies have demonstrated a negative impact on quality of life assessment associated with the presence of CIEDs. Patients with ICDs describe the sensation of a shock as a "lightning-like blow to the chest" or a feeling of "being kicked by a horse"; many patients develop an interest in joining a support group after receiving a shock [26]. In 2012, Czosek et al. assessed quality of life in a multicenter cross-sectional study comprised of 133 pediatric patients with pacemakers and 40 patients with ICDs. Utilizing the Pediatric Quality of Life Inventory, they found that the presence of an implanted device negatively affected an individual's self-perception. Quality of life scores in those patients with ICDs were lower than in patients with pacemakers, which were closer to the control group. History of a device shock (necessary or unnecessary) resulted in no significant difference in quality of life scores in this study [27]. Using the health-related quality of life scale, Cheng et al. demonstrated that patients with pacemakers had lower scores in psychosocial health, school functioning, social functioning, and emotional functioning relative to the general population [28]. Perceived quality of life of an athlete is often closely tied with participation in competitive sports. The negative psychological impact of a CIED can be exaggerated when the device is associated with an athlete's inability to participate in competitive sports.

For patients living with an ICD, there is anxiety associated with anticipation of both necessary and unnecessary shocks. Some patients develop post-traumatic stress disorder as a result of multiple shocks. An unnecessary shock can be associated with distrust of the device accuracy and has been associated with reduced mental well-being [29]. Anxiety and post-traumatic stress disorder can be debilitating and affect an athlete's performance, particularly, if the shock occurred during competitive play. It is important to balance the added quality of life that sports participation gives to the competitive athlete with potential adverse psychosocial effects associated with the device.

Team Huddle (*Shared Decision Making*)

Shared decision making is an essential component in the process of counseling an athlete with CIED regarding sports participation. The essential elements of this discussion and counseling are different for patients with pacemakers and patients with ICDs. In a patient with a pacemaker, it is important to discuss the possible need for additional surgical or interventional procedures, if their device were to be damaged during competitive play, particularly if the athlete is interested in a contact sport. Athletes who are pacemaker-dependent are at increased risk of injury if they were to lose capture and have syncope due to hemodynamically significant bradycardia with their underlying junctional or ventricular rhythm. If athletes can avoid sports with high-risk of impact to their device, the risks of device failure and associated injury appear to be low, though data are limited.

Counseling an athlete with an ICD should involve a more serious discussion of mortality risk. Athletes need to know that they might experience a ventricular arrhythmia and lose consciousness, placing them at risk for injury in any sport, particularly in those sports classified as dangerous (Table 13.2). The athlete needs to be counseled that a necessary ICD shock could fail to resuscitate them from cardiac arrest, and that an unnecessary shock can occur, causing discomfort, loss of consciousness, or even induction of a lethal arrhythmia. Risks of damage to the device and device leads need also to be discussed. The importance of recognizing device alarms and getting regular device checks should be emphasized. The shared decision making model requires that these risks be explained to the athlete's family (if under 18 years of age), coaches, trainers, overseeing sports organizations or school/university, and, in some circumstances, teammates.

Conclusion

Growing data suggests that some athletes with CIEDs can engage in competitive sports with a low incidence of adverse sequelae. A careful assessment of the athlete's underlying cardiac disease, indication for device placement, and the type and intensity of planned sport activity is necessary to provide appropriate recommendations regarding sport participation to an athlete with a CIED. Most recent ACC/AHA guidelines have left open the possibility for athletes, when deemed clinically allowable, to engage in more intensive sports through a shared decision making construct whereby the athlete assumes a portion of the potential risk for adverse events. Not only the athlete, but also the coaches, trainers, overseeing sports organizations or school/university surrounding the athlete, must understand and anticipate the unique risks to an athlete with a CIED, and the appropriate sideline preparations must be in place to promote the safest possible environment for sports participation.

References

1. Maron BJ, Mitchell JH, editors. 26th Bethesda Conference: recommendations for determining eligibility for competition in athletes with cardiovascular abnormalities, January 6 and 7, 1994. J Am Coll Cardiol. 1994;24:845–99.
2. Knapp v. Northwestern University. 101 F.3d 473 (7th Cir. 1996), cert. denied, 117 S.Ct. 2454 (1997).

3. Maron BJ, Mitten MJ, Quandt EF, Zipes DP. Competitive athletes with cardiovascular disease – the case of Nicholas Knapp. N Engl J Med. 1998;339(22):1632–5.
4. Lampert R, Cannom D, Olshansky B. Safety of sports participation in patients with implantable cardioverter defibrillators: a survey of Heart Rhythm Society members. J Cardiovasc Electrophysiol. 2006;17(1):11–5. https://doi.org/10.1111/j.1540-8167.2005.00331.x.
5. Maron BJ, Zipes DP. 36th Bethesda Conference: eligibility recommendations for athletes with cardiovascular abnormalities. J Am Coll Cardiol. 2005;45(8) https://doi.org/10.1159/000111411.
6. Saarel EV, Law I, Berul CI, et al. Safety of sports for young patients with implantable cardioverter-defibrillators. Circ Arrhythm Electrophysiol. 2018;11(11):e006305. https://doi.org/10.1161/CIRCEP.118.006305.
7. Saarel E, Pilcher T, Gamboa D, Etheridge S. Sports for young patients with implantable cardioverter-defibrillators: refining the risk. J Am Coll Cardiol. 2014;63(12):A529. https://doi.org/10.1016/s0735-1097(14)60529-5.
8. Epstein AE, DiMarco JP, Ellenbogen KA, et al. ACC/AHA/HRS 2008 guidelines for device-based therapy of cardiac rhythm abnormalities: executive summary. Circulation. 2008;117(21):2820–40. https://doi.org/10.1161/CIRCUALTIONAHA.108.189741.
9. Bennekers JH, Van Mechelen R, Meijer A. Pacemaker safety and long distance running. Neth Hear J. 2004;12(10):450–4.
10. Schuger CD, Mittleman R, Habbal B, Wagshal A, Huang SKS. Ventricular lead transection and atrial lead damage in a young softball player shortly after the insertion of a permanent pacemaker. Pacing Clin Electrophysiol. 1992;15(9):1236–9. https://doi.org/10.1111/j.1540-8159.1992.tb03132.x.
11. Zipes DP, Link MS, Ackerman MJ, Kovacs RJ, Myerburg RJ, Estes NAM 3rd. Eligibility and disqualification recommendations for competitive athletes with cardiovascular abnormalities: task force 9: arrhythmias and conduction defects: a scientific statement from the American Heart Association and American College of Cardiology. J Am Coll Cardiol. 2015;66(21):2412–23. https://doi.org/10.1016/j.jacc.2015.09.041.
12. Levine BD, Baggish AL, Kovacs RJ, Link MS, Maron MS, Mitchell JH. Eligibility and disqualification recommendations for competitive athletes with cardiovascular abnormalities: task force 1: classification of sports: dynamic, static, and impact: a scientific statement from the American Heart Association and American College of Cardiology. J Am Coll Cardiol. 2015;66(21):2350–5.
13. Kusumoto FM, Schoenfeld MH, Barrett C, et al. 2018 ACC/AHA/HRS guideline on the evaluation and management of patients with bradycardia and cardiac conduction delay. Circulation. 2019;140(8):e382–482. https://doi.org/10.1161/cir.0000000000000628.
14. Mulpuru SK, Madhavan M, McLeod CJ, Cha YM, Friedman PA. Cardiac pacemakers: function, troubleshooting, and management: part 1 of a 2-part series. J Am Coll Cardiol. 2017;69(2):189–210. https://doi.org/10.1016/j.jacc.2016.10.061.
15. Swerdlow CD, Ellenbogen KA. Implantable cardioverter-defibrillator leads: design, diagnostics, and management. Circulation. 2013;128(18):2062–71. https://doi.org/10.1161/CIRCULATIONAHA.113.003920.
16. Koneru JN, Swerdlow CD, Wood MA, Ellenbogen KA. Minimizing inappropriate or "unnecessary" implantable cardioverter-defibrillator shocks: appropriate programming. Circ Arrhythm Electrophysiol. 2011;4(5):778–90. https://doi.org/10.1161/CIRCEP.110.961243.
17. Lampert R, Olshansky B, Heidbuchel H, et al. Safety of sports for athletes with implantable cardioverter-defibrillators: results of a prospective, multinational registry. Circulation. 2013;127(20):2021–30. https://doi.org/10.1161/CIRCULATIONAHA.112.000447.
18. Poole JE, Johnson GW, Hellkamp AS, et al. Prognostic importance of defibrillator shocks in patients with heart failure. N Engl J Med. 2008;359(10):1009–17. https://doi.org/10.1056/nejmoa071098.
19. Zipes DP, Cobb LA, Garson A, et al. Task force VI: arrhythmias. J Am Coll Cardiol. 1985;6(6):1225–32. https://doi.org/10.1016/S0735-1097(85)80206-0.

20. Lampert R, Olshansky B, Heidbuchel H, et al. Safety of sports for athletes with implantable cardioverter-defibrillators. Circulation. 2017;135(23):2310–2. https://doi.org/10.1161/circulationaha.117.027828.
21. Saarel EV, Law I, Berul CI, et al. Safety of sports for young patients with implantable cardioverter-defibrillators: long-term results of the multinational ICD sports registry. Circ Arrhythm Electrophysiol. 2018;11:e006305. https://doi.org/10.1161/CIRCEP.118.006305.
22. Roston TM, Vinocur JM, Maginot KR, et al. Catecholaminergic polymorphic ventricular tachycardia in children: analysis of therapeutic strategies and outcomes from an international multicenter registry. Circ Arrhythm Electrophysiol. 2015;8(3):633–42. https://doi.org/10.1161/CIRCEP.114.002217.
23. AHA. 2005 American Heart Association guidelines for cardiopulmonary resuscitation and emergency cardiovascular care - Part 5: Electrical therapies: automated external defibrillators, defibrillation, cardioversion, and pacing. Circulation. 2005;112(24 Suppl):IV 35–46. https://doi.org/10.1161/CIRCULATIONAHA.105.166554.
24. McMullan J, Valento M, Attari M, Venkat A. Care of the pacemaker/implantable cardioverter defibrillator patient in the ED. Am J Emerg Med. 2007;25(7):812–22. https://doi.org/10.1016/j.ajem.2007.02.008.
25. Lamberti F. Sports practice in individuals with cardiac pacemakers and implantable cardioverter-defibrillators. In: Sports cardiology: from diagnosis to clinical management; 2012. p. 291–7. https://doi.org/10.2307/j.ctt1q1cr8b.30.
26. Duru F, Mattmann H, Candinas R, et al. How different from pacemaker patients are recipients of implantable cardioverter-defibrillators with respect to psychosocial adaptation, affective disorders, and quality of life? Heart. 2001;85(4):375–9.
27. Czosek RJ, Bonney WJ, Cassedy A, et al. Impact of cardiac devices on the quality of life in pediatric patients. Circ Arrhythm Electrophysiol. 2012;5(6):1064–72. https://doi.org/10.1161/CIRCEP.112.973032.
28. Cheng P, Gutierrez-Colina AM, Loiselle KA, et al. Health related quality of life and social support in pediatric patients with pacemakers. J Clin Psychol Med Settings. 2014;21(1):92–102. https://doi.org/10.1007/s10880-013-9381-0.
29. Sears SF, St Amant JB, Zeigler V. Psychosocial considerations for children and young adolescents with implantable cardioverter defibrillators: an update. Pacing Clin Electrophysiol. 2009;32:80–3.

Chapter 14
Diagnosis and Management of Coronary Artery Disease in Athletes

Prashant Rao and David Shipon

Introduction

It is well established that exercise is associated with a reduction in ischemic heart disease and acute coronary events [1–3]. However, the most common cause of exercise-related sudden cardiac death in athletes >35 years old is coronary artery disease (CAD) [4, 5]. Atherosclerotic CAD can also occur in younger athletes with familial dyslipidemia [6]. In the setting of underlying CAD, vigorous physical exertion may transiently increase the risk of an acute coronary event and sudden death [7–9]. Over the past decade, the scientific community has attempted to reconcile this apparent exercise paradox to ensure that athletes with CAD experience all the cardiovascular benefits that exercise affords while minimizing the risk of an adverse event.

What Is the Scope of the Problem?

Exercise-related SCD represents approximately 5–6% of the total cases of SCD in the population [10, 11], with an estimated incidence in the general population at approximately 0.46–0.76 cases per 100,000 person-years [12, 13]. The vast majority of exercise-related SCD occurs in those >35 years of age [12] and the annual incidence of exercise-related SCD in recreational middle-aged joggers is estimated at 13 cases per 100,000 joggers per year [14]. The most common cause of exercise-related sudden cardiac death in athletes >35 years old is CAD [4, 5].

P. Rao
Beth Israel Deaconess Medical Center, Harvard Medical School, Boston, MA, USA
e-mail: prao@bidmc.harvard.edu

D. Shipon (✉)
Thomas Jefferson University Hospital, Philadelphia, PA, USA
e-mail: David.M.Shipon@jefferson.edu

© Springer Nature Switzerland AG 2021
D. J. Engel, D. M. Phelan (eds.), *Sports Cardiology*,
https://doi.org/10.1007/978-3-030-69384-8_14

The burden of exercise-related SCD in those >35 years of age is likely to increase in the future. Over the past few decades, there has been an increase in participation rates in organized endurance sporting events, particularly among those >40 years of age with backgrounds markedly different to traditional competitive athletes [15–17]. Although speculative, it is possible that these "weekend warriors" have a higher risk of exercise-related SCD compared to traditional competitive athletes because of different underlying CAD risk profiles. While the commitment to exercise among individuals not accustomed to vigorous physical activity is to be commended, it is important to mitigate against the risk of adverse cardiac events among this group.

Managing CAD does not pertain only to nonathletes taking up rigorous exercise in later life but also to current and retired professional athletes. Evidence from active and retired National Football League (NFL) players indicates that professional athletes are not immune from traditional atherosclerotic risk factors. One-fifth of football linemen have cardiometabolic syndrome during their active career (defined as ≥3 of (1) elevated blood pressure, (2) elevated fasting glucose, (3) elevated triglycerides, (4) high waist circumference, and (5) low high-density lipoprotein cholesterol) [18]. After their professional careers, one-quarter have cardiometabolic disease [19] and nearly two-thirds of veteran linemen have established metabolic syndrome [20]. In addition to playing position, it is worth noting that the risk of CAD likely differs between different sports. Indeed, former NFL players have higher rates of cardiovascular mortality compared with former professional baseball players [21].

Mechanisms of Exercise-Related SCD due to CAD

Although the final pathway of exercise-related SCD due to CAD is likely to be an ischemic ventricular arrhythmia, the underlying causes remain uncertain. Potential mechanisms for the development of an exercise-induced ischemic ventricular arrhythmia may involve three distinct mechanisms. First is the traditional model of plaque rupture in the setting of underlying vulnerable plaque. Vulnerable plaque is lipid- and macrophage-rich atheromata with an overlying thin fibrous cap [22]. Plaque rupture may be precipitated by exercise-induced sympathetic activation, an acute increase in shear stress or activation of the hemostatic pathways. Postmortem analyses in men with severe CAD demonstrate a higher rate of acute plaque rupture in those cases where death was temporally linked to physical exertion or emotional stress as opposed to those who died at rest (68% versus 23% ($p < 0.001$)) [23].

Second, exercise-related ischemia may be caused by a demand-supply mismatch during vigorous physical activity. In support of this theory is the observation that immediate coronary angiography performed in a small number of marathon runners who survived cardiac arrest showed high-grade stenosis without evidence of plaque rupture [24].

Finally, the stress induced by high levels of vigorous exercise may lead to a model of chronic inflammation, endothelial dysfunction, and plaque erosion. The combination of these previously underappreciated mechanisms may contribute to the development of acute coronary syndromes [25, 26].

Management of CAD in Athletes

Preparticipation Screening

Often, asymptomatic athletes seek medical advice prior to the commencement of a training program. This may be due to a personal concern regarding exercise-related cardiac events or the need for medical clearance by a sporting body. Indeed, medical screening prior to mass community endurance races identifies individuals at high-risk for CAD and educational intervention decreases medical encounters during the race [27]. The purpose of a CAD screening assessment is to minimize the risk of myocardial ischemia or a cardiac event that may be triggered during exercise [28]. Mitigating the risk of exercise-induced ischemia in athletes centers not only on the underlying burden of atherosclerotic disease but also on the exercise dose (i.e., the intended intensity, duration, and volume of exercise). Indeed, every assessment and exercise prescription should be tailored on an individual basis.

We direct the reader to the European Society of Cardiology and the American Heart Association/American College of Cardiology consensus statements on the Eligibility and Disqualification Recommendations for Competitive Athletes With CAD [6, 29] (Table 14.1).

Of note, there are no randomized controlled trials in athletes with CAD and there is a paucity of evidence regarding the cause-and-effect relationship of high levels of exercise and the development of clinically significant CAD [17]. As a result, these documents are largely based on expert consensus and opinions.

The preparticipation screening is centered on the history and physical examination for the majority of asymptomatic athletes. The history should identify the presence of symptoms that may represent significant CAD such as chest pain, shortness of breath or palpitations during physical activity or a decrease in exercise capacity. In addition, chest pain present at the start of the workout that dissipates within 5 minutes of continued exertion, coined "warm-up angina" is another important feature of CAD in athletes [30]. The dissipation of pain after a few minutes of exercise is likely due to the result of systemic arterial vasodilation and reduction in left ventricular afterload, resulting in a decrease in myocardial oxygen consumption. The history should also include a detailed cardiovascular risk assessment. Components of a cardiovascular risk profile include obesity, hypertension, diabetes mellitus, smoking, and family history. Commonly used risk charts such as SCORE (http://www.heartscore.org/Pages/welcome.aspx), the Framingham risk score (http://hp2010.nhl-bihin.net/atpiii/calculator.asp), or the Global CV Risk score are valuable tools to estimate the risk of an ischemic event and should be used in athletes as well as the general population [31]. In addition to the traditional atherosclerotic risk factors, it is important to inquire about performance enhancing drugs, which are likely under-recognized among athletes. Early case reports published over 30 years ago linked

Table 14.1 American Heart Association/American College of Cardiology recommendations for the management of athletes with established CAD

Recommendation	Class	Level of evidence
Maximal exercise testing should be performed to evaluate exercise tolerance, the presence of inducible ischemia, and the presence of exercise- induced electrical instability. Maximal exercise testing should be performed on the patient's standard medical regimen	I	C
An assessment of left ventricular function should be performed	I	C
An informed shared decision model should be used to guide management, balancing the health and psychological benefits of exercise versus the estimated risk of an acute event	I	C
High-intensity statin therapy should be used to aggressively reduce the risk of plaque disruption	I	C
Participation in competitive activities are reasonable if they are asymptomatic, resting left ventricular ejection fraction is >50%, and there is no inducible ischemia or electrical instability	IIb	C
In those that do not fulfill the above criteria for participation in competitive sports, it is reasonable to restrict these patients to sports with low-dynamic and low-to-moderate static demands	IIb	C
It is reasonable to prohibit participation in competitive sports for at least 3 months after acute myocardial infarction or coronary revascularization procedure	IIb	C
It is reasonable to prohibit participation in competitive sports, if there is increasing frequency or worsening of myocardial ischemia	IIb	C

Adapted from American Heart Association/American College of Cardiology Scientific Statement on Eligibility and Disqualification Recommendations for Competitive Athletes with Cardiovascular Abnormalities: Task Force 8: Coronary Artery Disease [6]

supraphysiologic doses of illicit anabolic–androgenic steroids (AAS) to acute myocardial infarction in young men [32, 33]. Furthermore, AAS impair coronary vascular function [34] and markedly decrease HDL-cholesterol and increase LDL-cholesterol [35]. In line with these findings, male weightlifters using AAS demonstrate higher coronary artery plaque volume than nonusers and lifetime AAS dose is strongly associated with coronary atherosclerotic burden [36]. Other performance enhancing agents also increase the risk of atherothrombosis and infarction such as erythropoietin through an increase in blood viscosity and hypertension [37].

The physical examination should be directed to detect cardiac risk factors such as obesity, hypertension, vascular bruits, cardiac murmurs, corneal arcus, and xanthelasma (Table 14.2).

Investigations

Athletes with any cardiovascular risk factor or older athletes who wish to participate in competitive sport that has a moderate dynamic and/or static component should undergo an exercise ECG test [38, 39].

Table 14.2 Physical examination findings of risk factors associated with atherosclerosis

Xanthelasma
Tendon Xanthomata
Corneal Arcus
Vascular Bruits
Obesity
High waist circumference
Arteriosclerotic retinopathy
Reduced pedal pulses
Acanthosis nigricans

Table 14.3 Exercise findings associated with adverse prognosis and CAD

Low symptom-limiting exercise capacity
Angina Pectoris
Failure to increase systolic blood pressure or a sustained decrease ≥ 10 mmHg during progressive exercise
ST-segment depression, down sloping ST-segment with persistence into recovery
Exercise-induced ST-segment elevation
Reproducible sustained (>30s) or symptomatic ventricular tachycardia

Adapted from Bonow and Braunwald [40]

A classification of abnormal exercise test findings is outlined in Table 14.3.

Athletes with a low cardiovascular risk profile and normal maximal exercise test should be allowed to participate in competitive sports with annual follow-up [29]. In the setting of borderline exercise test findings or an uninterpretable electrocardiogram (e.g., pre-existing left bundle branch block or ventricular pacing), further investigations are required to mitigate against the risk of exercise-induced cardiac events. These include stress-echo/-CMR/PET/SPECT and the decision is often guided by an institution's local expertize and availability [29]. In the event of an abnormal exercise test, CT coronary angiography or a diagnostic coronary angiogram should be performed to better define the burden of atherosclerotic CAD [29] (Fig. 14.1).

Limitations of Exercise Testing in Athletes with CAD

Although a functional evaluation with exercise testing is important to evaluate the burden of CAD in athletes, it has significant limitations in this population. While exercise testing is able to detect flow limitation in the setting of increased cardiac output and high-grade stenosis, it is unable to identify vulnerable plaque. As such, exercise testing is useful in predicting angina but is a poor predictor of acute plaque rupture and infarction. Therefore, negative findings may be falsely reassuring when there is concern for an exercise-induced CAD event.

It should also be noted that performing and interpreting exercise tests in athletes differ from the general population. Athletes, particularly those in endurance sports,

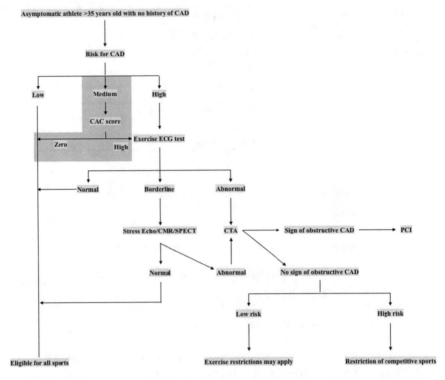

Fig. 14.1 An approach for CAD screening in an athlete without established CAD. (Adapted from Borjesson et al. [29])
*The red highlighted section refers to our practice and is not mentioned in the EAPC Position Statement. Caution should be used when using coronary artery calcium scores, particularly in older endurance athletes.

have a far greater exercise capacity than the general population. Furthermore, calculation of maximal heart rate has a wide standard deviation [41]. Taken together, exercise testing in athletes should be terminated based on maximal exercise capacity rather than heart rate criteria, as the latter will likely result in premature termination of the test. In addition, it is important to recognize that a "normal" workload in METs or maximal oxygen uptake may represent a relative functional impairment in the setting of a well-conditioned athlete.

Management of an Athlete with Established CAD

We define established CAD as proven either by a previous coronary event, cardiac CT, or coronary angiography. There is, however, ongoing debate regarding the clinical significance of coronary artery calcification in veteran endurance athletes, which we will address later in this chapter. The management of patients with established CAD is similar regardless of their athletic status. The definition of successful treatment is to reduce the risk of cardiovascular events, improve prognosis, and maximize health and function [42, 43]. Key principles of management include a combination of lifestyle modification, patient education, and evidence-based pharmacotherapy. Even in athletes, lifestyle modification programs and cardiac rehabilitation are of paramount importance.

Antiplatelet Therapy

Antiplatelet therapies are the cornerstone of medical management of CAD by decreasing platelet formation and preventing coronary thrombus formation.

Aspirin, which acts via platelet cyclooxygenase-1 (COX-1) inhibition and prevention of thromboxane production, is a well-established therapy in the prevention of ischemic events in the general population with established CAD [44]. Daily aspirin should be used in selected adults 40–70 years of age who are at higher CAD risk but not at increased risk of bleeding [45]. Among athletes, there is an important ongoing debate regarding the role of daily aspirin in low-risk veteran endurance athletes with incidental high coronary artery calcium (CAC) scores [46, 47]. More research is needed to assess the long-term health outcomes of these individuals to delineate whether high CAC scores portend the same prognosis as in the general population. We will address this question in more detail later in the chapter.

Clopidogrel, a thienopyridine, may be used in combination with aspirin as dual antiplatelet therapy (DAPT). Other commonly used thienopyridines for CAD include prasugrel and ticagrelor [48, 49]. DAPT is the standard of care in patients following ACS, as well as after PCI for stable CAD [50, 51]. While DAPT is critical in the secondary prevention of ACS and shorter courses of DAPT may be considered with newer generation drug eluting stents, they increase the risk of bleeding. In athletes, the risk of hemorrhage and major bleeding complications should be mitigated as best as possible with appropriate use of safety measures such as protective headgear. The precise-DAPT calculator is useful to provide a risk assessment of TIMI major and/or minor bleeding with DAPT therapy after stent implantation (http://www.precisedaptscore.com/predapt/webcalculator.html). It is important to note that the benefit of these drugs far outweighs the risk in patients with established CAD, particularly those with a history of ACS or revascularization. Taking into account the longer-term health of the athlete, the choice of stent and duration of DAPT therapy should be a shared decision between athlete and physician.

Hypertension and Antihypertensive Therapy

We refer the reader to Chap. 5 for a more detailed review of this topic. All young athletes diagnosed with hypertension require a detailed history and physical examination with a focus on causes of secondary hypertension, use of nonsteroidal anti-inflammatory drugs and performance enhancing drugs [52]. Laboratory testing should be kept to a minimum but should assess for dyslipidemia, glucose intolerance, diabetes mellitus, and chronic renal disease [52]. In some instances, a work-up for secondary hypertension may be required. According to the AHA/ACC eligibility and disqualification recommendations, all competitive athletes with hypertension should have a lipid profile, fasting serum glucose, electrolytes, and hemoglobin measured; as well as a urinary protein estimated by dipstick [52].

When commencing a medication regimen specific to competitive athletes, it is important to be cognizant of their respective sporting bodies' list of prohibited substances. Angiotensin-converting enzyme inhibitors (ACE-i), angiotensin receptor blockers (ARB), and calcium channel blockers are the preferred choice for blood pressure management in athletes with CAD. ACE-I and ARBs are particularly helpful in those with concomitant diabetes mellitus or LV dysfunction [42, 53, 54]. In addition, low-dose diuretics are often well-tolerated by athletes; however, they should be used with caution prior to endurance events or warm-weather training due to excessive volume depletion. It is important to note that diuretics may mask the presence of other banned substances and are included on The World AntiDoping Agency's (WADA) list of prohibited substances. Similarly, WADA prohibits the use of beta-blockers in-competition for certain sports including golf, archery, and billiards. In addition, beta-blockers may not be as well-tolerated in athletes due to symptoms of fatigue, a decreased maximal heart rate, and occasionally a decrease in maximal exercise capacity. Therefore, a shared decision with the athlete is required before instituting long-term beta-blockade, which improves survival following myocardial infarction [55].

Dyslipidemia and Lipid-Lowering Therapies

Young and veteran athletes are not immune from familial hyperlipidemias and developing dyslipidemias later in life [20]. In turn, screening policies for dyslipidemia should not be modified by virtue of athletic prowess. In those with established CAD, statin therapy is recommended irrespective of low-density lipoprotein cholesterol (LDL-C) levels (Class I, Level of Evidence A) [6, 42]. Statin therapy has pleiotropic effects, including modification and stabilization of coronary plaque, and regression of coronary atherosclerosis in patients with CAD [56–60]. Despite the benefits that statins afford, they are occasionally not well-tolerated by athletes [61]. Further, the combination of statin and exercise produces greater creatine kinase elevations than exercise alone [62, 63]. However, a substantial portion of statin-associated muscle symptoms likely represent nonspecific musculoskeletal pain unrelated to statin use [64]. Therefore, a rigorous approach is required for athletes with suspected statin intolerance and a formal diagnosis requires dechallenge and rechallenge phases to assess for temporal symptom causality. Alternative nonstatin pharmacotherapies include bile acid sequestrants, ezetimibe, and PCSK9 inhibitors [65–67]. However, more studies are required to assess the efficacy of these medications in athletes.

Return to Play After a Coronary Event

The decision as to whether an athlete can return to vigorous exercise after an acute coronary event or revascularization procedure is difficult. According to the ACC/ AHA guidelines, it is reasonable to prohibit athletes from competitive sports participation for at least 3 months after an acute myocardial infarction or coronary revascularization procedure (Class IIb, Level of Evidence C) [6]. Even after the 3-month period, the decision on return to play must be predicated on the ability to tolerate rehabilitation postevent, and detailed risk stratification for event recurrence. Some suggest that 2 years of aggressive lipid lowering therapy is required before a return to competitive sports to allow for optimal myocardial recovery and atherosclerotic plaque stabilization [68].

While competitive sports participation may be dangerous, exercise programs initiated early after myocardial infarction improves neurohormonal processes, preserves cardiac function, and is associated with a reduced mortality post-MI [69, 70]. Exercise programs also improve endothelial function, vascular remodeling, and skeletal muscle fuel utilization which are beneficial for patients with hypertension and diabetes [71, 72]. Cardiac rehabilitation is a valuable tool to not only safely engage athletes in exercise after an event, but also to challenge them in a controlled environment and in turn assess their eligibility for participation in more vigorous activities. Risk stratification for event recurrence should include assessment of resting left ventricular ejection fraction, exercise capacity, degree of exercise-induced ischemia, presence of residual coronary artery stenosis, and success of revascularization procedure [30]. Exercise prescription for the rehabilitation phase may be guided by a six-minute walk test, standard exercise stress test, or ideally by a cardiopulmonary exercise test (CPET). The CPET provides an objective measure of peak oxygen uptake, which may be used as a benchmark to assess the cardiovascular response to a specific training program. Furthermore, the shape of the oxygen-pulse curve, or direct measurement of cardiac output at varying VO2 levels may act as a surrogate marker of ischemia in the appropriate setting. In turn, this can guide nonischemia-inducing work rates for the individual. If the athlete is planning to increase the intensity of training after rehabilitation, repeat cardiopulmonary and exercise ECG testing are important to evaluate the degree of adaptation and cardiovascular remodeling. This repeat assessment also provides critical information regarding future safety of exercise training at greater intensities.

Coronary Artery Calcification in Endurance Athletes

There has been fierce debate regarding the role of exercise in the development of CAC in athletes, and its clinical significance. Coronary CT scans in male veteran marathon runners reveal a greater degree of CAC compared to age- and risk factor-matched controls [73]. A deeper analysis of this study, however, demonstrated that half of the marathon runners were former smokers. Furthermore, of the four individuals with high CAC scores that had ischemic coronary events, three were former smokers, had a history of hypertension, and two had dyslipidemia. The prevalence of these atherosclerotic risk factors clearly blurs the complex relationship between high levels of exercise and coronary artery disease.

When veteran endurance athletes are more rigorously screened for atherosclerotic risk factors, the findings consistently demonstrate a higher burden of CAC and luminal irregularities compared to sedentary controls matched for age and risk factors [74, 75]. Furthermore, in a longitudinal study of eight participants of the Race Across the USA (a 140-day foot race), four runners showed increases in noncalcified plaque volume after the race, all of whom had coronary atherosclerosis at baseline [76]. This increase in plaque volume was not observed in runners without baseline coronary atherosclerosis. These findings highlight the potential for an acceleration of coronary plaque development among vulnerable individuals performing extreme levels of endurance exercise.

While these data provide a strong case-linking CAC to high levels of exercise in male athletes, the clinical significance of increased plaque formation in athletes must be questioned. First, the majority of veteran endurance athletes do not have CAC and, if present, the morphology of coronary artery plaques is predominantly calcific [74, 75]. In nonathletic cohorts, calcific plaque is understood to protect against plaque rupture and coronary events [77, 78]. While it is conceivable that CAC in athletes may represent an increased risk of exercise-induced ischemic events, it is equally plausible that calcific plaque represents the exercise-induced remodeling of previously vulnerable plaque in individuals predisposed to CAD [17]. As multimodality imaging of coronary artery disease continues to improve, it may be possible to gain a deeper insight into the clinical significance of this phenotype in the future.

It is also important to recognize that while CAC is strongly associated with risk of future cardiovascular events [79, 80]; exercise impacts the relationship between CAC and mortality. Among asymptomatic patients with high CAC scores, exercise appears to play a protective role, whereas minimal to no exercise substantially increases mortality risk [81]. In support of this thesis, Radford et al. showed a reduction of 11% reduction in cardiovascular disease events for each additional MET of fitness when adjusting for CAC categories (scores of 0, 1–99, 100–399, and$\geq$400) [82].

Interestingly, no differences in CAC scores are seen between athletic and sedentary females [74], and some data show a lower prevalence of coronary atherosclerosis in female athletes compared with controls [83]. It should be noted, however, that there is a paucity of data on the association between exercise dose and coronary artery disease among female athletes and findings from studies of predominantly male athletes cannot be extrapolated to females [84].

Finally, as our understanding of the etiology of atherogenesis develops, it is possible that in the future we appreciate CAD risk factors that have not been captured by these previous observational studies. For example, psychosocial/emotional stressors, fat and carbohydrate consumption, sleep quality, genetic, proteomic, and metabolomic factors not captured on traditional risk assessments may contribute to the development of atherosclerosis. Of utmost importance, future research should aim to provide longitudinal prospective outcome data to determine the mechanistic relationship between high levels of exercise and clinically relevant CAD.

Summary

The most common cause of exercise-related sudden cardiac death in athletes >35 years old is CAD. While for decades, there have been huge efforts to research atherosclerotic coronary disease in the general population; we have only recently begun to address this disease in the athlete population. Assessing CAD in athletes is increasingly common in sports cardiology practice and is often challenging given the uncertainties in this field. While future research may validate the increasing use of multimodality imaging and wearable technologies to guide management, it is important in today's practice that physicians engage in shared decision making with athletes and are open about the lack of definitive data in this field. Of utmost importance, physicians should be aware that athletes are not immune from this disease and should use traditional risk scores to guide lifestyle and pharmacologic recommendations, as we would do for our nonathletic patients.

References

1. Soares-Miranda L, Siscovick DS, Psaty BM, Longstreth WTJ, Mozaffarian D. Physical activity and risk of coronary heart disease and stroke in older adults: the cardiovascular health study. Circulation. 2016;133:147–55.
2. Powell KE, Thompson PD, Caspersen CJ, Kendrick JS. Physical activity and the incidence of coronary heart disease. Annu Rev Public Health. 1987;8:253–87.
3. Thompson PD, Buchner D, Pina IL, et al. Exercise and physical activity in the prevention and treatment of atherosclerotic cardiovascular disease: a statement from the Council on Clinical Cardiology (Subcommittee on Exercise, Rehabilitation, and Prevention) and the Council on Nutrition, Physical. Circulation. 2003;107:3109–16.
4. Chugh SS, Weiss JB. Sudden cardiac death in the older athlete. J Am Coll Cardiol. 2015;65:493–502.
5. Webner D, DuPrey KM, Drezner JA, Cronholm P, Roberts WO. Sudden cardiac arrest and death in United States marathons. Med Sci Sports Exerc. 2012;44:1843–5.
6. Thompson PD, Myerburg RJ, Levine BD, Udelson JE, Kovacs RJ. Eligibility and disqualification recommendations for competitive athletes with cardiovascular abnormalities: task force 8: coronary artery disease: a scientific statement from the American Heart Association and American College of Cardiology. Circulation. 2015;132:e310–4.
7. Giri S, Thompson PD, Kiernan FJ, Clive J, Fram DB, Mitchel JF, Hirst JA, McKay RG, Waters DD. Clinical and angiographic characteristics of exertion-related acute myocardial infarction. JAMA. 1999;282:1731–6.
8. Mittleman MA, Maclure M, Tofler GH, Sherwood JB, Goldberg RJ, Muller JE. Triggering of acute myocardial infarction by heavy physical exertion. Protection against triggering by regu-

lar exertion. Determinants of Myocardial Infarction Onset Study Investigators. N Engl J Med. 1993;329:1677–83.

9. Siscovick DS, Weiss NS, Fletcher RH, Lasky T. The incidence of primary cardiac arrest during vigorous exercise. N Engl J Med. 1984;311:874–7.

10. Berdowski J, de Beus MF, Blom M, et al. Exercise-related out-of-hospital cardiac arrest in the general population: incidence and prognosis. Eur Heart J. 2013;34:3616–23.

11. Reddy PR, Reinier K, Singh T, Mariani R, Gunson K, Jui J, Chugh SS. Physical activity as a trigger of sudden cardiac arrest: the Oregon Sudden Unexpected Death Study. Int J Cardiol. 2009;131:345–9.

12. Marijon E, Tafflet M, Celermajer DS, et al. Sports-related sudden death in the general population. Circulation. 2011;124:672–81.

13. Landry CH, Allan KS, Connelly KA, Cunningham K, Morrison LJ, Dorian P. Sudden cardiac arrest during participation in competitive sports. N Engl J Med. 2017;377:1943–53.

14. Thompson PD, Funk EJ, Carleton RA, Sturner WQ. Incidence of death during jogging in Rhode Island from 1975 through 1980. JAMA. 1982;247:2535–8.

15. Lepers R, Cattagni T. Do older athletes reach limits in their performance during marathon running? Age (Dordr). 2012;34:773–81.

16. Haskell WL, Lee I-M, Pate RR, Powell KE, Blair SN, Franklin BA, Macera CA, Heath GW, Thompson PD, Bauman A. Physical activity and public health: updated recommendation for adults from the American College of Sports Medicine and the American Heart Association. Circulation. 2007;116:1081–93.

17. Rao P, Hutter AMJ, Baggish AL. The limits of cardiac performance: can too much exercise damage the heart? Am J Med. 2018. https://doi.org/10.1016/j.amjmed.2018.05.037.

18. Selden MA, Helzberg JH, Waeckerle JF, Browne JE, Brewer JH, Monaco ME, Tang F, O'Keefe JH. Cardiometabolic abnormalities in current National Football League players. Am J Cardiol. 2009;103:969–71.

19. Churchill TW, Krishnan S, Weisskopf M, Yates BA, Speizer FE, Kim JH, Nadler LE, Pascual-Leone A, Zafonte R, Baggish AL. Weight gain and health affliction among former National Football League players. Am J Med. 2018;131:1491–8.

20. Miller MA, Croft LB, Belanger AR, Romero-Corral A, Somers VK, Roberts AJ, Goldman ME. Prevalence of metabolic syndrome in retired National Football League players. Am J Cardiol. 2008;101:1281–4.

21. Nguyen VT, Zafonte RD, Chen JT, et al. Mortality among professional American-Style Football players and professional American Baseball Players Mortality among US NFL players and MLB Players Mortality among US NFL players and MLB players. JAMA Netw Open. 2019;2:e194223.

22. Libby P, Pasterkamp G. Requiem for the "vulnerable plaque". Eur Heart J. 2015;36:2984–7.

23. Burke AP, Farb A, Malcom GT, Liang Y, Smialek JE, Virmani R. Plaque rupture and sudden death related to exertion in men with coronary artery disease. JAMA. 1999;281:921–6.

24. Kim JH, Malhotra R, Chiampas G, et al. Cardiac arrest during long-distance running races. N Engl J Med. 2012;366:130–40.

25. Sugiyama T, Yamamoto E, Bryniarski K, Xing L, Lee H, Isobe M, Libby P, Jang I-K. Nonculprit plaque characteristics in patients with acute coronary syndrome caused by plaque erosion vs plaque rupture: a 3-vessel optical coherence tomography study. JAMA Cardiol. 2018;3:207–14.

26. Crea F, Libby P. Acute coronary syndromes: the way forward from mechanisms to precision treatment. Circulation. 2017;136:1155–66.

27. Schwellnus M, Swanevelder S, Derman W, Borjesson M, Schwabe K, Jordaan E. Prerace medical screening and education reduce medical encounters in distance road races: SAFER VIII study in 153 208 race starters. Br J Sports Med. 2019;53:634–9.

28. Thompson PD, Franklin BA, Balady GJ, et al. Exercise and acute cardiovascular events placing the risks into perspective: a scientific statement from the American Heart Association Council on Nutrition, Physical Activity, and Metabolism and the Council on Clinical Cardiology. Circulation. 2007;115:2358–68.

29. Borjesson M, Dellborg M, Niebauer J, et al. Recommendations for participation in leisure time or competitive sports in athletes-patients with coronary artery disease: a position statement from the Sports Cardiology Section of the European Association of Preventive Cardiology (EAPC). Eur Heart J. 2018. https://doi.org/10.1093/eurheartj/ehy408.
30. Parker MW, Thompson PD. Assessment and management of atherosclerosis in the athletic patient. Prog Cardiovasc Dis. 2012;54:416–22.
31. Sytkowski PA, Kannel WB, D'Agostino RB. Changes in risk factors and the decline in mortality from cardiovascular disease. The Framingham Heart Study. N Engl J Med. 1990;322:1635–41.
32. McNutt RA, Ferenchick GS, Kirlin PC, Hamlin NJ. Acute myocardial infarction in a 22-year-old world class weight lifter using anabolic steroids. Am J Cardiol. 1988;62:164.
33. Ferenchick GS, Adelman S. Myocardial infarction associated with anabolic steroid use in a previously healthy 37-year-old weight lifter. Am Heart J. 1992;124:507–8.
34. Tagarakis CV, Bloch W, Hartmann G, Hollmann W, Addicks K. Testosterone-propionate impairs the response of the cardiac capillary bed to exercise. Med Sci Sports Exerc. 2000;32:946–53.
35. Thompson PD, Cullinane EM, Sady SP, Chenevert C, Saritelli AL, Sady MA, Herbert PN. Contrasting effects of testosterone and stanozolol on serum lipoprotein levels. JAMA. 1989;261:1165–8.
36. Baggish AL, Weiner RB, Kanayama G, Hudson JI, Lu MT, Hoffmann U, Pope HGJ. Cardiovascular toxicity of illicit anabolic-androgenic steroid use. Circulation. 2017;135:1991–2002.
37. Lunghetti S, Zaca V, Maffei S, Carrera A, Gaddi R, Diciolla F, Maccherini M, Chiavarelli M, Mondillo S, Favilli R. Cardiogenic shock complicating myocardial infarction in a doped athlete. Acute Card Care. 2009;11:250–1.
38. Gibbons RJ, Balady GJ, Bricker JT, et al. ACC/AHA 2002 guideline update for exercise testing: summary article. A report of the American College of Cardiology/American Heart Association Task Force on Practice Guidelines (Committee to Update the 1997 Exercise Testing Guidelines). J Am Coll Cardiol. 2002;40:1531–40.
39. Mitchell JH, Haskell W, Snell P, Van Camp SP. Task Force 8: classification of sports. J Am Coll Cardiol. 2005;45:1364–7.
40. Mann DL, Zipes DP, Libby P, Bonow RO, Braunwald E. Braunwald's heart disease: a textbook of cardiovascular medicine. In: Elsevier Saunders. Amsterdam, Netherlands; 2015. p. 155–78.
41. Laukkanen JA, Makikallio TH, Rauramaa R, Kiviniemi V, Ronkainen K, Kurl S. Cardiorespiratory fitness is related to the risk of sudden cardiac death: a population-based follow-up study. J Am Coll Cardiol. 2010;56:1476–83.
42. Fihn SD, Gardin JM, Abrams J, et al. 2012 ACCF/AHA/ACP/AATS/PCNA/SCAI/STS Guideline for the diagnosis and management of patients with stable ischemic heart disease: a report of the American College of Cardiology Foundation/American Heart Association Task Force on Practice Guidelines, and the American College of Physicians, American Association for Thoracic Surgery, Preventive Cardiovascular Nurses Association, Society for Cardiovascular Angiography and Interventions, and Society of Thoracic Surgeons. J Am Coll Cardiol. 2012;60:e44–e164.
43. Members TF, Montalescot G, Sechtem U, et al. 2013 ESC guidelines on the management of stable coronary artery disease The Task Force on the management of stable coronary artery disease of the European Society of Cardiology. Eur Heart J. 2013;34:2949–3003.
44. Berger JS, Roncaglioni MC, Avanzini F, Pangrazzi I, Tognoni G, Brown DL. Aspirin for the primary prevention of cardiovascular events in women and men: a sex-specific meta-analysis of randomized controlled trials. JAMA. 2006;295:306–13.
45. Arnett DK, Blumenthal RS, Albert MA, et al. 2019 ACC/AHA guideline on the primary prevention of cardiovascular disease. Circulation. 2019;CIR0000000000000678.
46. Siegel AJ, Noakes TD. Aspirin to prevent sudden cardiac death in athletes with high coronary artery calcium scores. Am J Med. 2018. https://doi.org/10.1016/j.amjmed.2018.09.015.
47. Rao P, Hutter AM, Baggish AL. The reply. Am J Med. 2019; https://doi.org/10.1016/j.amjmed.2018.12.012.

224 P. Rao and D. Shipon

48. Wiviott SD, Braunwald E, McCabe CH, Montalescot G, Ruzyllo W, Gottlieb S, Neumann F-J, Ardissino D, De Servi S, Murphy SA. Prasugrel versus clopidogrel in patients with acute coronary syndromes. N Engl J Med. 2007;357:2001–15.
49. Cannon CP, Harrington RA, James S, et al. Comparison of ticagrelor with clopidogrel in patients with a planned invasive strategy for acute coronary syndromes (PLATO): a randomised double-blind study. Lancet (London, England). 2010;375:283–93.
50. Hamm CW, Bassand J-P, Agewall S, et al. ESC Guidelines for the management of acute coronary syndromes in patients presenting without persistent ST-segment elevation: the Task Force for the management of acute coronary syndromes (ACS) in patients presenting without persistent ST-segment elevatio. Eur Heart J. 2011;32:2999–3054.
51. Yusuf S, Zhao F, Mehta SR, Chrolavicius S, Tognoni G, Fox KK, Clopidogrel in Unstable Angina to Prevent Recurrent Events Trial Investigators. Effects of clopidogrel in addition to aspirin in patients with acute coronary syndromes without. N Engl J Med. 2001;345:494–502.
52. Black HR, Sica D, Ferdinand K, White WB. Eligibility and disqualification recommendations for competitive athletes with cardiovascular abnormalities: task force 6: hypertension: a scientific statement from the American Heart Association and the American College of Cardiology. Circulation. 2015;132:e298–302.
53. Fox KM. Investigators EUtOrocewPiscAd. Efficacy of perindopril in reduction of cardiovascular events among patients with stable coronary artery disease: randomised, double-blind, placebo-controlled, multicentre trial (the EUROPA study). Lancet. 2003;362:782–8.
54. Yusuf S, Sleight P, Pogue J. Effects of an angiotensin-converting-enzyme inhibitor, ramipril, on cardiovascular events in high-risk patients. The Heart Outcomes Prevention Evaluation Study Investigators. Engl J Med. 2000;342:145–53.
55. Gottlieb SS, McCarter RJ, Vogel RA. Effect of beta-blockade on mortality among high-risk and low-risk patients after myocardial infarction. N Engl J Med. 1998;339:489–97.
56. Group SSSS. Randomised trial of cholesterol lowering in 4444 patients with coronary heart disease: the Scandinavian Simvastatin Survival Study (4S). Lancet. 1994;344:1383–9.
57. Sacks FM, Pfeffer MA, Moye LA, et al. The effect of pravastatin on coronary events after myocardial infarction in patients with average cholesterol levels. Cholesterol and Recurrent Events Trial investigators. N Engl J Med. 1996;335:1001–9.
58. LaRosa JC, Grundy SM, Waters DD, Shear C, Barter P, Fruchart J-C, Gotto AM, Greten H, Kastelein JJP, Shepherd J. Intensive lipid lowering with atorvastatin in patients with stable coronary disease. N Engl J Med. 2005;352:1425–35.
59. Nissen SE, Nicholls SJ, Sipahi I, et al. Effect of very high-intensity statin therapy on regression of coronary atherosclerosis: the ASTEROID trial. JAMA. 2006;295:1556–65.
60. Nicholls SJ, Ballantyne CM, Barter PJ, et al. Effect of two intensive statin regimens on progression of coronary disease. N Engl J Med. 2011;365:2078–87.
61. Sinzinger H, O'Grady J. Professional athletes suffering from familial hypercholesterolaemia rarely tolerate statin treatment because of muscular problems. Br J Clin Pharmacol. 2004;57:525–8.
62. Thompson PD, Zmuda JM, Domalik LJ, Zimet RJ, Staggers J, Guyton JR. Lovastatin increases exercise-induced skeletal muscle injury. Metabolism. 1997;46:1206–10.
63. Meador BM, Huey KA. Statin-associated myopathy and its exacerbation with exercise. Muscle Nerve. 2010;42:469–79.
64. Rosenson RS, Baker S, Banach M, et al. Optimizing cholesterol treatment in patients with muscle complaints. J Am Coll Cardiol. 2017;70:1290–301.
65. Moriarty PM, Thompson PD, Cannon CP, et al. Efficacy and safety of alirocumab vs ezetimibe in statin-intolerant patients, with a statin rechallenge arm: the ODYSSEY ALTERNATIVE randomized trial. J Clin Lipidol. 2015;9:758–69.
66. Nissen SE, Stroes E, Dent-Acosta RE, et al. Efficacy and tolerability of evolocumab vs ezetimibe in patients with muscle-related statin intolerance: the GAUSS-3 randomized clinical trial. JAMA. 2016;315:1580–90.
67. Sabatine MS, Giugliano RP, Keech AC, et al. Evolocumab and clinical outcomes in patients with cardiovascular disease. N Engl J Med. 2017;376:1713–22.

68. Fernandez AB, Thompson PD. Exercise training in athletes with heart disease. Prog Cardiovasc Dis. 2017;60:121–9.
69. Wan W, Powers AS, Li J, Zhang JQ, Ji L, Erikson JM. Effect of post–myocardial infarction exercise training on the renin-angiotensin-aldosterone system and cardiac function. Am J Med Sci. 2007;334:265–73.
70. Lawler PR, Filion KB, Eisenberg MJ. Efficacy of exercise-based cardiac rehabilitation post-myocardial infarction: a systematic review and meta-analysis of randomized controlled trials. Am Heart J. 2011;162:571–584.e2.
71. Hambrecht R, Wolf A, Gielen S, Linke A, Hofer J, Erbs S, Schoene N, Schuler G. Effect of exercise on coronary endothelial function in patients with coronary artery disease. N Engl J Med. 2000;342:454–60.
72. Burstein R, Polychronakos C, Toews CJ, MacDougall JD, Guyda HJ, Posner BI. Acute reversal of the enhanced insulin action in trained athletes: association with insulin receptor changes. Diabetes. 1985;34:756–60.
73. Mohlenkamp S, Lehmann N, Breuckmann F, et al. Running: the risk of coronary events : prevalence and prognostic relevance of coronary atherosclerosis in marathon runners. Eur Heart J. 2008;29:1903–10.
74. Merghani A, Maestrini V, Rosmini S, et al. Prevalence of subclinical coronary artery disease in masters endurance athletes with a low atherosclerotic risk profile. Circulation. 2017;136:126–37.
75. Aengevaeren VL, Mosterd A, Braber TL, Prakken NHJ, Doevendans PA, Grobbee DE, Thompson PD, Eijsvogels TMH, Velthuis BK. Relationship between lifelong exercise volume and coronary atherosclerosis in athletes. Circulation. 2017;136:138–48.
76. Lin J, DeLuca JR, Lu MT, Ruehm SG, Dudum R, Choi B, Lieberman DE, Hoffman U, Baggish AL. Extreme endurance exercise and progressive coronary artery disease. J Am Coll Cardiol. 2017;70:293–5.
77. Criqui MH, Denenberg JO, Ix JH, McClelland RL, Wassel CL, Rifkin DE, Carr JJ, Budoff MJ, Allison MA. Calcium density of coronary artery plaque and risk of incident cardiovascular events. JAMA. 2014;311:271–8.
78. Ahmadi N, Nabavi V, Hajsadeghi F, Flores F, French WJ, Mao SS, Shavelle D, Ebrahimi R, Budoff M. Mortality incidence of patients with non-obstructive coronary artery disease diagnosed by computed tomography angiography. Am J Cardiol. 2011;107:10–6.
79. Bamberg F, Sommer WH, Hoffmann V, Achenbach S, Nikolaou K, Conen D, Reiser MF, Hoffmann U, Becker CR. Meta-analysis and systematic review of the long-term predictive value of assessment of coronary atherosclerosis by contrast-enhanced coronary computed tomography angiography. J Am Coll Cardiol. 2011;57:2426–36.
80. Budoff MJ, Mayrhofer T, Ferencik M, et al. Prognostic value of coronary artery calcium in the PROMISE study (prospective multicenter imaging study for evaluation of chest pain). Circulation. 2017;136:1993–2005.
81. Arnson Y, Rozanski A, Gransar H, Hayes SW, Friedman JD, Thomson LEJ, Berman DS. Impact of exercise on the relationship between CAC scores and all-cause mortality. JACC Cardiovasc Imaging. 2017;10:1461–8.
82. Radford NB, DeFina LF, Leonard D, Barlow CE, Willis BL, Gibbons LW, Gilchrist SC, Khera A, Levine BD. Cardiorespiratory fitness, coronary artery calcium, and cardiovascular disease events in a cohort of generally healthy middle-age men: results from the Cooper Center Longitudinal Study. Circulation. 2018;137:1888–95.
83. Roberts WO, Schwartz RS, Kraus SM, et al. Long-term marathon running is associated with low coronary plaque formation in women. Med Sci Sports Exerc. 2017;49:641–5.
84. Aengevaeren VL, Mosterd A, Sharma S, Prakken NHJ, Möhlenkamp S, Thompson PD, Velthuis BK, Eijsvogels TMH. Exercise and coronary atherosclerosis: observations, explanations, relevance, and clinical management. Circulation. 2020;141:1338–50.

Chapter 15
Marfan Syndrome and Other Genetic Aortopathies

Jeffrey S. Hedley and Dermot M. Phelan

Introduction

The adaptive changes in the heart resulting from the hemodynamic stress of regular and intensive exercise have long been recognized and resulted in coining of the term "Athlete's Heart". Less appreciated, however, is the effect that this lifestyle has on the aorta. Factors that induce aortic wall stress, such as chronically elevated blood pressure, result in an increased risk of aortic dilation, aneurysm, and dissection in some individuals. Strength-type sports induce repetitive spikes in blood pressure during muscle contraction while endurance-type sports result in prolonged increases in cardiac output that are translated to the aorta as wall stress. It is perhaps not surprising, therefore, that athletes have slightly larger aortas compared to sedentary controls. This is unlikely to translate to any increased risk for the majority of athletes. However, particular concern is given to those athletes with inherited conditions such as the collagen vascular disorders or a bicuspid aortic valve (BAV), which independently predispose to aortopathy. Therefore, a nuanced understanding of the intimate interplay of baseline predisposition and the hemodynamic stress of exercise is required to care for such athletes.

Despite concerns about the hemodynamic stress of exercise on the aorta, data suggest that acute aortic syndrome (AAD = aortic dissection and rupture for the purposes of this chapter) is a relatively rare cause of sudden cardiac death (SCD) in athletes, accounting for roughly 0–4.6% of cases [1–4].

J. S. Hedley
Department of Cardiovascular Medicine, Section of Cardiac Pacing and Electrophysiology, Cleveland Clinic Foundation, Cleveland, OH, USA
e-mail: hedleyj@ccf.org

D. M. Phelan (✉)
Sports Cardiology Center, Hypertrophic Cardiomyopathy Center, Atrium Health Sanger Heart & Vascular Institute, Charlotte, NC, USA
e-mail: dermot.phelan@atriumhealth.org

© Springer Nature Switzerland AG 2021
D. J. Engel, D. M. Phelan (eds.), *Sports Cardiology*,
https://doi.org/10.1007/978-3-030-69384-8_15

227

Data from the International Registry of Aortic Dissection (IRAD) reveal that the average age of a patient with dissection is 63 years and that hypertension is the most common risk factor for dissection, being present in roughly 75% of patients. However, in those patients under 40 years of age, 59% of patients with AAD had either Marfan Syndrome (MFS) or a bicuspid aortic valve (BAV). Regarding the size of the aorta, the mean aortic diameter at the time of AAD was 5.31 cm, and an aortic diameter of >5.5 cm conveyed a mortality odds ratio of 3.06 [5, 6]. These data help us to focus our evaluation of a young athlete with a dilated aorta and counsel them on surgical timing.

This chapter will focus on the impact of sporting participation on the aorta and the unique aspects of care of the athlete with aortopathy.

The Normal Aorta

Beginning with a bulb-shaped aortic root, the aorta has a candy-cane shape as it ascends in the chest, arches, while giving off branches to the head and arms, and descends through the thorax and abdomen before bifurcating in the pelvis (Fig. 15.1). The aorta is the largest blood vessel in the body. The aortic wall is composed of three layers – the intima, the media, and the adventitia. While the aortic wall has high tensile strength, its properties allow it to be distensible and elastic to allow the aorta to act as both a reservoir and a conduit for the boluses of blood ejected from the heart with each cardiac cycle. The aging aorta progressively loses these elastic

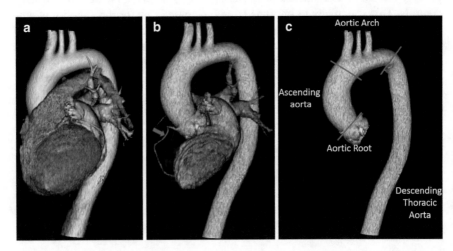

Fig. 15.1 Gated computed tomographic angiogram with 3D volume rendered reconstruction of the thoracic aorta. **Panel 1a** shows the thoracic aorta with full heart in situ. **Panel 1b** shows the same image with removal of the right heart to reveal the aortic root with visualization of the right coronary artery arising from the right coronary cusp (arrow). **Panel 1c** shows the same image with removal of all other structures to define the segments of the thoracic aorta

properties with a resultant increase in pulse pressure and dilation of the aorta. An area of ongoing research is the differential effect of sport type on the elastic properties of the aorta.

Providing normal ranges for the aorta is fraught with challenges. Aortic size is highly dependent on age and body size, in particular height. For example, the upper limit of normal for an 18 year-old female with a body surface area (BSA) of 1.7 m² is 3.3 cm, while the upper limit of normal is 4.2 cm for a 70 year-old man with a BSA of 2.0 m² [7]. Gender and age-specific nomograms for different body sizes are available for the general population but not in the athletic population [8, 9]. Z-scores, which describe the number of standard deviations above or below the predicted mean aortic size, are particularly important when evaluating the pediatric population but have not been adapted for athletic individuals. A Z-score ≥2 is classified as abnormal.

Defining normal ranges of aortic size is also hampered by variability in measurement techniques. Using echocardiography, the aortic root should be measured from a parasternal long-axis view in end-diastole from leading edge-to-leading edge according to ASE guidelines [10] (Fig. 15.2a); using images obtained in systole or different edges will result in different values. The optimal technique using tomographic imaging such as gated computed tomographic angiography (CTA) or cardiac magnetic resonance imaging (CMR) is even less well defined. We recommend following the ASE guidelines which suggest averaging the three sinus to sinus measurements in end-diastole at the level of the Sinus of Valsalva (SoV) plane (Fig. 15.2b) [10]. Asymmetric roots are particularly problematic. The current

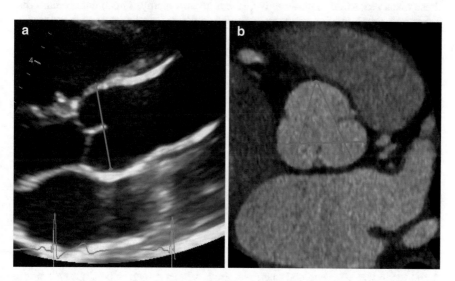

Fig. 15.2 Measurement techniques for the aortic root. **Panel A:** The aortic root is measured from leading edge-to-leading-edge at end-diastole in a parasternal long-axis view on transthoracic echocardiography. **Panel B:** The average of three inner-edge measurements from sinus-to-sinus in end-diastole is recommended for gated computed tomographic angiography. This same method should be employed for cardiac magnetic resonance imaging

American Heart Association/American College of Cardiology (AHH/ACC) eligibility and disqualification recommendations for competitive athletes with cardiovascular disorders suggest reporting the largest diameter that has been measured using the recommended methodologies [11]. We recommend also reporting the aortic cross-sectional area to body height ratio which is strongly predictive of outcomes [12]. Irrespective of the technique used, being consistent in methodology should be a priority, and comparing side-by-side images with prior studies is important when evaluating for progression over time.

Normal Population vs Athletes

Despite the above-mentioned limitations, there are a number of important observations that can be made regarding aortic dimensions in athletes. First, athletes have slightly larger aortas compared to their nonathlete counterparts. In a meta-analysis by Iskandar et al., aortic diameters were larger by 3.2 mm at the aortic root (sinus of Valsalva) compared to sedentary controls [13]. Second, while these data suggest some adaptation of the aorta to the hemodynamic stress of exercise, it is important to note that the aortic measurements in young athletes rarely exceed normal ranges for the general population [13, 14]. In most studies involving athletes, an aortic root size >40 mm in men or >34 mm in women is exceedingly rare, in the order of 0.5–1.8% [13–15]. Therefore, particular attention should be paid to athletes above these observed aortic diameters to rule out an aortopathy. Third, data remain discrepant as to whether strength or endurance training results in greater degrees of aortic enlargement. Strength training does appear to result in increased aortic stiffness while endurance sports increase aortic distensibility; these features may have important implications for the masters' athlete [14, 16–18]. Finally, there appears to be a plateauing of the relationship between aortic dimensions and body size at the extremes of body morphometrics with even the tallest male athletes rarely exceeding an aortic root size of 40 mm as elegantly described by Engel et al. in their study of National Association Basketball players [14, 19].

Masters Athlete

Available data on normal ranges of aortic size in athletes almost exclusively relate to young (<35 years) athletes. There is little data addressing the natural history of aortic dilation in the middle aged and older athletes. Recognizing that the aorta increases in size with age and that the aorta has been shown to be slightly larger in young athletes compared to sedentary controls, the question arises whether the aorta stays on the same age-related growth curve as the general population. Using the example of the 70 year-old man with a BSA of 2.0 m^2, in the normal population, the upper limit of normal indexed to age, gender, and BSA is expected to be 42 mm but if that individual were an athlete whose aorta was 3.2 mm larger as a youth, then perhaps the upper limit of normal for that individual would be ~45.2 mm. One might also anticipate that the athlete who continues to expose the aorta to the same increased hemodynamic stress that resulted in a slightly larger aorta in youth would see greater rates of growth in the aorta. Furthermore, according to the law of LaPlace, even small increases in size of the aorta in youth will translate to greater wall stress on the aorta throughout that athlete's life. A study looking at retired National League Football (NFL) players compared to an age, gender, and racially matched population-based control group from the Dallas Heart Study compared aortic size between the two groups. A significantly higher number of former NFL players had aortic diameters >40 mm (29.6% versus 8.6%; $p < 0.0001$) and even after adjusting for age, race, BSA, systolic blood pressure, history of hypertension, current smoking, diabetes, and lipid profile, the former NFL players were still twice as likely to have a dilated aorta [20]. A more recent study from Churchill et al. examined this question in a broader range of athletes. They examined the aortic size in 442 veteran rowers and runners with a mean age of 61 years and revealed that 24% had at least one Z-score of 2 or more, indicating an ascending aortic measurement >2 standard deviations above the population mean. In this cohort, 21% had an aortic root >40 mm [21]. Whether these data translate to other masters athletes or an increased risk of dissection in this cohort has yet to be defined.

Inherited Etiologies of Aortopathy

Bicuspid Aortic Valve (BAV)

BAV, a common congenital valve defect, is associated with early valve degeneration, manifest as either aortic regurgitation or stenosis in isolation or combined. In young athletes, BAV is usually identified by a murmur auscultated at the time of pre-participation screening, on medical history intake if there is a family history of BAV, or because of symptoms if there is advanced valve disease. Aortic enlargement is present in roughly half of those individuals with BAV, a process that begins in childhood [22, 23]. The prevalence of this valvulopathy in the general population (0.5–2%) is similar to the prevalence seen in trained athletes (0.8–2.5%), and in both populations, an approximate 3:1 male predominance exists [24, 25]. Some cases of BAV are hereditary, often autosomal dominant secondary to mutations in the transcription factor NOTCH1 [26–28]. 9–12% of first-degree family members can be affected; therefore, first-degree relatives should be screened. BAV with a dilated aorta can also be seen in other genetic disorders such as Turner Syndrome (~30%), Loeys-Dietz Syndrome (2.5–17%), and familial thoracic aortic aneurysm syndromes (3%). BAV can also be associated with coarctation of the aorta where the risk of dissection can be higher and treatment strategies and sporting recommendations will differ. Referral to a geneticist and a center of excellence in the treatment of aortopathy should be considered if clinical features of any of these disorders exist or if there is severe aortic enlargement in a younger individual (<35 years).

BAV-associated aortopathy is usually isolated to the aortic root, ascending aorta, and proximal aortic arch. The etiology for aortic enlargement is thought to be related to a combination of hemodynamic stress created by flow as blood ejects through a BAV and defects at a cellular level in the aortic wall itself. Regarding the former, four-dimensional MRI flow analysis has revealed disordered blood flow with exaggerated and sometimes reversed helical flow. The exact nature of the flow derangements depends upon the anatomical subtype of the bicuspid valve [29, 30]. Fusion of the right and left coronary cusps, which is the most common BAV variation (Fig. 15.3), results in dilation of the tubular ascending aorta with some root involvement while fusion of the right and noncoronary cusps affects the distal ascending aorta with relative sparing of the root. On a cellular level, cystic medial necrosis stemming, at least in part, from decreased fibrillin-1 and increased metalloproteinase activity has been described [31–34]. These changes can mimic aortic changes seen in MFS.

The aforementioned changes, and their resultant increase in aortic diameter, place those with BAV at an increased risk of dissection compared with the general population, roughly eight-fold in magnitude [35]. Despite these data, the overall incidence of dissection or rupture in BAV remains low at ~0.4% [36].

There are an estimated eight million young athletes participating in structured sports in the USA [37]. Assuming a prevalence of BAV of 1–2% of the population, there are ~80,000–160,000 young athletes with BAV participating in sports, many with associated aortopathy [38]. The number of athletes who die each year from dissection in the USA is estimated to be between 0.7 and 2.5/year. Based on IRAD data, dissections in those individuals <40 years of age were related to BAV only 9% of the time – the majority of dissections in this age group were related to

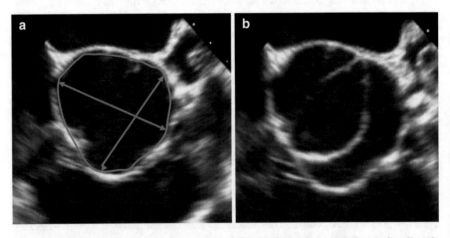

Fig. 15.3 Bicuspid aortic valve with an asymmetric root. Bicuspid aortic valve during diastole (**panel A**) and systole (**panel B**) showing fusion of the right and left coronary cusps and an asymmetric aortic root

MFS. Therefore, BAV-associated aortopathy is common while dissection is rare. When discussing risk of participating in sports with young athletes with BAV and aortopathy, it is important to contextualize this risk.

Both the size of the aorta and the rate of enlargement are validated clinical metrics that assist in the prediction of future adverse events. Wall stress is directly related to aortic size; therefore, the larger the aorta the faster the growth rate. The question arises as to whether participation in sports results in an accelerated growth rate. Boraita et al. utilized a database of 5136 athletes to compare 41 BAV athletes to a control of 41 BAV nonathletes and found no difference in either aortic diameter or annual growth rate [24]. This study reported average growth rates in BAV athletes of 0.04–0.21 mm/year, depending on the aortic segment, which is comparable to the general population. Galanti et al. followed 88 athletes with BAV for 5 years and similarly found aortic growth rates comparable to the general population [25]. Therefore, the limited available data suggests no difference in aortic growth rate between those who participate in athletics and sedentary individuals.

Marfan Syndrome

Marfan Syndrome is a connective tissue disorder due to mutations in the FBN1 gene that encodes fibrillin-1. There have been ~500 mutations identified in this gene, not all associated with the same cardiovascular risk. The condition exhibits autosomal dominant inheritance but can often arise de novo. Fibrillin-1 is a glycoprotein integral to the extracellular matrix, and mutations in this glycoprotein result in connective tissue fragility. This fragility manifests in multiple organ systems, and thus, a scoring system known as the "Systemic Score" is used to aid in the diagnosis of MFS (Table 15.1) [39].

Diagnostic criteria for MFS are summarized in the 2010 Revised Ghent Nosology [39]. When using this diagnostic criterion, an integral starting point in the evaluation of an individual for potential MFS is establishing whether or not there is a family history of confirmed MFS. With a confirmed family history of MFS, the diagnosis is made in presence of any of the following:

- Ectopia Lentis (lens dislocation)
- Systemic score ≥ 7
- Aortic root dilation (Z-score ≥ 2 above 20 years old, ≥3 below 20 years old)

Absent a family history of MFS, the diagnosis is made in presence of the following:

- Aortic root dilation and ectopia lentis.
- Aortic root dilation and FBN1 mutation.
- Aortic root dilation and systemic score ≥ 7.
- Ectopia lentis and an FBN1 mutation with known association with aortic dilation.

Table 15.1 Marfan syndrome systemic score

Feature	Points
Wrist and thumb sign	3
Wrist or thumb sign	1
Pectus carinatum deformity	2
Pectus excavatum or chest asymmetry	1
Hindfoot deformity	2
Plain pes planus	1
Pneumothorax	2
Lumbosacral dural ectasia	2
Protusio acetabuli	2
Reduced upper-segment to lower-segment ratio (<0.85 in white adults; <0.78 in black adults) and increased arm span-to-height ratio (>1.05) and no severe scoliosis	1
Scoliosis or throacolumbar kyphosis	1
Reduced elbow extension	1
Facial features (3 of 5): dolichocephaly, enophthalmos, down slanting palpebral fissures, malar hypoplasia, retrognathia	1
Skin striae	1
Myopia (>3 diopters)	1
Mitral valve prolapse	1

Reprinted with permission from Loeys et al. [39], BMJ Publishing Group, Ltd
Maximum total 20 points: score > 7 indicates systemic involvement

A common manifestation of patients with MFS is tall stature and large wingspan. It is easy to see how this physique is rewarded in sports where height is an advantage. Thus, it is quite possible that MFS may be overrepresented in athletics.

Aortopathy with dissection or rupture is the most serious complication associated with MFS. In fact, 93% of all deaths in patients with MFS are from cardiovascular causes. Of those, 80% were aortic dissection [40]. IRAD data show MFS accounts for 4% of all aortic dissections and 21.5% of recurrent cases of dissection. In patients <40 years old, MFS accounted for ~50% of dissections [41].

Other Inherited Aortopathies

Loeys-Dietz Syndrome (LDS) is an autosomal dominant connective tissue disorder similar to MFS in pathophysiology. Derangements in transforming growth factor beta (TGFβ) signaling are known to contribute to MFS. LDS is caused by mutations in genes encoding TGFβ receptors (TGFBR1 and TGFBR2) as well as SMAD3, a TGFβ transcription modulator. Characteristic phenotypic findings of LDS consist of hypertelorism, cleft palate, bifid uvula, and craniosynostosis. Aortic aneurysmal disease is the most common cardiovascular manifestation of LDS and aortic dissection is the most dreaded complication. These dissections in LDS often occur at a young age and classically involve the sinuses of Valsalva.

Table 15.2 Most common genetic aortopathies with implicated genes and clinical manifestations

Inherited condition	Implicated gene	Clinical features
Marfan syndrome (MFS)	FBN1	Aneurysm of the aortic root, dilatation of the pulmonary artery, and aortic dissection
Ehlers-Danlos syndrome (EDS)	COL5A1, COL5A2, and COL3A1	Arterial mid-sized rupture, specially involving thoracic vasculature
Loeys-Dietz syndrome (LDS)	TGFBR1, TGFBR2, SMAD3, TGFB2, TGFB3	Premature and aggressive aneurysm and dissection; aneurysm may involve aortic segments other than the root
Familial aortic aneurysm and/or dissection syndromes (FAAD)	TGFBR2, MYH11, PRKG1, MYLK, ACTA2	Thoracic aortic aneurysm and dissection; associated vascular disease (e.g., patent ductus arteriosus)
Bicuspid aortic valve (BAV)	Unknown (may be associated with ACTA2, MYH11, syndromic connective tissue diseases)	Aortic dilation typically involving the aortic root and ascending aorta
Autosomal dominant polycystic kidney disease (ADPKD)	PKD1 and PKD2	Dilatation of the aortic root and dissection of the thoracic aorta
Turner syndrome	45,X	Thoracic aortic aneurysms and dissections, bicuspid aortic valve, aortic coarctation

Reprinted from Cury et al. [58], Hindawi (https://creativecommons.org/licenses/by/3.0/)

Familial thoracic aortic aneurysm and dissection (FTAAD) is yet another autosomal dominant condition predisposing to aortic enlargement and dissection. TGFBR1, TGFBR2, and SMAD3 are once again implicated, but mutations in several other genes have also been described such as ACTA2 and MYH11.

Vascular Ehlers Danlos syndrome Type IV (vEDS) is a particularly aggressive autosomal dominant disorder leading to arterial aneurysms and rupture. It is reported that 80% of patients with vEDS will experience a complication by the age of 40 [42]. The condition results from mutations in the COL3A1 gene which encodes type III procollagen.

A summary of the most common genetic aortopathies, implicated genes, and clinical manifestations is shown in Table 15.2.

Management of Aortic Diseases in Athletes

Screening and Monitoring

Dilation of the thoracic aorta is generally asymptomatic, and diagnosis requires imaging of the aorta. Widespread screening for aortopathy is generally regarded as impractical at this time due to the cost of imaging, lack of expertise, relative low incidence of disease, and false-negative results due to lack of visualization of the entire aorta with echocardiography. Rather, the impetus for screening an athlete must derive from a careful history and physical exam. Transthoracic echocardiogram should be obtained as a screening exam for aortopathy in each of the following scenarios:

- A known family history of aortopathy or predisposing familial conditions.
- Recognition of phenotypic characteristics consistent with a systemic connective tissue disorder associated with aortopathy.
- Auscultation of murmurs or extra heart sounds suggestive of either BAV (opening snap or murmur of aortic stenosis or regurgitation) or mitral valve prolapse which can be seen in connective tissue disorders associated with aortopathy.

If an aortopathy is discovered in a young athlete, then screening of first-degree relatives is advised and genetic testing may be considered. Frequency of surveillance imaging does depend on the underlying etiology, size of the aorta, and duration of documented stability, but screening is generally recommended every 6–12 months for active athletes.

Medical Management

Most evidence to date regarding medical interventions for the management of thoracic aortic dilation stems from research on either mouse models of thoracic aortic aneurysm or on humans with MFS. There is no research on medical management of a dilated aorta in athletic populations. Thus, guidance almost universally reflects extrapolation and expert opinion.

Traditionally, beta-blockers have been the cornerstone of medical management for patients with aortopathy. This treatment is grounded in several lines of evidence. First, beta-blockers are a mainstay of management of acute aortic syndromes as they reduce left ventricular contractility and the resultant shear stress in the aorta. Additionally, trials utilizing propranolol and atenolol seemed to show decreased rate of aortic growth in pediatric patients with MFS when compared with placebo [43]. However, two recent meta-analyses have challenged this age-old assertion. Both analyses found that, while rate of growth may decrease, rate of aortic dissection and final aortic diameter were unchanged [44, 45].

Angiotensin receptor blockers (ARBs) have also been shown to reduce the rate of aortic growth in patients with MFS [46, 47]. This approach appears to have firm physiologic rationale given that ARBs have been shown to decrease TGFβ levels [48, 49] which, as previously described, is involved in the aberrant TGFβ signaling seen in many genetic aortopathies. By extension, and through additional dedicated trials, angiotensin converting enzyme inhibitors (ACEi) have also entered the armamentarium [50].

Current ACC guideline recommendations suggest using beta-blockers, angiotensin receptor blockers, or ACE-Inhibitors to achieve the lowest tolerated blood pressure without adverse side effects – ideally with systolic blood pressure in the 105–120 mmHg range (Class IIa, Level of evidence: B) [51]. In addition, lipid profile optimization and smoking cessation are also strongly advocated. Statins in particular have been linked to reduced aortic growth and should be considered [52].

Surgical Management

Indications for elective surgical repair depend largely on three factors: underlying etiology and dissection risk, maximum aortic diameter, and rate of growth. The following are Class I recommendations with a level of evidence C and apply to all patients with ascending thoracic aortic aneurysms:

- Elective aortic repair/replacement should be performed for all suitable candidates with an aortic diameter ≥5.5 cm.
- Elective aortic repair/replacement should be performed for all suitable candidates if there is a rapid rate of growth (>5 mm/year).
- Patients with an aortic diameter >4.5 cm undergoing cardiac surgery for other reasons should have concomitant repair/replacement performed.

Thresholds for surgical replacement for patients with BAV have been controversial with major differences between guidelines published in 2010 and subsequently in 2014 [53]. A statement of clarification was published in 2016 which gave a Class I recommendation for surgery if the ascending aorta was ≥5.5 cm and a Class IIa recommendation if the aorta is ≥5.0 cm with an additional risk factor (including a family history of dissection or a growth rate of ≥0.5 cm) [54].

For patients with genetically mediated thoracic aortic aneurysm such as MFS, LDS, vEDS, and Turner syndrome, the surgical thresholds are generally lower (4–5 cm). The threshold does depend on the underlying condition and concomitant clinical factors. If patients with a genetic condition have an aortic area to body height ratio >10 cm/m^2, there is a IIa (Level of Evidence C) recommendation for aortic surgery. This recommendation stems from research indicating that risk stratification is improved when aortic measurements are indexed for height [12].

Considerations for the Athlete with Aortopathy

Exercise Guidance in the Athlete with Aortopathy

There are little data to guide exercise training in athletes with aortopathy. Recommendations must be individualized to the specific athlete and should be based on the demands of their training and competition, their individual blood pressure response to these demands, and the risk of bodily collision. In general, aerobic exercise leads to modest increases in mean arterial pressure (MAP), but systolic and diastolic blood pressure and MAP increase dramatically and rapidly with resistance exercise (isotonic and isometric) [55]. The extent of the increase correlates with the relative intensity of the exercise, technique used (Valsalva) as well as the level of fatigue (MAP rise is greatest for the last 2–3 reps prior to fatigue). We feel that no absolute "cut-off" weight restriction for athletes with aortopathy can or should be promoted. Furthermore, the data supporting commonly espoused weightlifting restrictions are not available. There are some data to support a restriction to half of the patient's lean body weight, but even this restriction would elicit discrepant MAP responses for a variety of weightlifting maneuvers (i.e. lateral abduction of the arm vs. seated leg press).

There are reports of astoundingly high blood pressure recordings (as high as 400 mmHg systolic) with low repetitions of maximum weights using large muscle groups [55]. These findings have prompted physicians to counsel patients with aortopathy to avoid heavy lifting with Valsalva; however, this advice is controversial. In concert with systolic blood pressure, the effect of Valsalva must also be considered. Haykowsky et al. first described this intriguing interplay [56]. Five healthy volunteers performed submaximal and maximal leg press exercises with simultaneous monitoring of both intravascular and intrathoracic pressures. Aortic transmural pressure is equal to intravascular pressure minus extravascular (intrathoracic) pressure. With leg press and brief Valsalva, the intrathoracic pressure increased from an average of 1.7 mmHg to roughly 112 mmHg. The left ventricular end-systolic pressure increased from 120 to 255 mmHg. Therefore, the aortic transmural pressure (intraventricular end-systolic pressure minus intrathoracic pressure) was ~120 mmHg at rest and ~ 143 mmHg when lifting with Valsalva. Consequently, there was no substantial increase in aortic transmural wall stress despite the dramatically elevated systolic blood pressure [56]. Not only is more research required, but the classic advice of Valsalva avoidance may be misguided and we must consider the heart–lung interaction when considering aortic wall stress.

Sport Participation Guidelines

Aortic dissection or rupture occurs when hemodynamic forces exceed the strength of the degenerating aortic wall. The two primary aims when considering restriction from sports participation are: (1) avoidance of precipitating an acute aortic syndrome/SCD, and (2) prevent acceleration of aortic enlargement. The most recent guidelines can be found in the 2015 Eligibility and Disqualification for Competitive Athletes with Cardiovascular Abnormalities championed by the American Heart Association and the American College of Cardiology [57]. These guidelines are summarized below and in Table 15.3.

Athletes with mildly enlarged aortic dimensions but no known history of genetic aortopathy or causal valvular disease should undergo a comprehensive assessment to assess for an underlying connective tissue or cardiovascular disorder. If no such

Table 15.3 Sport participation guidelines for athletes with aortopathies

Condition	Frequency of imaging monitoring	Clinical scenario of aortic root diameter	Eligibility and disqualification recommendations
MFS	Every 6–12 mos.	All	Avoid bodily collision
		Normal aorta—no risk factors[a]	IA/IIA permitted
		+ Risk factors	Avoid all competitive sports
BAV	No specific recommendation	Normal aorta	All sports permitted
	Every 6–12 mos.	Men: 40–42 mm; women: 36–39 mm; Z-score: 2–3.5	IA-C; IIA-C permitted. Avoid bodily collision. Avoid intense weight training
		40–45 mm	IA sports permitted. Avoid bodily collision
		>45 mm	Avoid all competitive sports
Other familial/ genetic aortopathies (LDS vEDS, FTAAD)	Every 6–12 mos.	FTAAD—normal aorta and no risk factors[b]	IA permitted. Avoid bodily collision
		LDS or vEDS – Normal Aorta & No Risk Factors[c]	IA permitted
Unexplained aortic dilation	Every 6–12 mos.	Men: 40–41 mm; women: 35–37 mm	All sports permitted after thorough evaluation. Avoid intense weight training
Successful surgical correction	Every 6–12 mos.	No remaining dilation	IA permitted. Avoid bodily collision
Chronic dissection	No specific recommendation	All	Avoid all competitive sports

Reprinted with permission from Hedley and Phelan [59], Springer Nature
Abbreviations: *MFS* Marfan syndrome, *BAV* bicuspid aortic valve, *LDS* Loeys-Dietz syndrome, *vEDS* vascular Ehlers-Danlos syndrome, *FTAAD* familial thoracic aorta aneurysm and dissection
[a]MFS risk factors: aortic root dilatation (>40 mm in adults or Z-score > 2 in adolescents <15 years old); moderate to severe mitral regurgitation: left ventricular ejection fraction <40%; family history of aortic dissection at aortic diameter less than 50 mm
[b]FTAAD risk factors: aortic root dilatation (>40 mm in adults or Z-score > 2 in adolescents <15 years old); moderate to severe mitral regurgitation; family history of aortic dissection; cerebrovascular disease; branch vessel aneurysm or dissection
[c]LDS/vEDS risk factors: aortic enlargement (Z-score >2) or dissection, or branch vessel enlargement; moderate to severe mitral regurgitation; extracardiac organ system involvement that makes participation hazardous

etiology is discovered, these athletes can freely participate in all sports, save for intense weight training. Athletes with BAV but normal aortic dimensions can also freely participate in all sports.

On the opposite end of the spectrum are those athletes with not only known aortic disease, but also high-risk features. Athletes with chronic aortic or branch vessel aneurysm and/or dissection, and athletes with BAV and aortic size >45 mm, are recommended not to participate in any competitive sports. Once the dissection or aneurysm has been surgically addressed (assuming no residual pathology remains), athletes can reasonably resume participation in IA athletics which do not involve bodily collision. It should be noted that some high-profile professional athletes have returned to competition after surgery but these decisions must be individualized and are against current guideline recommendations. Also considered high risk are athletes with MFS and certain risk factors. These risk factors are: aortic root dilatation (>40 mm in adults or Z-score >2 in adolescents <15 years old), moderate to severe mitral regurgitation, left ventricular ejection fraction <40%, and family history of aortic dissection at aortic diameter less than 50 mm. It is recommended that athletes with MFS and risk factors avoid all competitive sports.

More difficult is the discussion pertaining to those athletes who are neither very high nor low risk. Athletes with BAV and aortic dimensions which are no longer normal but <45 mm can participate in IA-C and IIA-C sports but are recommended to avoid intense weight training. Athletes with MFS but lacking risk factors can participate in IA and IIa sports, but all athletes with MFS should avoid any sport with potential for bodily collision. Lastly are those athletes with either LDS, vEDS, FTAAD, or an otherwise unexplained TAA. These athletes can reasonably participate in IA and IIA sports. However, if such athletes possess certain high-risk features, they should also avoid sports with bodily collision. For FTAAD, these risk factors include: aortic root dilatation (>40 mm in adults or Z-score > 2 in adolescents <15 years old), moderate to severe mitral regurgitation, left ventricular ejection fraction <40%, and family history of aortic dissection, cerebrovascular disease, branch vessel aneurysm, or dissection. Risk factors for LDS and vEDS include: aortic enlargement (Z-score > 2) or dissection, branch vessel enlargement, moderate to severe mitral regurgitation, and extracardiac organ system involvement that makes participation hazardous.

As with all guidance provided to athletes, these recommendations are largely based on expert opinion and require individual consideration and shared decision-making.

Conclusion

When performing pre-participation cardiac evaluations of athletes, aortic diseases need to be considered in the spectrum of cardiovascular disorders that have the potential to place an athlete at risk for an exercise-triggered emergency. Clinical assessments for conditions associated with aortic enlargement, such as a bicuspid aortic valve or a connective tissue disorder, are required to identify an athlete that could have an aortopathy. It is essential to be familiar with normative data for aortic diameters in athletic and nonathletic populations when performing and reviewing aortic imaging tests in athletes. Given the relative paucity of prospective data on athletes with aortopathy, recommendations for sport participation for athletes with aortic diseases should be aligned with current AHA/ACC guidelines, and individualized decisions utilizing shared decision-making are required for those athletes who do not have high-risk features.

References

1. Chandra N, Bastiaenen R, Papadakis M, Sharma S. Sudden cardiac death in young athletes: practical challenges and diagnostic dilemmas. J Am Coll Cardiol. 2013;61(10):1027–40.
2. Finocchiaro G, Papadakis M, Robertus JL, et al. Etiology of sudden death in sports: insights from a United Kingdom regional registry. J Am Coll Cardiol. 2016;67(18):2108–15.
3. Maron BJ. Sudden death in young athletes. N Engl J Med. 2003;349(11):1064–75.
4. Maron BJ, Haas TS, Murphy CJ, Ahluwalia A, Rutten-Ramos S. Incidence and causes of sudden death in U.S. college athletes. J Am Coll Cardiol. 2014;63(16):1636–43.
5. Evangelista A, Maldonado G, Gruosso D, Teixido G, Rodriguez-Palomares J, Eagle K. Insights from the international registry of acute aortic dissection. Glob Cardiol Sci Pract. 2016;2016(1):e201608.
6. Pape LA, Awais M, Woznicki EM, et al. Presentation, diagnosis, and outcomes of acute aortic dissection: 17-year trends from the international registry of acute aortic dissection. J Am Coll Cardiol. 2015;66(4):350–8.
7. Devereux RB, de Simone G, Arnett DK, et al. Normal limits in relation to age, body size and gender of two-dimensional echocardiographic aortic root dimensions in persons >/=15 years of age. Am J Cardiol. 2012;110(8):1189–94.
8. Campens L, Demulier L, De Groote K, et al. Reference values for echocardiographic assessment of the diameter of the aortic root and ascending aorta spanning all age categories. Am J Cardiol. 2014;114(6):914–20.
9. Roman MJ, Devereux RB, Kramer-Fox R, O'Loughlin J. Two-dimensional echocardiographic aortic root dimensions in normal children and adults. Am J Cardiol. 1989;64(8):507–12.
10. Goldstein SA, Evangelista A, Abbara S, et al. Multimodality imaging of diseases of the thoracic aorta in adults: from the American Society of Echocardiography and the European Association of Cardiovascular Imaging: endorsed by the Society of Cardiovascular Computed Tomography and Society for Cardiovascular Magnetic Resonance. J Am Soc Echocardiogr. 2015;28(2):119–82.
11. Braverman AC, Harris KM, Kovacs RJ, Maron BJ. Eligibility and disqualification recommendations for competitive athletes with cardiovascular abnormalities: task force 7: aortic diseases, including Marfan syndrome: a scientific statement from the American Heart Association and American College of Cardiology. Circulation. 2015;132(22):e303–9.
12. Masri A, Kalahasti V, Svensson LG, et al. Aortic cross-sectional area/height ratio and outcomes in patients with a trileaflet aortic valve and a dilated aorta. Circulation. 2016;134(22):1724–37.
13. Iskandar A, Thompson PD. A meta-analysis of aortic root size in elite athletes. Circulation. 2013;127(7):791–8.
14. Boraita A, Heras ME, Morales F, et al. Reference values of aortic root in male and female white elite athletes according to sport. Circ Cardiovasc Imaging. 2016;9(10).
15. Pelliccia A, Di Paolo FM, Quattrini FM. Aortic root dilatation in athletic population. Prog Cardiovasc Dis. 2012;54(5):432–7.
16. D'Andrea A, Cocchia R, Riegler L, et al. Aortic stiffness and distensibility in top-level athletes. J Am Soc Echocardiogr. 2012;25(5):561–7.
17. D'Andrea A, Cocchia R, Riegler L, et al. Aortic root dimensions in elite athletes. Am J Cardiol. 2010;105(11):1629–34.
18. Kasikcioglu E, Kayserilioglu A, Oflaz H, Akhan H. Aortic distensibility and left ventricular diastolic functions in endurance athletes. Int J Sports Med. 2005;26(3):165–70.
19. Engel DJ, Schwartz A, Homma S. Athletic cardiac remodeling in US professional basketball players. JAMA Cardiol. 2016;1(1):80–7.
20. Gentry JL 3rd, Carruthers D, Joshi PH, et al. Ascending aortic dimensions in former National Football League athletes. Circ Cardiovasc Imaging. 2017;10(11):e006852.
21. Churchill TW, Groezinger E, Kim JH, et al. Association of ascending aortic dilatation and long-term endurance exercise among older masters-level athletes. JAMA Cardiol. 2020;5:522.
22. Siu SC, Silversides CK. Bicuspid aortic valve disease. J Am Coll Cardiol. 2010;55(25):2789–800.

23. Beroukhim RS, Kruzick TL, Taylor AL, Gao D, Yetman AT. Progression of aortic dilation in children with a functionally normal bicuspid aortic valve. Am J Cardiol. 2006;98(6):828–30.
24. Boraita A, Morales-Acuna F, Marina-Breysse M, et al. Bicuspid aortic valve behaviour in elite athletes. Eur Heart J Cardiovasc Imaging. 2019;20(7):772–80.
25. Galanti G, Stefani L, Toncelli L, Vono MC, Mercuri R, Maffulli N. Effects of sports activity in athletes with bicuspid aortic valve and mild aortic regurgitation. Br J Sports Med. 2010;44(4):275–9.
26. Huntington K, Hunter AG, Chan KL. A prospective study to assess the frequency of familial clustering of congenital bicuspid aortic valve. J Am Coll Cardiol. 1997;30(7):1809–12.
27. Clementi M, Notari L, Borghi A, Tenconi R. Familial congenital bicuspid aortic valve: a disorder of uncertain inheritance. Am J Med Genet. 1996;62(4):336–8.
28. Garg V, Muth AN, Ransom JF, et al. Mutations in NOTCH1 cause aortic valve disease. Nature. 2005;437(7056):270–4.
29. Bissell MM, Hess AT, Biasiolli L, et al. Aortic dilation in bicuspid aortic valve disease: flow pattern is a major contributor and differs with valve fusion type. Circ Cardiovasc Imaging. 2013;6(4):499–507.
30. Hope MD, Hope TA, Meadows AK, et al. Bicuspid aortic valve: four-dimensional MR evaluation of ascending aortic systolic flow patterns. Radiology. 2010;255(1):53–61.
31. Boyum J, Fellinger EK, Schmoker JD, et al. Matrix metalloproteinase activity in thoracic aortic aneurysms associated with bicuspid and tricuspid aortic valves. J Thorac Cardiovasc Surg. 2004;127(3):686–91.
32. Fedak PW, de Sa MP, Verma S, et al. Vascular matrix remodeling in patients with bicuspid aortic valve malformations: implications for aortic dilatation. J Thorac Cardiovasc Surg. 2003;126(3):797–806.
33. Fedak PW, Verma S, David TE, Leask RL, Weisel RD, Butany J. Clinical and pathophysiological implications of a bicuspid aortic valve. Circulation. 2002;106(8):900–4.
34. Ikonomidis JS, Jones JA, Barbour JR, et al. Expression of matrix metalloproteinases and endogenous inhibitors within ascending aortic aneurysms of patients with bicuspid or tricuspid aortic valves. J Thorac Cardiovasc Surg. 2007;133(4):1028–36.
35. Michelena HI, Della Corte A, Prakash SK, Milewicz DM, Evangelista A, Enriquez-Sarano M. Bicuspid aortic valve aortopathy in adults: incidence, etiology, and clinical significance. Int J Cardiol. 2015;201:400–7.
36. Masri A, Svensson LG, Griffin BP, Desai MY. Contemporary natural history of bicuspid aortic valve disease: a systematic review. Heart. 2017;103(17):1323–30.
37. National Federation of State High School Associations. http://www.nfhs.org/content.aspx?id¼43282. Accessed 8 Dec 2013.
38. National Collegiate Athletic Association. Latest news: participation rates continue to rise. http://www.ncaapublications.com/productdownloads/PR2014.pdf. Accessed.
39. Loeys BL, Dietz HC, Braverman AC, et al. The revised Ghent nosology for the Marfan syndrome. J Med Genet. 2010;47(7):476–85.
40. Murdoch JL, Walker BA, Halpern BL, Kuzma JW, McKusick VA. Life expectancy and causes of death in the Marfan syndrome. N Engl J Med. 1972;286(15):804–8.
41. Isselbacher EM, Bonaca MP, Di Eusanio M, et al. Recurrent aortic dissection: observations from the international registry of aortic dissection. Circulation. 2016;134(14):1013–24.
42. Pepin M, Schwarze U, Superti-Furga A, Byers PH. Clinical and genetic features of Ehlers-Danlos syndrome type IV, the vascular type. N Engl J Med. 2000;342(10):673–80.
43. Shores J, Berger KR, Murphy EA, Pyeritz RE. Progression of aortic dilatation and the benefit of long-term beta-adrenergic blockade in Marfan's syndrome. N Engl J Med. 1994;330(19):1335–41.
44. Koo HK, Lawrence KA, Musini VM. Beta-blockers for preventing aortic dissection in Marfan syndrome. Cochrane Database Syst Rev. 2017;11:CD011103.
45. Krishnamoorthy P. Effect of beta-blockers on progressive aortic dilatation in patients with Marfan's syndrome. J Am Coll Cardiol. 2015;65(10 Suppl):62106–62104.

46. Brooke BS, Habashi JP, Judge DP, Patel N, Loeys B, Dietz HC 3rd. Angiotensin II blockade and aortic-root dilation in Marfan's syndrome. N Engl J Med. 2008;358(26):2787–95.
47. Teixido-Tura G, Forteza A, Rodriguez-Palomares J, et al. Losartan versus atenolol for prevention of aortic dilation in patients with Marfan syndrome. J Am Coll Cardiol. 2018;72(14):1613–8.
48. el-Agroudy AE, Hassan NA, Foda MA, et al. Effect of angiotensin II receptor blocker on plasma levels of TGF-beta 1 and interstitial fibrosis in hypertensive kidney transplant patients. Am J Nephrol. 2003;23(5):300–6.
49. Nataatmadja M, West J, Prabowo S, West M. Angiotensin II receptor antagonism reduces transforming growth factor Beta and SMAD signaling in thoracic aortic aneurysm. Ochsner J. 2013;13(1):42–8.
50. Ahimastos AA, Aggarwal A, D'Orsa KM, et al. Effect of perindopril on large artery stiffness and aortic root diameter in patients with Marfan syndrome: a randomized controlled trial. JAMA. 2007;298(13):1539–47.
51. Hiratzka LF, Bakris GL, Beckman JA, et al. 2010 ACCF/AHA/AATS/ACR/ASA/SCA/SCAI/SIR/STS/SVM guidelines for the diagnosis and management of patients with thoracic aortic disease. A Report of the American College of Cardiology Foundation/American Heart Association Task Force on Practice Guidelines, American Association for Thoracic Surgery, American College of Radiology, American Stroke Association, Society of Cardiovascular Anesthesiologists, Society for Cardiovascular Angiography and Interventions, Society of Interventional Radiology, Society of Thoracic Surgeons, and Society for Vascular Medicine. J Am Coll Cardiol. 2010;55(14):e27–e129.
52. Salata K, Syed M, Hussain MA, et al. Statins reduce abdominal aortic aneurysm growth, rupture, and perioperative mortality: a systematic review and meta-analysis. J Am Heart Assoc. 2018;7(19):e008657.
53. Nishimura RA, Otto CM, Bonow RO, et al. 2014 AHA/ACC guideline for the management of patients with valvular heart disease: a report of the American College of Cardiology/American Heart Association Task Force on Practice Guidelines. J Am Coll Cardiol. 2014;63(22):e57–185.
54. Hiratzka LF, Creager MA, Isselbacher EM, et al. Surgery for aortic dilatation in patients with bicuspid aortic valves: a statement of clarification from the American College of Cardiology/American Heart Association Task Force on Clinical Practice Guidelines. Circulation. 2016;133(7):680–6.
55. Mayerick C, Carre F, Elefteriades J. Aortic dissection and sport: physiologic and clinical understanding provide an opportunity to save young lives. J Cardiovasc Surg. 2010;51(5):669–81.
56. Haykowsky M, Taylor D, Teo K, Quinney A, Humen D. Left ventricular wall stress during leg-press exercise performed with a brief Valsalva maneuver. Chest. 2001;119(1):150–4.
57. Braverman AC, Harris KM, Kovacs RJ, Maron BJ. Eligibility and disqualification recommendations for competitive athletes with cardiovascular abnormalities: task force 7: aortic diseases, including Marfan syndrome: a scientific statement from the American Heart Association and American College of Cardiology. J Am Coll Cardiol. 2015;66(21):2398–405.
58. Cury M, Zeidan F, Lobato A. Aortic disease in the young: genetic aneurysm syndromes, connective tissue disorders, and familial aortic aneurysms and dissections. Int J Vasc Med. 2013;2013:267215.
59. Hedley JS, Phelan D. Athletes and the aorta: normal adaptations and the diagnosis and management of pathology. Curr Treat Options Cardio Med. 2017;19:88.

Chapter 16
Congenital Heart Disease: Approach to Evaluation, Management, and Physical Activity

Silvana Molossi and Hitesh Agrawal

Introduction

Congenital heart disease (CHD) consists of a spectrum of abnormalities with varying severity, progression, and hemodynamic consequence. CHD affects an estimated 0.8–1% of live-births. Specific congenital diseases, based on the pathophysiology and degree of hemodynamic compromise, can predispose to various cardiac problems including heart failure, arrhythmias, myocardial ischemia, and vascular compromise. The altered physiology inherent in many forms of CHD will affect the heart's ability to compensate for the increased work and demand that is required for vigorous physical activity and intensive exercise, and as such, all patients with CHD require a pre-participation medical evaluation prior to engaging in competitive sports. The type of sport and the intended degree of intensity must be factored into decision-making regarding sports participation for patients with CHD. The dynamic and static components of exercise place differential loads on the heart. High-intensity dynamic exercise elicits a large increase in heart rate and stroke volume causing a volume load on the left ventricle, while high-intensity static exercise elicits a significant increase in arterial pressure and wall stress on the left ventricle causing a pressure load [1]. Risk of impact in a given sport is another factor to consider as some CHDs require patients to be on antiplatelet/anticoagulant drugs. It is crucial to incorporate the patient's anatomy in the context of the desired

S. Molossi (✉)
Department of Pediatric Cardiology, Texas Children's Hospital, Baylor College of Medicine, Houston, TX, USA
e-mail: smolossi@bcm.edu

H. Agrawal
Pediatric Interventional Cardiology, Le Bonheur Children's Hospital, The University of Tennessee Health Science Center, St Jude Children's Research Hospital, Memphis, TN, USA

Department of Pediatric Cardiology, University of Texas, Austin, TX, USA
e-mail: hagrawal@uthsc.edu

© Springer Nature Switzerland AG 2021
D. J. Engel, D. M. Phelan (eds.), *Sports Cardiology*,
https://doi.org/10.1007/978-3-030-69384-8_16

physical activity to help determine the specific diagnostic investigations needed to thoroughly assess patients and their risk for sports participation. Commonly used tests in CHD patients to define precise anatomy and functional status include electrocardiogram (ECG), echocardiogram (TTE), exercise stress test (EST), cardiac magnetic resonance imaging (CMR), and computed tomographic angiography (CTA). Patients with CHD ultimately require a multidisciplinary, individualized, and shared decision-making approach for evaluation and management, and for recommendations regarding sports participation. This chapter will review the most common forms of structural CHD (congenital valvular heart disease is reviewed in chapters 6 and 15) and congenital coronary artery anomalies, with emphasis on pathophysiology, diagnostic evaluation and management, and recommendations for sport participation.

Common Congenital Defects and Recommendations for Sports Participation

Atrial Septal Defect (ASD)

Anatomy/Physiology

ASD is a deficiency in the atrial septum leading to blood flow between the atrial chambers. The direction and amount of shunting between atria is determined by the downstream resistance and the size of the defect. ASDs generally lead to left-to-right shunting that causes an increase in pulmonary blood flow and reduction in cardiac output. In the long term, increased pulmonary blood flow can cause pulmonary congestion which is responsible for associated symptoms such as shortness of breath and easy fatigability. Hemodynamically significant ASDs should be closed. Hemodynamic significance is defined by the presence of right ventricular volume overload, right ventricular systolic dysfunction, and/or elevation of right-sided pressures as a consequence of left-to-right atrial level shunting [2].

Surgical/Interventional Repair

Small (<5 mm in diameter) and medium-sized (5–8 mm) secundum ASDs diagnosed in early infancy tend to close spontaneously within the first 2 years of life. If the defects are ≥8 mm and persist beyond 2 years of life with favorable rims, these ASDs can be closed using occluder devices during interventional cardiac catheterization (Fig. 16.1). Sinus venosus defects and primum ASDs do not close spontaneously and require surgical repair, given their location, which can be performed at around 1 year of age [3].

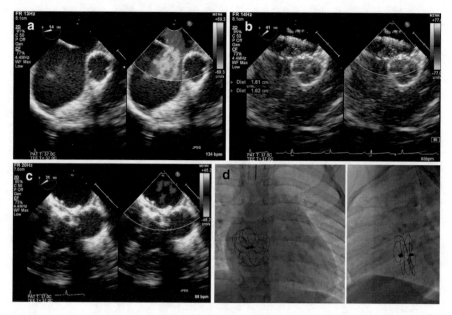

Fig. 16.1 Two-year-old female with a large ostium secundum atrial septal defect (ASD) and dilation of the right atrium and ventricle. Transesophageal echo short-axis color compare image showing a large ASD (**panel A**); On balloon sizing, stop flow showed a 16 mm defect (**panel B**); A 32 mm Gore ASD occluder device was deployed (**panels C and D**) with no residual shunt. (© 2020 Le Bonheur Children's Hospital (reprinted with permission))

Exercise Recommendations

Patients with ASDs that have normal right ventricular volume and no pulmonary hypertension can participate in all sports. Patients with ASDs that have mild pulmonary hypertension should participate in low-intensity competitive sports (class IA) only. However, ASD patients with associated moderate-to-severe pulmonary hypertension with cyanosis and right-to-left shunting should be restricted from all competitive sports. Following ASD closure, patients can be released to full activity 3–6 months post-procedure if there is no evidence of pulmonary hypertension, ventricular dysfunction, arrhythmia, or heart block. Those patients post-ASD closure with pulmonary hypertension, arrhythmias, or myocardial dysfunction can be considered for participation in low-intensity (class IA) sports [4].

Ventricular Septal Defect (VSD)

Anatomy/Physiology

VSDs can be classified based on their location in the interventricular septum as perimembranous, inlet, muscular, or outlet types. VSDs can be categorized as small, moderate, or large based on size. The degree of shunting depends on the size of the defect and the downstream resistance. Due to high pulmonary vascular resistance in newborns, left-to-right shunting associated with VSDs may not initially be significant. However, in the next 4–6 weeks of life, pulmonary vascular resistance drops and pulmonary over-circulation can develop, leading to dilation of the pulmonary arteries, left atrium, and left ventricle. In the setting of large VSDs, the right ventricle and the pulmonary arteries will be subjected to systemic pressures. If this physiology is left untreated, the pulmonary arterioles will develop irreversible vascular changes and resultant pulmonary hypertension with right-to-left shunting and cyanosis (Eisenmenger's syndrome) [5].

Surgical Repair

Small/restrictive VSDs in asymptomatic patients can be followed observationally over time. Hemodynamically significant VSDs, however, causing left-sided volume overload, failure to thrive, or recurrent respiratory infections need surgical closure. Patients with uncomplicated repaired VSDs typically enjoy normal quality of life thereafter.

Exercise Recommendations

Patients with an unrepaired VSD and normal pulmonary artery pressure can participate in all sports, while those patients with large VSDs and pulmonary hypertension should participate in low-intensity class IA sports only. Following 3–6 months post-VSD closure, patients can participate in competitive sports if they have no evidence of pulmonary hypertension, ventricular or atrial tachyarrhythmias, or myocardial dysfunction. Athletes with mild-to-moderate pulmonary hypertension or ventricular dysfunction should refrain from competitive sports, with the possible exception of low-intensity (class IA) sports. Symptomatic athletes with atrial or ventricular tachyarrhythmias or second- or third-degree atrioventricular (AV) block should not participate in competitive sports until further evaluation by an electrophysiologist [4].

Atrioventricular Septal Defect (AVSD)

Anatomy/Physiology

AVSDs comprise a spectrum of anomalies that result from maldevelopment of embryonic endocardial cushion tissue. These lesions are divided into partial and complete forms. In partial AVSD, a primum ASD is present and there are two distinct but contiguous, right and left atrioventricular valves. The inlet VSD component is small/absent and the left atrioventricular (AV) valve has a cleft. The complete form includes a primum ASD, a large inlet VSD with a single orifice common AV valve [6]. The pathophysiology is remarkable for a large left-to-right shunt from a combination of ASD, VSD, and additional AV valve regurgitation. As pulmonary vascular resistance drops in the first few weeks of life, pulmonary over-circulation and failure to thrive can develop. If left untreated, pulmonary vascular obstructive disease and pulmonary hypertension ensue.

Surgical Repair

The majority of patients with balanced defects (adequate size ventricles) can undergo complete biventricular repair between 6 and 12 weeks of age. Children with hypoplasia of one of the ventricles (unbalanced) will require staged single ventricle palliation.

Exercise Recommendations

Patients with biventricular repair of AVSD with normal pulmonary artery pressure and no significant AV valve stenosis/regurgitation can participate in unrestricted exercise 3–6 months post-surgery [7]. Individualized recommendations should be made for patients with residual or persistent lesions. Exercise recommendations for patients that undergo single ventricle palliation are discussed later in this chapter.

Tetralogy of Fallot (TOF)

Anatomy/Physiology

TOF is a spectrum of anomalies that result from anterior-cephalad deviation of the infundibular septum. The four basic components of TOF are:

(a) large VSD
(b) pulmonary stenosis
(c) overriding aorta
(d) right ventricular hypertrophy

The pulmonary stenosis/right ventricular outflow tract (RVOT) obstruction causes increased resistance to blood flow into the pulmonary circulation. Hence, there is right-to-left shunting across the VSD and into the overriding aorta resulting in cyanosis, depending on the degree of RVOT obstruction [8].

Surgical Repair

Cyanotic newborns if <5 kg will either undergo a palliative shunt/ductal stent/RVOT stent or a transventricular complete repair in the neonatal period. Following palliative shunt/stent placement, patients can undergo complete repair at 4–6 months once the branch pulmonary arteries have attained interval growth. If patients are able to grow to ~5 kg without interval procedures, they can undergo infundibular sparing repair (transatrial/transpulmonary repair of VSD, RVOT resection, and limited incision across the pulmonary valve annulus).

Exercise Recommendations

Patients with repaired TOF need a comprehensive clinical assessment, ECG, assessment of ventricular function, measurement of RV volume, and exercise testing prior to consideration of participation in competitive sports. Children status-post repair of TOF can be cleared for moderate-to-high-intensity sports participation (class II to III) if ventricular function is preserved (ejection fraction >50%), and if exercise-induced arrhythmias or RVOT obstruction is not present. Athletes with severe ventricular dysfunction (ejection fraction <40%), severe RVOT obstruction, or recurrent or uncontrolled atrial or ventricular arrhythmias should be restricted from all competitive sports, with the exception of low-intensity (class IA) sports [4].

D-Transposition of the Great Arteries (D-TGA)

Anatomy/Physiology

D-TGA is a cyanotic condition where there is discordant ventriculo-arterial connection (aorta arises from the right ventricle and pulmonary artery from the left ventricle). The circulatory pattern is such that deoxygenated blood from systemic veins is circulated back to the body and oxygenated pulmonary venous blood is returned back to the lungs, in parallel circulations. This can lead to profound cyanosis, and oxygenation is dependent on mixing of blood which can happen at either the atrial, ventricular, or ductus arteriosus levels [9].

Surgical Repair

Patients are started on prostaglandin infusion at birth and typically undergo balloon atrial septostomy in the first few days of life followed by an arterial switch operation a few days later. The coronary arteries are removed from the native aortic root with a button of tissue and are translocated into the neo-aorta [9]. Until recently, the preferred surgical technique was the atrial switch procedure (Mustard or Senning operation, leaving the morphologic RV as the systemic ventricle connected to the aorta), and thus, there are many living adults who have undergone such repairs. These patients are particularly prone to atrial arrhythmias, severe tricuspid regurgitation, and heart failure.

Exercise Recommendations

Patients who have undergone repair of D-TGA require yearly evaluation with ECG and TTE, and functional stress imaging every 3–4 years with EST or CMR. Asymptomatic patients with normal ventricular function, normal exercise capacity as assessed by EST, and no tachyarrhythmia can participate in all sports. Athletes with more than mild hemodynamic abnormalities or ventricular dysfunction, with normal exercise capacity, and no exercise-induced ischemia can participate in low- and moderate-intensity competitive sports (classes IA, IB, IIA, and IIB). Athletes with severe systemic RV dysfunction, severe RV outflow tract obstruction, or recurrent or uncontrolled atrial or ventricular arrhythmias should be restricted from all competitive sports, with the exception of low-intensity (class IA) sports [4].

Coarctation of the Aorta (CoAo)

Anatomy/Physiology

Coarctation of the aorta is a spectrum of narrowing in the aortic arch ranging from hypoplasia of a segment to discrete narrowing. Newborns with coarctation can be asymptomatic in the setting of a patent ductus arteriosus. However, signs of shock can develop with closure of the ductus depending on the severity of coarctation. Older children with milder forms of coarctation may develop collaterals and be detected later in life due to hypertension, murmur, or decreased lower extremity pulses [10].

Surgical/Interventional Repair

Neonatal CoAo is treated via a surgical approach following stabilization with prostaglandin infusion. Postsurgical re-coarctation is usually treated with balloon angioplasty/stenting depending on the patient's size and anatomy. Patients diagnosed during adolescent years are typically treated with endovascular stenting as the primary therapy as their vessel size allows placement of adult size stents (Fig. 16.2).

Exercise Recommendations

Treated patients require follow up with physical exam, TTE, and EST to assess for a residual coarctation gradient, ventricular hypertrophy and systolic function, hypertension, and the blood pressure response with exercise. CMR or CTA is recommended to evaluate the entire aortic arch. These patients also require screening for intracranial aneurysms by magnetic resonance angiography or CTA [11]. Three

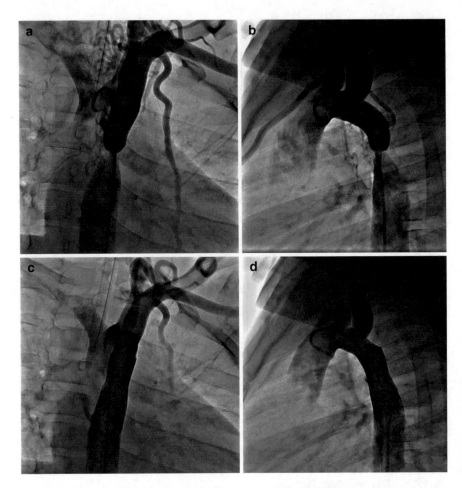

Fig. 16.2 Seventeen-year-old male with hypertension and diminished pedal pulses was found to have severe coarctation of the aorta. Angiogram showing severe coarctation of the aortic isthmus with extensive collateralization (**panels A and B**); Angiogram post-implantation of a Cordis Palmaz XL P4010 stent on a 16 mm balloon shows good position of the stent and no residual stenosis (**panel C and D**). (© 2020 Le Bonheur Children's Hospital (reprinted with permission))

months following intervention for CoAo, patients without significant residual/recurrent narrowing of the aortic arch (<20 mm Hg arm/leg systolic gradient), and normal blood pressure during rest and exercise can participate in those sports that do not involve a large static load. If these conditions continue to be met beyond 1 year post-intervention, patients may then advance to competitive sports. Athletes with evidence of aortic dilation, aortic wall thinning, or aneurysm formation should be restricted to low-intensity (class IA) sports [7].

Single Ventricle Spectrum

Anatomy/Physiology

Single ventricle refers to a variety of cyanotic heart diseases comprising of two atria communicating with a primitive ventricle. The single ventricle connects to an outlet chamber via a bulboventricular foramen. The pulmonary artery and aorta can be normally related or transposed. The clinical presentation and initial management are determined by the extent of compromise to the pulmonary or systemic blood flow.

Surgical Repair

Staged surgical palliation is typically the common approach. The first stage may include (pending associated anatomy):

(a) Severe pulmonary stenosis: There is severe restriction to pulmonary blood flow resulting in cyanosis. These patients are treated with prostaglandin and will require a shunt or ductal stent to maintain pulmonary blood flow.
(b) No pulmonary stenosis: Such patients will have pulmonary over-circulation and heart failure requiring a pulmonary artery band to restrict pulmonary blood flow.
(c) Severe left heart hypoplasia: These patients will have compromised systemic blood flow and will require the pulmonary artery to be connected with the systemic outflow. Pulmonary blood flow is maintained via a systemic to pulmonary shunt.

Regardless of the initial palliation, the second stage of palliation is to perform a partial cavopulmonary connection (superior vena cava to pulmonary artery, so-called Glenn shunt) at 3–6 months of age, aiming at diverting deoxygenated blood directly to the pulmonary circulation. The third stage is the total cavopulmonary connection (Fontan operation) usually performed at 2–4 years of age. This involves connecting the inferior vena cava to the pulmonary circulation either via baffle within the right atrium or an extracardiac conduit. At this stage, all deoxygenated blood is diverted to the pulmonary circulation passively.

Exercise Recommendations

Patients with unrepaired cyanotic heart disease should only be allowed to participate in low-intensity (class IA) sports. Many studies have reported limited exercise capacity and reduced cardiac output in patients at rest and during exercise following Fontan palliation [12, 13]. Patients, especially with a lateral tunnel baffle, are at risk of developing atrial arrhythmias. Patients should undergo comprehensive evaluation, including EST with measurement of oxygen saturation prior to any sports participation. Athletes palliated with Fontan who have no symptomatic heart failure or significantly abnormal intravascular hemodynamics can participate in low-intensity class IA sports [4]. Individualized decisions to participate in other sports can be made based on the athlete's ability to complete an exercise test without evidence of exercise-induced arrhythmias, hypotension, ischemia, or other concerning clinical symptoms [4]. As mortality in repaired congenital heart disease ranges 1–2% in centers of excellence, there is a growing population of adults with congenital heart disease and many with single ventricle physiology that will need to be counseled prior to exercise participation, often by adult cardiologists [11]. Additional consultation with an adult congenital cardiologist should be obtained.

Congenital Coronary Anomalies

Congenital coronary artery anomalies, though not common, can pose substantial risk for myocardial ischemia in the athlete, both as children and young adults as well as later in adult life. The congenital anomalies that this section will focus on include anomalous origin of the right or left coronary artery from the pulmonary artery (ARCAPA/ALCAPA) and anomalous aortic origin of a coronary artery (AAOCA) from the opposite sinus of Valsalva with or without an intraseptal/intramyocardial course. Overall aspects of anatomy and physiology, repair, and exercise recommendations will be reviewed for these two entities.

Anomalous Origin from the Pulmonary Artery (ARCAPA/ALCAPA)

Anatomy, Pathophysiology, and Clinical Presentation

The first described congenital coronary anomaly was the left coronary artery originating from the pulmonary artery, most commonly arising from the left posterior sinus of the pulmonary valve. This anomaly is also known as Bland-White-Garland syndrome given its first report relating clinical and autopsy findings in a 3-month-old infant by Bland et al. [14]. This anomaly is known to affect 1 in every 300,000 births [15].

In fetal life, pressure and oxygen saturations are similar in both the aorta and pulmonary artery, thus myocardial prefusion is presumably normal, and no stimulus occurs for the development of collateral circulation. Following birth, with a decrease in pulmonary arterial pressure over time, deoxygenated blood perfuses the affected coronary circulation and varying degrees of myocardial ischemia develops. Stimuli for neoangiogenesis with collateral circulation occurs and patients may either present with severe ventricular dysfunction and heart failure or they may continue to compensate over time until presentation in later years or even adult life [16]. This progressive dilation of coronary vessels and growth of collaterals affect both right and left systems. It is incompletely understood why some patients advance into adulthood without evidence of myocardial ischemia, even when exercising at high levels, whereas other patients succumb to varying degrees of ischemia and consequent ventricular dysfunction. Approximately 87% of patients present during infancy and the other 13% at later ages/adulthood [17].

The ECG hallmark of ALCAPA is the presence of Q waves in the anterolateral leads, specifically leads I and aVL. The Q waves may also be seen in V4-V6, though in children this finding in lateral precordial leads may be a normal finding and Q wave depth should be compared with age-specific normative ECG data. In adults, varying signs of myocardial ischemia may be present on the resting ECG. Variable degrees of mitral regurgitation may also be seen depending on the ischemic burden and effect on the mitral valve apparatus. Clinical presentation includes the presence of a murmur, chest pain and/or dyspnea upon exertion, syncope, congestive heart failure, or sudden death [18–23]. Many patients can also be asymptomatic. Diagnosis can be made by TTE (retrograde flow in the affected coronary artery seen by color Doppler) as well as advanced imaging including CMR and CTA. Cardiac catheterization with angiography can also be utilized, though less invasive techniques are preferred in the younger population.

The incidence of ARCAPA is considerably less than ALCAPA, approximating 1/10 of ALCAPA cases [24]. These patients can be asymptomatic or present clinically in a similar fashion as with ALCAPA, including the presence of a murmur or symptoms of myocardial ischemia such as angina, syncope, heart failure, or sudden death [25]. There are no specific diagnostic findings on the ECG for ARCAPA. Diagnostic imaging using TTE, CMR, CTA, or cardiac catheterization is similarly utilized as with ALCAPA.

Surgical Repair

Surgical repair is indicated upon diagnosis. In the younger population, options for ALCAPA repair include direct reimplantation of the anomalous left coronary with a button from the pulmonary artery/sinus into the correct sinus of Valsalva [18, 26–28], or performing the Takeuchi repair [18, 29] in which an aortopulmonary window is created and a tunnel is formed to direct blood from the aorta to the coronary ostium. In adults, there may be a need for bypass grafting if reimplantation is not possible [20, 30]. Depending on the degree of papillary muscle ischemia/infarction, residual mitral regurgitation may be a problem and is a cause for re-intervention in these patients. In ARCAPA patients, direct reimplantation is the preferred surgical technique. It is important to mention that in adults, direct ligation/closure of the anomalous coronary in the PA may be a reasonable option given the prolific development of collateral circulation over time and sufficient flow to maintain myocardial demands without evidence of ischemia [23, 31].

Exercise Recommendations

Pursuant to the latest recommendations from the American Heart Association (AHA) and American College of Cardiology Foundation (ACC) Scientific Statement on eligibility and disqualification recommendations for competitive athletes with cardiovascular abnormalities: Task Force 4 [4], individuals with nonrepaired ALCAPA or ARCAPA should be restricted from exercise and sports participation except for low-intensity Class IA sports (Class I; Level of Evidence C). Those individuals with repaired ALCAPA or ARCAPA, decision-making regarding exercise and sports participation will depend on the presence of sequelae of the lesion, such as myocardial infarction or ventricular dysfunction (Class IIb; Level of Evidence C).

Anomalous Origin from the Aorta (AAOCA)

Anomalous aortic origin of a coronary artery (AAOCA) is a congenital anomaly of the origin or course of a coronary artery that arises from the aorta. The estimated frequency of anomalous aortic origin of the left coronary artery (AAOLCA) is estimated at 0.03–0.15% live-births, while that of anomalous aortic origin of the right coronary artery (AAORCA) is estimated to be 0.28–0.92% [32, 33]. Although the true prevalence of AAOCA is yet unknown, given that most studies have focused primarily on symptomatic patients, recent studies by Angelini et al. have tried to establish the prevalence in the general population [34, 35].

For many years, congenital coronary anomalies were shown to be the second identifiable leading cause of sudden cardiac death (SCD) in the young, second to hypertrophic cardiomyopathy [36–38]. However, in two recent publications on rates of SCD, coronary abnormalities comprised the number one identifiable cause of SCD, second to undetermined/unknown cause [39, 40]. Although the estimated risk, based on available data, for SCD in young athletes is low at approximately 0.5–1 athletes per 100,000 athletes per year [39], and potentially higher in certain populations [40], these events have tremendous impact on families, communities, and organized sports at large. In fact, these estimates may not truly reflect this at-risk population given the lack of universal reporting of numbers of sudden cardiac arrest (SCA), which may be higher [41]. Exercise activity appears to trigger SCA, but events also may occur at rest and, in fact, contemporary studies have highlighted a higher incidence of SCA events either during night time or noncompetitive physical activities [39, 42]. Moreover, it is unknown why individuals susceptible to SCA can exercise at high intensity and competitive levels for many years until the sentinel event occurs.

Anatomy and Pathophysiology

Multiple anatomic subtypes of AAOCA have been described with varying degrees of perceived risk for sudden adverse events (Fig. 16.3). The anomalous coronary arising from the opposite sinus of Valsalva and taking an intramural [course within the media (muscular) layer of the aorta] and/or interarterial (segment traveling between the aorta and pulmonary artery) course carries the highest risk for compromising myocardial perfusion and inducing myocardial ischemia. Often the origin of the anomalous coronary is close to the commissure and higher in the opposite sinus, or close to or above the sinotubular junction. Particularly in the case of AAOLCA, a variant where the coronary travels within the conal septum and has an additional intramyocardial component – a classified intraseptal course – previously thought to be a benign entity, [43] has recently been shown to cause myocardial ischemia in a

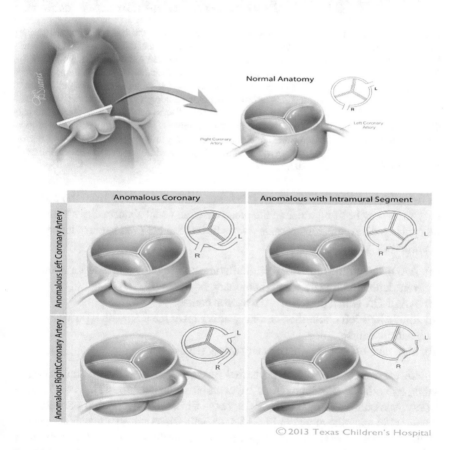

© 2013 Texas Children's Hospital

Fig. 16.3 Diagram illustrating normal coronary artery origins and anomalous aortic origin of a left and right coronary artery from the opposite sinus of Valsalva with and without an intramural course. (© 2013 Texas Children's Hospital (reprinted with permission) Published in Molossi and Sachdeva [57])

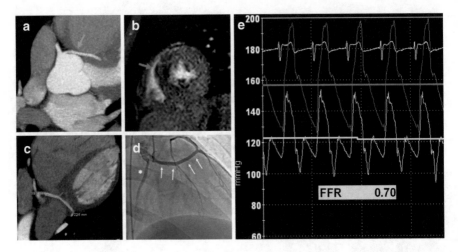

Fig. 16.4 Representative images of anomalous aortic origin of the left main coronary artery (AAOLCA) with an intraspetal course. (**a**) Anomalous aortic origin of the left main coronary artery (orange arrow) from the right sinus of Valsalva on computerized tomography angiography. (**b**) Presence of an inducible subendocardial perfusion defect by Dobutamine stress cardiac magnetic resonance imaging in the superior portion of the interventricular septum. (**c**) Intraseptal course of the left main coronary artery on computerized tomography angiography. (**d**) Coronary angiogram delineating the right coronary artery (white asterisk), the adjacent origin of the left main coronary artery, length of the intraseptal course of the left main coronary (white arrows), and distal bifurcation to the left anterior descending and left circumflex coronary arteries. (**e**) Fractional flow reserve tracings in the intraseptal segment demonstrating compromised flow. (© 2019 Texas Children's Hospital (reprinted with permission))

subset of patients [44] (Fig. 16.4). Likewise, AAOLCA arising from the noncoronary sinus may be of high risk in the presence of an ostial abnormality and intramural course [45]. Anomalous coronary variants that are believed to carry low risk and classified as "benign" include:

(a) AAOLCA with an anterior – pre-pulmonic course (coursing anterior to the right ventricular outflow tract and pulmonary valve).
(b) AAOLCA with a posterior – retroaortic course.
(c) anomalous left circumflex coronary artery (AAOCxCA) with a posterior – retroaortic course.
(d) high take-off of the right coronary artery (RCA).

However, there are some reports that link some of these anomalous coronary subtypes with the development of myocardial ischemia [46, 47]. The Coronary Artery Anomalies Program (CAAP) at Texas Children's Hospital has developed a topographic map, illustrated in Fig. 16.5, to delineate precisely the ostium location of the anomalous coronary as it relates to the aortic sinuses and commissures. Additionally, the ostial geometry of the coronaries is of importance.

To date, there is an incomplete understanding of the mechanisms leading to myocardial ischemia and potential SCD in AAOCA, particularly during exercise [48,

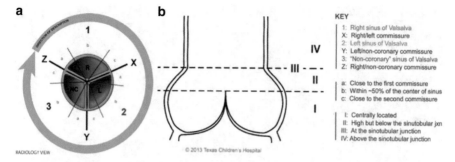

Fig. 16.5 Standardized nomenclature map used to describe the origin of the coronary arteries by CT angiography or surgical findings. (© 2013 Texas Children's Hospital (reprinted with permission) Published in Agrawal et al. [93])

49]. Much knowledge has been acquired to delineate multiple variations of coronary anatomy though there remains continued uncertainty regarding the anatomic variants that carry the highest risk for SCD and the physiologic conditions predisposing to severe compromise of myocardial perfusion through the anomalous coronary. Several pathophysiologic mechanisms have been postulated, including occlusion and/or compression of the anomalous artery during its intramural segment and/or interarterial course, and ostial abnormalities such as slit-like (acute angle of take-off), stenotic, and/or hypoplastic ostium which may obstruct/collapse particularly during dynamic changes occurring with exercise [50, 51] (Fig. 16.6). Sudden decrease in perfusion to the territory supplied by the anomalous coronary presumably leads to myocardial ischemia and development of (potentially lethal) ventricular arrhythmias [49].

Clinical Presentation

The clinical presentation on AAOCA varies from asymptomatic individuals diagnosed serendipitously to occurrence of SCA or SCD. Several studies have reported up to 50% of patients being asymptomatic at the time of diagnosis. Growing numbers of children and adolescents are diagnosed following routine pre-participation screening due to the presence of a heart murmur or "abnormal ECG" [45, 49, 52]. Molossi et al. [45] recently reported that only 21% of a cohort of 163 AAOCA patients followed prospectively presented with symptoms upon exertion, and 3% presented following SCA or shock. Significant exertional symptoms included chest pain and syncope. In a study by Basso et al. [53], only 10 (36%) of 27 cases presenting with SCD (23 AAOLCA and 4 AAORCA) had symptoms including syncope, chest pain, or palpitations, prior to the arrest. Anatomic features in this study suggestive of a high-risk lesion included acute angle take off and a slit-like ostium. Eckart et al. [54] reported 11 (52%) of 21 military recruits with SCD and AAOCA had prior symptoms of syncope, chest pain, and dyspnea.

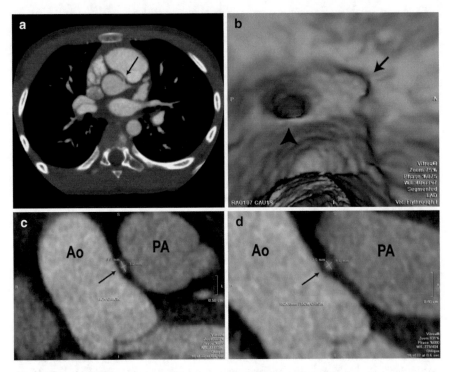

Fig. 16.6 Computerized tomographic angiography demonstrating an anomalous right coronary artery. (**a**) The anomalous right coronary arises from the left sinus with an intramural course as it courses in between the aorta and the pulmonary artery. (**b**) Virtual angioscopy shows a normal left coronary ostium (arrowhead) and the anomalous right coronary with a stenotic slit-like ostium arising just above and to the left of the intercoronary commissure. (**c**) The anomalous coronary (arrow) has an oval shape on its intramural segment compared to (**d**) the round shape of the distal coronary past its intramural segment. Ao: aorta; PA: pulmonary artery. (© 2014 Texas Children's Hospital (reprinted with permission) Published in Molossi and Sachdeva [57])

The initial diagnosis of AAOCA is typically made by TTE with imaging that identifies the sinus of origin and the interarterial course, and possibly the presence or absence of an intramural course [52, 55]. Sachdeva and colleagues found TTE was able to diagnose AAOCA in more than 95% of their cohort, and TTE findings were consistent with the surgical descriptions of the anatomy [56]. Lorber and colleagues found variable agreement between TTE and surgical findings [55]. However, TTE is inadequate to fully evaluate ostial morphology, to precisely define the length of an intramural course, and to demonstrate intraseptal and intramyocardial courses [57]. Advanced imaging modalities are essential to provide detailed anatomy of the anomalous coronary, including ostial morphology and the presence of an interarterial, intramural, or intramyocardial course. CTA or CMR is the preferred mode of imaging, and we have found CTA being superior in defining with precision the intramural length and extent of intraseptal/intramyocardial courses [43–45, 58–61].

In recent studies, about 50% of patients with AAOCA have been noted to be asymptomatic at the time of diagnosis [37, 49, 56, 62–64]. An increasing number of children and adolescents are being diagnosed with AAOCA following routine pre-participation screening, evaluating the presence of a murmur or an abnormal ECG [54, 63]. Typical presenting symptoms that have been reported in association with AAOCA are exertional chest pain, palpitations, syncope, as well as SCA [63, 64].

Evaluation and Management

1. Diagnostic evaluation

Despite significant advances in the understanding of AAOCA subtypes, clinical presentations, and ischemic risks, much remains to be established for appropriate risk stratification for this condition. There is significant variability in the approach to diagnosis, evaluation, and management of patients with AAOCA among providers [65]. Many questions and uncertainties persist, including the best approach for management and long-term outcomes of AAOCA patients according to management strategy. These uncertainties have prompted some institutions to develop dedicated multidisciplinary programs to evaluate and manage patients with AAOCA [45, 66], providing a platform for prospective data gathering following a standardized approach. Figure 16.7 depicts the current algorithm at Texas Children's Hospital.

ECG-gated CTA has demonstrated great accuracy in determining the precise anatomy of the anomalous coronary. The presence and length of an intramural course is determined using cross-sectional shape of the lumen and the peri-coronary fat sign [57, 58, 67], and the ostial location in relation to the aortic sinuses and commissures is defined based on a topography map (Fig. 16.5). The standardized report thus includes all details in every type of AAOCA.

A functional assessment should be performed in all patients with AAOCA to determine the presence of inducible myocardial ischemia, with an exception for those patients presenting with SCA, and for young children with no concerning symptoms. A cardiopulmonary exercise stress test is typically performed, though ischemic changes are rarely encountered, as demonstrated in several reports [44, 45, 53, 68, 69]. The validity of exercise stress testing remains to be determined for this condition.

Assessment of myocardial perfusion is an integral part of the evaluation of patients with AAOCA for risk stratification. Stress echocardiography to identify wall motion abnormalities is utilized in some centers and may be of value [70]. Caution should be taken, though, in centers or programs where this modality is not routinely performed and where reader expertise may be lacking to appropriately identify abnormalities in wall motion. Stress nuclear perfusion imaging (sNPI) is another tool used to determine perfusion abnormalities under provocative stress and this modality may be helpful in some centers depending on the type of sNPI utilized. In the cohort reported by Molossi et al., sNPI was unreliable to truly detect

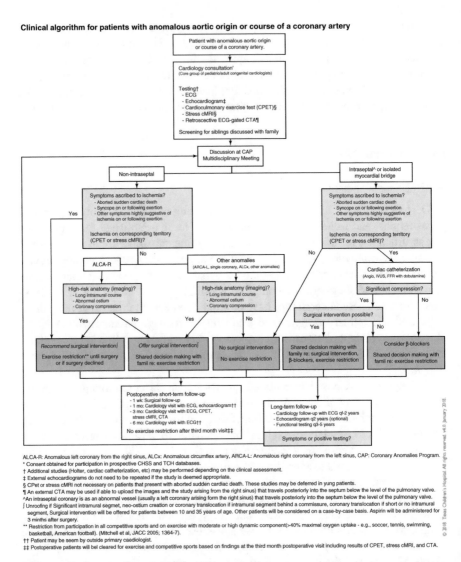

Clinical algorithm for patients with anomalous aortic origin or course of a coronary artery

ALCA-R: Anomalous left coronary from the right sinus, ALCx: Anomalous circumflex artery, ARCA-L: Anomalous right coronary from the left sinus, CAP: Coronary Anomalies Program.
* Consent obtained for participation in prospective CHSS and TCH databases.
† Additional studies (Holter, cardiac catheterization, etc) may be performed depending on the clinical assessment.
‡ External echocardiograms do not need to be repeated if the study is deemed appropriate.
§ CPet or stress cMRI not necessary on patients that present with aborted sudden cardiac death. These studies may be deferred in yung patients.
¶ An external CTA may be used if able to upload the images and the study arising from the right sinus) that travels posteriorly into the septum below the level of the pulmonary valve.
^An intraseptal coronary is as an abnormal vessel (usually a left coronary arising form the right sinus) that travels posteriorly into the septum below the level of the pulmonary valve.
∫ Unroofing if Significant intramural segmet, neo-ostium creation or coronary translocation if intramural segment behind a commissure, coronary translocation if short or no intramural segment, Surgical intervention will be offered for patients between 10 and 35 years of age. Other patients will be considered on a case-by-case basis. Aspirin will be administered for 3 mirths after surgery.
** Restriction from participation in all competitive sports and on exercise with moderate or high dynamic component(>40% maximal oxygen uptake - e.g., soccer, tennis, swimming, basketball, American football). (Mitchell et al, JACC 2005; 1364-7).
†† Patient may be seem by outside primary caediologist.
‡‡ Postoperative patients will bel cleared for exercise and competitive sports based on findings at the third month postoperative visit including results of CPET, stress cMRI, and CTA.

Fig. 16.7 Algorithm for the evaluation and management of patients with coronary anomalies in the Coronary Anomalies Program at Texas Children's Hospital. (© 2018 Texas Children's Hospital (reprinted with permission) Published in Mery et al. [47])

abnormalities related to the territory supplied by the anomalous coronary [45, 68]. sNPI in this study was associated with a high incidence of false-positive and false-negative findings, decreased spatial resolution, attenuation artifacts related to the body wall and diaphragm movement, and utilization of ionizing radiation.

Stress CMR (sCMR) has become a valuable tool in evaluating perfusion abnormalities in this patient population. Moreover, information on wall motion abnormalities and myocardial viability is advantageous, especially for following these patients over time, regardless of management strategy. Some of sCMR's advantageous qualities include high-quality cardiac imaging with excellent spatial resolution [71], feasibility and safety in children [72], lack of ionizing radiation, and improved sensitivity and specificity when compared to sNPI in young AAOCA patients [68]. Provocative stress is achieved with the administration of dobutamine, the preferred agent given the presumed important dynamic component for the mechanism believed to lead to myocardial ischemia in AAOCA. Dobutamine induces increased chronotropy and inotropy, with achievement of high heart rate levels, mimicking physiologic exercise conditions [72–74]. The use of atropine may be indicated in some cases to achieve the desired heart rate increase to 85% predicted peak heart rate. Doan et al. recently presented data in 250 sCMR studies in 204 patients with AAOCA and myocardial bridges, establishing the feasibility and safety in children with mean age of 14.1 ± 3.4 years and mean weight of 60.6 ± 22.0 kg. Inducible perfusion abnormalities were seen in 16% of all studies and half of these cases also showed wall motion abnormalities. No major adverse event occurred but there were minor adverse events in 11% of the cohort, including severe hypertension, chest pain, nausea/vomiting, anxiety, and dyspnea [75]. The implications of sCMR results on risk stratification remain to be determined with respect to long-term clinical outcomes in this patient population.

A subset of patients may require additional determination of coronary blood flow compromise for risk stratification, such as in the setting of equivocal findings on functional studies, when there remains significant clinical concern after negative myocardial functional studies, or when there is complex anatomy including a long intraseptal/intramyocardial course [76]. Invasive assessment of coronary flow can be made during cardiac catheterization with measurement of fractional flow reserve (FFR). FFR is a reference standard for coronary flow given that is not affected by heart rate, myocardial contractility, or blood pressure [77, 78]. Selective coronary angiography with FFR assessment upon administration of dobutamine +/− adenosine (with similar target heart rates as with sCMR) is performed, along with intravascular ultrasound in some cases to estimate the degree of obstruction during the cardiac cycle [76, 79]. Agrawal et al. recently reported good correlation between sCMR results and FFR measurement in a cohort of patients with AAOCA, suggesting that these modalities positively correlate with abnormalities in myocardial coronary blood flow [80].

2. Clinical decision-making

Counseling patients and families with AAOCA has proven to be a difficult task given the many unknowns surrounding these anomalies. These factors include an unknown true risk of sudden death which relates to incompletely understood mechanisms leading to sudden death, and anatomic/dynamic factors contributing to this risk. It is largely unknown why some patients may exercise strenuously for several years until the first presentation with SCA or SCD. Additionally, SCD can occur at rest or during sleep, though less frequently so. Approximately half of AAOCA patients are diagnosed serendipitously, with the other half presenting with some form of symptoms [45], including those presenting with SCD/SCA [53].

The lack of long-term data on outcomes of both repaired and unrepaired AAOCA patients challenges decision-making regarding the most appropriate management. Current AHA/ACC statements [4] and American Association for Thoracic Surgery guidelines [81] have differentiated the classified high-risk interarterial AAOLCA and the classified low-risk interarterial AAORCA, with no mention of ostial morphology or intramurality. Recommendations suggest no need for intervention in asymptomatic patients with AAORCA in the presence of a normal EST, although Basso and colleagues [53] have reported cases of patients with normal EST prior to suffering SCD. The data in our institution has also demonstrated that patients may present with inducible myocardial ischemia on dobutamine sCMR in the presence of a normal EST [45]. Moreover, patients with AAOCA and intraseptal course have presented with ischemia, in up to 50% of cases, without developing ischemic changes on EST [44]. Optimal risk stratification remains the pursued golden treasure in the scientific community [82]. We have developed a standardized approach in the CAAP in which the algorithm depicts risk stratification according to low- and high-risk categories. Figure 16.7 depicts the most current algorithm in use. Quality assurance multidisciplinary meetings are held every 18–24 months to evaluate the acquired data acquired and to discuss potential changes in the standardized approach, based on the prospective gathering of these data [45, 47].

3. Management

Management remains controversial in AAOCA, despite recommendations put forth by different societies [4, 81], especially with emerging new data on multiple anatomic subtypes and strategies to determine inducible myocardial ischemia. Shared decision-making is essential with a detailed review of what is known and what remains unknown in this condition, including the risk of sudden death in repaired and unrepaired patients, the risk factors predisposing to myocardial ischemia, and associated factors that place the younger population at higher risk for sudden events.

A proposed management algorithm (Fig. 16.7) is also included in the CAAP in our institution.

Patients with AAOLCA and high-risk anatomy are offered surgical intervention:

(a) origin from the opposite sinus with interarterial and/or intramural course.
(b) commissural origin with ostial abnormalities.
(c) intramural course in the setting of inducible myocardial ischemia.

Patients with AAORCA from the opposite sinus are offered surgical intervention:

(a) in the setting of symptoms ascribed to myocardial ischemia.
(b) an abnormal myocardial perfusion study.
(c) clinical suspicion for high-risk anatomy such as a long intramural course and ostial abnormalities.
(d) in the setting of persistent symptoms, following shared decision-making with the family.

Our initial data recently reported an intramural length of around 5 mm correlating with a high-risk lesion [45]. More recently, as our experience with dobutamine sCMR grows and more reliably assesses for inducible myocardial perfusion abnormalities upon provocative pharmacologic stress [75], the indications for considering surgical intervention have become more refined from simply the length of an intramural course.

AAOCA with an intraseptal/intramyocardial course is especially challenging as surgical intervention may not be possible without significant morbidity given the long segment within the myocardium that may extend beyond the conal septum. Exercise restriction may be an alternative for symptomatic patients with evidence of inducible myocardial ischemia, though there are no data if this strategy alters the risk for SCA or SCD. We have placed some patients on beta-blocker therapy and thus far these patients have remained free of recurrent symptoms after several years. Recently, Doan et al. [83] reported on a patient with an intraseptal course of the AAOLCA and prior myocardial infarction, inducible myocardial ischemia on dobutamine sCMR, and abnormal FFR in the intraseptal segment on cardiac catheterization, who underwent surgical intervention and evaluation post intervention. The previously seen inducible perfusion defect resolved. Others have also reported on surgical results with intraseptal AAOLCA, including in adults presenting with ischemia [84, 85].

Surgical techniques utilized in the repair of AAOCA include the unroofing procedure [86], coronary translocation with reimplantation into the correct sinus [87], neo-ostium creation [88], and pulmonary translocation [89, 90]. Mery et al. published the surgical experience in our institution in 44 patients, with 80% being AAORCA and 20% AAOLCA [47]. In the total cohort of patients with AAORCA, 25% underwent surgical intervention, with most undergoing the unroofing procedure. Bonilla et al. reported recent experience with translocation of the anomalous coronary in those patients in which unroofing would not provide complete re-establishment of the ostium into the correct sinus [91]. This surgical procedure is safe in experienced hands with a low incidence of complications. Post-cardiotomy syndrome was seen more frequently in this cohort (9%) [47]. Jegatheeswaran et al. reported significant complications associated with variable procedures in the large Registry of the Congenital Heart Surgeons' Society [92]. It remains unknown if surgical intervention modifies the potential for SCD/SCA over time in this population.

Patients should be followed at specific time intervals, even after surgical intervention, for monitoring of changes in clinical status. Those patients undergoing surgery are re-evaluated at 1 month postoperatively with ECG and TTE, and at 3 months postoperatively with ECG, myocardial functional studies, CTA (same studies performed on initial presentation), as well as repeat cardiac catheterization with IVUS/FFR. Patients are allowed to return to full exercise activities and competitive sports participation, following a reconditioning period, when no concerns are raised by postoperative studies.

Exercise restriction with respect to surgical intervention is only recommended for patients:

(a) awaiting surgical intervention.
(b) during the first 3 months postoperatively.
(c) for patients with high-risk lesions who have declined recommendations for surgical intervention.
(d) those patients deemed unsuitable for the current surgical options given a long intraseptal/intramyocardial course.

All other patients deemed to have low-risk lesions are not offered surgical intervention and are allowed unrestricted exercise activities.

Exercise Recommendations

The 2015 AHA/ACC eligibility and disqualification recommendations for competitive athletes with cardiovascular abnormalities: Task Force 4 [4] state the following:

(a) *"Athletes with an anomalous origin of a right coronary artery from the left sinus of Valsalva should be evaluated by an exercise stress test. For those without either symptoms or a positive exercise stress test, permission to compete can be considered after adequate counseling of the athlete and/or the athlete's parents (in the case of a minor) as to risk and benefit, taking into consideration the uncertainty of accuracy of a negative stress test (Class IIa; Level of Evidence C)."*
(b) *"Nonoperated athletes with an anomalous origin of a right coronary artery from the left sinus of Valsalva who exhibit symptoms, arrhythmias, or signs of ischemia on exercise stress test should be restricted from participation in all competitive sports, with the possible exception of class IA sports, before a surgical repair (Class III; Level of Evidence C)."*
(c) *"After successful surgical repair of an anomalous origin from the wrong sinus, athletes may consider participation in all sports 3 months after surgery if the patient remains free of symptoms and an exercise stress test shows no evidence of ischemia or cardiac arrhythmias (Class IIb; Level of Evidence C)."*
(d) *"Athletes with an anomalous origin of a left coronary artery from the right sinus of Valsalva, especially when the artery passes between the pulmonary artery and aorta, should be restricted from participation in all competitive sports, with the possible exception of class IA sports, before surgical repair. This recommendation applies whether the anomaly is identified as a consequence of symptoms or discovered incidentally (Class III; Level of Evidence B)."*

However, a few points must be considered:

1. AAORCA is viewed as safe if asymptomatic and with negative EST, but these patients may have inducible perfusion abnormalities with advanced imaging in the presence of normal EST and in the absence of significant symptoms [45].
2. Following successful repair and with no symptoms and negative EST, AAOCA patients may return to athletic activities, though there is no mention in the guidelines of evaluation by imaging or myocardial functional studies to assess for

inducible perfusion abnormalities, again weighing heavily on the EST that has been shown to be have low sensitivity [53, 68].
3. No guidance is given for those patients with more complex anatomy that involves an intraseptal/intramyocardial course.

Shared decision-making is essential to guide exercise activities in these patients. Exercise benefits cardiovascular health, including and particularly in the young, as exercise patterns in childhood will shape exercise patterns in adulthood. A thorough discussion of what is known and what is unknown in AAOCA, including the multi-faceted expression of these anomalies both anatomically and functionally, needs to be shared with patients and families.

Conclusions

Congenital heart disease affects 0.8–1% of all live-births and is becoming more prevalent across lifespan as mortality is greatly reduced, leading to an ever-growing number of adults with these conditions. Substantial knowledge has been acquired in AAOCA, but significant gaps remain, especially as it relates to the risk and safety of exercise activity in the repaired and unrepaired patient population. Conservative approaches may hurt more than benefit these patients, as cardiovascular health is essential for longevity and quality of life, and extending the boundaries to foster exercise activity must continue to be pursued.

References

1. Levine BD, Baggish AL, Kovacs RJ, Link MS, Maron MS, Mitchell JH. Eligibility and disqualification recommendations for competitive athletes with cardiovascular abnormalities: Task Force 1: classification of sports: dynamic, static, and impact: a scientific statement from the American Heart Association and American College of Cardiology. J Am Coll Cardiol. 2015;66:2350–5.
2. Feltes TF, Bacha E, Beekman RH, Cheatham JP, Feinstein JA, Gomes AS, Hijazi ZM, Ing FF, de Moor M, Morrow WR, Mullins CE, Taubert KA, Zahn EM. Indications for cardiac catheterization and intervention in pediatric cardiac disease: a scientific statement from the American Heart Association. Circulation. 2011;123:2607–52.
3. Abdulla R-I, Hanrahan A. Atrial septal defect. In: Abdulla R-I, editor. Heart diseases in children Berlin, Germany: Springer Science Business Media, LLC; 2011. p. 91–102.
4. Van Hare GF, Ackerman MJ, Evangelista J-AK, Kovacs RJ, Myerburg RJ, Shafer KM, Warnes CA, Washington RL. Eligibility and disqualification recommendations for competitive athletes with cardiovascular abnormalities: Task Force 4: congenital heart disease: a scientific statement from the American Heart Association and American College of Cardiology. J Am Coll Cardiol. 2015;66:2372–84.
5. Rubio AE, Lewin MB. Ventricular septal defects. In: Allen HD, Shaddy RE, Penny DJ, Feltes TF, Cetta F, editors. Moss and Adams' heart disease in infants, children, and adolescents: including the fetus and young adult; 2013. p. 713–21.

6. Cetta F, Truong D, Minich LL, Maleszewski JJ, O'Leary PW, Dearani JA, Burkhart HM. Atrioventricular septal defects. In: Allen HD, Shaddy RE, Penny DJ, Feltes TF, Cetta F, editors. Moss and Adams' heart disease in infants, children, and adolescents: including the fetus and young adult; 2013. p. 691–712.

7. Graham TP Jr, Driscoll DJ, Gersony WM, Newburger JW, Rocchini A, Towbin JA. Task force 2: congenital heart disease. J Am Coll Cardiol. 2005;45:1326–33.

8. Roche SL, Greenway SC, Redington AN. Tetralogy of Fallot with pulmonary stenosis and Tetralogy of Fallot with absent pulmonary valve. In: Allen HD, Shaddy RE, Penny DJ, Feltes TF, Cetta F, editors. Moss and Adams' heart disease in infants, children, and adolescents: including the fetus and young adult; 2013. p. 969–89.

9. Villafane J, Lantin-Hermoso MR, Bhatt AB, Tweddell JS, Geva T, Nathan M, Elliott MJ, Vetter VL, Paridon SM, Kochilas L, Jenkins KJ, Bekkman RH III, Wernovsky G, Towbin JA. D-transposition of the great arteries: hot topics in the current era of the arterial switch operation. J Am Coll Cardiol. 2014;64(5):498–511.

10. Beekman RA III. Coarctation of the aorta. In: Allen HD, Shaddy RE, Penny DJ, Feltes TF, Cetta F, editors. Moss and Adams' heart disease in infants, children, and adolescents: including the fetus and young adult; 2013. p. 1044–60.

11. Stout KK, Daniels CJ, Aboulhosn JA, Bozkurt B, Broberg CS, Colman JM, Crumb SR, Dearani JA, Fuller S, Gurvitz M, Khairy P, Landzberg MJ, Saidi A, Valente AM, Van Hare GF. 2018 AHA/ACC guideline for the management of adults with congenital heart disease: a report of the American College of Cardiology/American Heart Association Task Force on Clinical Practice Guidelines. Circulation. 2019;139:e698–800.

12. McCrindle BW, Williams RV, Mital S, Clark BJ, Russell JL, Klein G, Eisenmann JC. Physical activity levels in children and adolescents are reduced after the Fontan procedure, independent of exercise capacity, and are associated with lower perceived general health. Arch Dis Child. 2007;92:509–14.

13. Shachar GB, Fuhrman BP, Wang Y, Lucas RV, Lock JE. Rest and exercise hemodynamics after the Fontan procedure. Circulation. 1982;65:1043–8.

14. Bland EF, White PD, Garland J. Congenital anomalies of the coronary arteries: report of an unusual case associated with cardiac hypertrophy. Am Heart J. 1933;8:787–801.

15. Marwaha B, Idris O, Mahmood M, Gundabolu A, Sohail S, Kanaan T, Singh H. Sudden cardiac arrest in adult due to anomalous origin of left main coronary artery from pulmonary artery. JACC Cardiovasc Interv. 2018;11(24):e203–5.

16. Moodie DS, Fyfe D, Gill CC, Cook SA, Lytle BW, Taylor PC, Fitzgerald R, Sheldon WC. Anomalous origin of the left coronary artery from the pulmonary artery (Bland-White-Garland syndrome) in adult patients: long-term follow-up after surgery. Am Heart J. 1983;106(2):381–8.

17. Lim DS, Matherne GP. Congenital anomalies of the coronary vessels and the aortic root. In: Allen HD, Shaddy RE, Penny DJ, Feltes TF, Cetta F, editors. Moss and Adams' heart disease in infants, children, and adolescents: including the fetus and young adult; 2013. p. 746–57.

18. Cabrera AG, Chen DW, Pignatelli RH, Khan MS, Jeewa A, Mery CM, McKenzie ED, Fraser CD Jr. Outcomes of anomalous left coronary artery from pulmonary artery repair: beyond normal function. Ann Thorac Surg. 2015;99:1342–7.

19. Marwaha B, Idris O, Mahmood M, Gundabolu A, Ali SS, Kanaan T, Singh H. Sudden cardiac arrest in adult due to anomalous aortic origin of left main coronary artery from pulmonary artery. JACC Cardiovasc Interv. 2018;11(24):e203–5.

20. Purut CM, Sabiston DC Jr. Origin of the left coronary artery from the pulmonary artery in older adults. J Thorac Cardiovasc Surg. 1991;102:566–70.

21. Wesselhoeft H, Fawcett JS, Johnson AL. Anomalous origin of the left coronary artery from the pulmonary trunk: its clinical spectrum, pathology, and pathophysiology, based on a review of 140 cases with seven further cases. Circulation. 1968;38:403–25.

22. Yau JM, Singh R, Halpern EJ, Fischman D. Anomalous origin of the left coronary artery from the pulmonary artery in adults: a comprehensive review of 151 adult cases and a new diagnosis in a 53-year-old woman. Clin Cardiol. 2011;34:204–10.

23. Boutsikou M, Shore D, Li W, Rubens M, Pijuan A, Gatzoulis MA, Babu-Narayan SV. Anomalous left coronary artery from the pulmonary artery (ALCAPA) diagnosed in adulthood: varied clinical presentation, therapeutic approach and outcome. Int J Cardiol. 2018;261:49–53.
24. Ogden JA. Congenital anomalies of the coronary arteries. Am J Cardiol. 1970;25:474–9.
25. Yao CT, Wang JN, Yeh CN, Huang SC, Yang YR, Wu JM. Isolated anomalous origin of right coronary artery from the main pulmonary artery. J Card Surg. 2005;20:487–9.
26. Lange R, Vogt M, Horer J, Cleuziou J, Menzel A, Holper K, Hess J, Schreiber C. Long term results of repair of anomalous origin of the left coronary artery from the left pulmonary artery. Ann Thorac Surg. 2007;83(4):1463–71.
27. Ben Ali W, Metton O, Roubertie F, Pouard P, Sidi D, Raisky O, Vouhe PR. Anomalous origin of the left coronary artery from the pulmonary artery: late results with special attention to the mitral valve. Eur J Cardiothorac Surg. 2009;36(2):244–8.
28. Imamura M, Dossey AM, Jaquiss RD. Reoperation and mechanical circulatory support after repair of anomalous origin of the left coronary artery from the pulmonary artery: a twenty-year experience. Ann Thorac Surg. 2011;92(1):167–72.
29. Takeuchi S, Imamura H, Katsumoto K, Hayashi I, Katohgi T, Yozu R, Ohkura M, Inoue T. J Thorac Cardiovasc Surg. 1979;78(1):7–11.
30. Rajbanshi BG, Burkhart HM, Schaff HV, Daly RC, Phillips SD, Dearani JA. Surgical strategies for anomalous origin of coronary artery from pulmonary artery in adults. J Thorac Cardiovasc Surg. 2014;148(1):220–4.
31. Ortiz de Salazar A, Juanena C, Aramendi JI, Castellanos E, Cabrera A, Agosti J. Anomalous origin of the left coronary artery from the pulmonary artery: surgical alternatives depending on the age of the patient. J Cardiovasc Surg (Torino). 1990;31:1801–4.
32. Paolo A, Antonio VJ, Scott F. Coronary anomalies. Circulation. 2002;105(20):2449–54.
33. Angelini P. Coronary artery anomalies: an entity in search of an identity. Circulation. 2007;115(10):1296–305.
34. Angelini P, Vidovich MI, Lawless CE, Elayda MA, Lopez JA, Wolf D, Willerson JT. Preventing sudden cardiac death in athletes: in search of evidence-based, cost-effective screening. Tex Heart Inst J. 2013;40(2):148–55.
35. Angelini P, Cheong BY, Lenge De Rosen VV, Lopez A, Uribe C, Masso AH, Ali SW, Davis BR, Muthupillai R, Willerson JT. High-risk cardiovascular conditions in sports-related sudden death: prevalence in 5,169 schoolchildren screened via cardiac magnetic resonance. Tex Heart Inst J. 2018;45(4):205–13.
36. Maron BJ. Sudden death in young athletes. N Engl J Med. 2003 Sep 11;349(11):1064–75.
37. Maron BJ, Doerer JJ, Haas TS, Tierney DM, Mueller FO. Sudden deaths in young competitive athletes: analysis of 1866 deaths in the United States, 1980-2006. Circulation. 2009;119(8):1085–92.
38. Maron BJ, Haas TS, Ahluwalia A, Murphy CJ, Garberich RF. Demographics and epidemiology of sudden deaths in young competitive athletes: from the United States National Registry. Am J Med. 2016;129(11):1170–7.
39. Bagnall RD, Weintraub RG, Ingles J, Duffiou J, Yeates L, Lam L, David AM, Thompson T, Connell V, Wallace J, Naylor C, Crawford J, Love DR, Hallam L, White J, Lawrence C, Lynch M, Morgan N, James P, du Sart D, Puranik R, Langlois N, Vohra J, Winship I, Atherton J, McGaughran J, Skinner JR, Semsarian C. A prospective study of sudden cardiac death among children and young adults. N Engl J Med. 2016;374(25):2441–52.
40. Harmon KG, Asif IM, Klossner D, Drezner JA. Incidence of sudden cardiac death in National Collegiate Athletic Association athletes. Circulation. 2011;123(15):1594–600.
41. Atkins DL, Everson-Stewart S, Sears GK, Daya M, Osmond MH, Warden CR, Berg RA. Resuscitation Outcomes Consortium Investigators. Epidemiology and outcomes from out-of-hospital cardiac arrest in children: the Resuscitation Outcomes Consortium Epistry-Cardiac Arrest. Circulation. 2009;119(11):1484–91.
42. Landry CH, Allan KS, Connelly KA, Cunningham K, Morrison LJ, Dorian P, Rescu Investigators. Sudden cardiac arrest during participation in competitive sports. N Engl J Med. 2017;377(18):1943–53.

43. Brothers JA, Whitehead KK, Keller MS, Fogel MA, Paridon SM, Weinberg PM, Harris MA. Cardiac MRI and CT: differentiation of normal ostium and intraseptal course from slitlike ostium and interarterial course in anomalous left coronary artery in children. Am J Roentgenol. 2015;204(1):W104–9.
44. Doan T, Zea-Vera R, Masand P, Reaves-O'Neal D, Agrawal H, Mery C, Krishnamurthy R, Masand P, Noel C, Qureshi A, Sexon-Tejtel S, Fraser CD Jr, Molossi S. Myocardial ischemia in children with anomalous aortic origin of a coronary artery with intraseptal course. Circ Cardiovasc Interv. 2020;13(3):e008375.
45. Molossi S, Agrawal H, Mery CM, Krishnamurthy R, Masand P, Sexson-Tejtel SK, Noel CV, Qureshi AM, Jadah SP, McKenzie ED, Fraser CD Jr. Outcomes in anomalous aortic origin of a coronary artery following a prospective standardized approach. Circ Cardiovasc Interv. 2020;13(2):e008445.
46. Murphy DA, Roy DL, Sohal M, Chandler BM. Anomalous origin of left main coronary artery from anterior sinus of Valsalva with myocardial infarction. J Thorac Cardiovasc Surg. 1978;75:282–5.
47. Mery CM, De León LE, Molossi S, Sexson-Tejtel S, Agrawal H, Krishnamurthy R, Masand P, Qureshi A, McKenzie E, Fraser CD Jr. Outcomes of surgical intervention for anomalous aortic origin of a coronary artery: a large contemporary prospective cohort study. J Thorac Cardiovasc Surg. 2018;155(1):305–19.
48. Cheitlin MD, MacGregor J. Congenital anomalies of coronary arteries: role in the pathogenesis of sudden cardiac death. Herz. 2009;34:268–79.
49. Molossi S, Martínez-Bravo LE, Mery CM. Anomalous aortic origin of a coronary artery. Methodist Debakey Cardiovasc J. 2019;15(2):111–21.
50. Angelini P, Villason S, Chan AV Jr, Diez JG. Normal and anomalous coronary arteries in humans. In: Angelini P, editor. Coronary artery anomalies. Philadelphia: Lippincott Williams & Wilkins; 1999. p. 27–150.
51. Angelini P, Uribe C, Monge J, Tobis JM, Elayda MA, Willerson JT. Origin of the right coronary artery from the opposite sinus of Valsalva in adults: characterization by intravascular ultrasonography at baseline and after stent angioplasty. Catheter Cardiovasc Interv. 2015;86:199–208.
52. Frommelt PC, Berger S, Pelech AN, Bergstrom S, Williamson JG. Prospective identification of anomalous origin of left coronary artery from the right sinus of valsalva using transthoracic echocardiography: importance of color Doppler flow mapping. Pediatr Cardiol. 2001;22(4):327–32.
53. Basso C, Maron BJ, Corrado D, Thiene G. Clinical profile of congenital coronary artery anomalies with origin from the wrong aortic sinus leading to sudden death in young competitive athletes. J Am Coll Cardiol. 2000;35(6):1493–501.
54. Eckart RE, Scoville SL, Campbell CL, Shry EA, Stajduhar KC, Potter RN, Pearse LA, Virmani R. Sudden death in young adults: a 25-year review of autopsies in military recruits. Ann Intern Med. 2004;141(11):829–34.
55. Lorber R, Srivastava S, Wilder TJ, McIntyre S, DeCampli WM, Williams WG, Frommelt PC, Parness IA, Blackstone EH, Jacobs ML, Mertens L, Brothers JA, Herlong JR, AAOCA Working Group of the Congenital Heart Surgeons Society. Anomalous aortic origin of coronary arteries in the young: echocardiographic evaluation with surgical correlation. JACC Cardiovasc Imaging. 2015;8(11):1239–49.
56. Sachdeva S, Frommelt MA, Mitchell ME, Tweddell JS, Frommelt PC. Surgical unroofing of intramural anomalous aortic origin of a coronary artery in pediatric patients: single-center perspective. J Thorac Cardiovasc Surg. 2018;155(4):1760–8.
57. Molossi S, Sachdeva S. Anomalous coronary arteries: what is known and what remains to be learned? Curr Opin Cardiol. 2020;35(1):42–51.
58. Krishnamurthy R, Masand P, Jadhav S, Zhang W, Molossi S, Sexson K, McKenzie D, Fraser C, Mery C. Diagnostic accuracy of CT angiography (CTA) for critical pathologic features in anomalous aortic origin of the coronary arteries (AAOCA) in children: a comparative study with surgery in a single center. J Am Coll Cardiol. 2015;65(10 Suppl):A1304.

59. de Jonge GJ, van Ooijen PM, Piers LH, Dikkers R, Tio RA, Willems TP, van den Heuvel AF, Zijlstra F, Oudkerk M. Visualization of anomalous coronary arteries on dual-source computed tomography. Eur Radiol. 2008;18(11):2425–32.
60. Su JT, Chung T, Muthupillai R, Pignatelli RH, Kung GC, Diaz LK, Vick GW 3rd, Kovalchin JP. Usefulness of real-time navigator magnetic resonance imaging for evaluating coronary artery origins in pediatric patients. Am J Cardiol. 2005;95(5):679–82.
61. Aljaroudi WA, Flamm SD, Saliba W, Wilkoff BL, Kwon D. Role of CMR imaging in risk stratification for sudden cardiac death. JACC Cardiovasc Imaging. 2013;6(3):392–406.
62. Mainwaring RD, Reddy VM, Reinhartz O, Petrossian E, Punn R, Hanley FL. Surgical repair of anomalous aortic origin of a coronary artery. Eur J Cardiothorac Surg. 2014;46(1):20–6.
63. Molossi S, Agrawal H. Clinical evaluation of anomalous aortic origin of a coronary artery (AAOCA). Congenit Heart Dis. 2017;12(5):607–9.
64. Mainwaring RD, Murphy DJ, Rogers IS, Chan FP, Petrossian E, Palmon M, Hanley FL. Surgical repair of 115 patients with anomalous aortic origin of a coronary artery from a single institution. World J Pediatr Congenit Heart Surg. 2016;7(3):353–9.
65. Agrawal H, Mery C, Day P, Sexson-Tejtel S, Mckenzie E, Fraser C, Qureshi A, Molossi S. Current practices are variable in the evaluation and management of patients with anomalous aortic origin of a coronary artery: results of a survey. Congenit Heart Dis. 2017;12(5):610–4.
66. Mery CM, Lawrence SM, Krishnamurthy R, Sexton-Tejtel SK, Carberry K, McKenzie ED, Fraser C. Anomalous aortic origin of a coronary artery: toward a standardized approach. Semin Thorac Cardiovasc Surg. 2014;26(2):110–22.
67. Angelini P. Novel imaging of coronary artery anomalies to assess their prevalence, the causes of clinical symptoms, and the risk of sudden cardiac death. Circ Cardiovasc Imaging. 2014;7:747–54.
68. Agrawal H, Mery C, Krishnamurthy R, Sexson-Tejtel SK, Noel C, Masand P, Jadhav S, McKenzie E, Qureshi A, Fraser CD Jr, Molossi S. Stress myocardial perfusion imaging in anomalous aortic origin of a coronary artery: Results following a standardized approach. J Am Coll Cardiol. 2017;69(11_S):1616.
69. Brothers J, Carter C, McBride M, Spray T, Paridon S. Anomalous left coronary artery origin from the opposite sinus of Valsalva: evidence of intermittent ischemia. J Thorac Cardiovasc Surg. 2010;140:e27–9.
70. Brothers JA, McBride MG, Seliem MA, Marino BS, Tomlinson RS, Pampaloni MH, Gaynor JW, Spray TL, Paridon SM. Evaluation of myocardial ischemia after surgical repair of anomalous aortic origin of a coronary artery in a series of pediatric patients. J Am Coll Cardiol. 2007;50(21):2078–82.
71. Pennell DJ, Sechtem UP, Higgins CB, Manning WJ, Pohost GM, Rademakers FE, van Rossum AC, Shaw LJ, Yucel EK, European Society of Cardiology; Society for Cardiovascular Magnetic Resonance. Clinical indications for cardiovascular magnetic resonance (CMR): Consensus Panel report. Eur Heart J. 2004;25(21):1940–65.
72. Noel Cory V, Krishnamurthy R, Silvana M, Moffett B, Mery C, Krishnamurthy R. Cardiac MR stress perfusion with regadenoson or dobutamine in children: single center experience in repaired and unrepaired congenital and acquired heart disease. Circulation. 2016;134(suppl_1):A19899.
73. Asrress KN, Schuster A, Ali NF, Williams R, Kutty S, Lockie T, Yousuff M, De Silva K, Danford DA, Beerbaum P, Marber M, Plein S, Nagel E, Redwood S. Myocardial hemodynamic response to dobutamine stress compared to physiological exercise during cardiac magnetic resonance imaging. J Cardiovasc Magn Reson. 2013;15(Suppl 1):P16.
74. Escaned J, Cortés J, Flores A, Goicolea FA, Alfonso F, Hernandez R, Fernandez-Ortiz A, Sabate M, Banuelos C, Macaya C. Importance of diastolic fractional flow reserve and dobutamine challenge in physiologic assessment of myocardial bridging. J Am Coll Cardiol. 2003;42:226–33.
75. Doan T, Molossi S, Sachdeva S, Wilkinson J, Loar R, Weigand J, Schlingmann T, Reaves-O'Neal D, Pednekar A, Masand P, Noel C. Dobutamine stress-cardiac magnetic resonance

imaging in children with anomalous aortic origin of a coronary artery and myocardial bridge. Circ Cardiovasc Imaging. 2020: Submitted in press.

76. Agrawal H, Molossi S, Alam M, Sexon-Tejtel S, Mery C, McKenzie E, Fraser CD Jr, Qureshi A. Anomalous coronary arteries and myocardial bridges: risk stratification in children using novel cardiac catheterization techniques. Pediatr Cardiol. 2017;38(3):624–30.

77. Tonino PA, De Bruyne B, Pijls NH, Siebert U, Ikeno F, van't Veer M, Klauss V, Maniharan G, Engstrom T, Oldroyd KG, Ver Lee PN, MacCarthy PA, Fearon WF, FAME Study Investigators. Fractional flow reserve versus angiography for guiding percutaneous coronary intervention. N Engl J Med. 2009;360:213–24.

78. De Bruyne B, Bartunek J, Sys SU, Pijls NH, Heyndrickx GR, Wijns W. Simultaneous coronary pressure and flow velocity measurements in humans. Feasibility, reproducibility, and hemodynamic dependence of coronary flow velocity reserve, hyperemic flow versus pressure slope index, and fractional flow reserve. Circulation. 1996;94:1842–9.

79. Doan T, Wilkinson J, Agrawal H, Molossi S, Alam M, Mery C, Qureshi A. Instantaneous wave-free ratio (iFR) correlates with fractional flow reserve (FFR) assessment of coronary artery stenoses and myocardial bridges in children. J Invas Cardiol. 2020;13(3):e008375.

80. Agrawal H, Noel C, Qureshi A, Masand P, Mery C, Sexson-Tejtel SK, Fraser CD Jr, Molossi S. Impaired myocardial perfusion on stress cardiovascular magnetic resonance imaging correlates with invasive fractional flow reserve in children with anomalous aortic origin of a coronary artery and/or myocardial bridges. Circulation. 2017;136(Suppl_1):A15784.

81. Brothers JA, Frommelt MA, Jaquiss RDB, Myerburg RJ, Fraser CD Jr, Tweddell JS. Expert consensus guidelines: anomalous aortic origin of a coronary artery. J Thorac Cardiovasc Surg. 2017;153:1440–57.

82. Molossi S, Mery C. The search for the Holy Grail: risk stratification in anomalous aortic origin of a coronary artery. J Thorac Cardiovasc Surg. 2018;155:1758–9.

83. Doan T, Molossi S, Qureshi A, McKenzie E. Intraseptal anomalous coronary artery with myocardial infarction: novel surgical approach. Ann Thorac Surg. 2020;110(4):e271–4.

84. Mainwaring RD, Hanley FL. Surgical treatment of anomalous left main coronary artery with an intraconal course. Congenit Heart Dis. 2019;14(4):504–10.

85. Najm HK, Ahmad M. Transconal unroofing of anomalous left main coronary artery from right sinus with transseptal course. Ann Thorac Surg. 2019;108:e383–6.

86. Romp RL, Herlong JR, Landolfo CK, Sanders SP, Miller CE, Ungerleider RM, Jaggers J. Outcome of unroofing procedure for repair of anomalous aortic origin of left or right coronary artery. Ann Thorac Surg. 2003;76(2):589–95; discussion 595–6.

87. Law T, Dunne B, Stamp N, Ho KM, Andrews D. Surgical results and outcomes after reimplantation for the management of anomalous aortic origin of the right coronary artery. Ann Thorac Surg. 2016;102(1):192–8.

88. Karamichalis JM, Vricella LA, Murphy DJ, Reitz BA. Simplified technique for correction of anomalous origin of left coronary artery from the anterior aortic sinus. Ann Thorac Surg. 2003;76(1):266–7.

89. Rodefeld MD, Culbertson CB, Rosenfeld HM, Hanley FL, Thompson LD. Pulmonary artery translocation: a surgical option for complex anomalous coronary artery anatomy. Ann Thorac Surg. 2001;72(6):2150–2.

90. Mainwaring RD, Reddy VM, Reinhartz O, Petrossian R, MacDonald M, Nasirov T, Miyake CY, Hanley FL. Anomalous aortic origin of a coronary artery: medium-term results after surgical repair in 50 patients. Ann Thorac Surg. 2011;92(2):691–7.

91. Bonilla-Ramirez C, Binsalamh Z, Masand P, Sachdeva S, Reaves-O'Neal D, Caldarone C, Molossi S. Outcomes in anomalous aortic origin of a coronary artery following surgical reimplantation in a prospective cohort. Circulation. 2019;140(Suppl_1):A11820.

92. Jegatheeswaran A, Devlin PJ, Williams WG, Brothers JA, Jacobs ML, DeCampli WM, Fleishman CE, Kirklin JK, Mertens L, Mery CM, Molossi S, Caldarone CA, Aghaei N, Lorber RO, McCrindle BW. Outcomes after anomalous aortic origin of a coronary artery repair: A Congenital Heart Surgeons' Society Study. J Thorac Cardiovasc Surg. 2020; 160(3):757–71. e5. https://doi.org/10.1016/j.jtcvs.2020.01.114. Epub 2020 Apr 13.
93. Agrawal H, Mery CM, Krishnamurthy R, Molossi S. Anatomic types of anomalous aortic origin of a coronary artery: A pictorial summary. Congen Heart Dis. 2017;104(3):e265–7. https://doi.org/10.1111/chd.12518.

Chapter 17
Sleep Disorders in Athletes

Meeta Singh, Michael Workings, Christopher Drake, and Thomas Roth

Introduction

Sleep is essential for optimal physiological and psychological health; and for athletes, optimizing sleep is becoming recognized as a critical tool for enhancing athletic performance. Unrecognized and untreated sleep disorders compromise athletic health and performance. The major categories of sleep disorders include sleep-related breathing disorders, insomnia, central disorders of hypersomnolence, circadian rhythm sleep-wake disorders, parasomnias, and sleep-related movement disorders. Of these, some are more relevant and common among athletes and will be discussed in further detail. Prior to discussing these specific sleep disorders, its essential to point out that insufficient sleep among athletes is very common [130, 131] and may be attributable to scheduling constraints and the low priority of sleep relative to other training demands, as well as a lack of awareness of the role of sleep in optimizing athletic performance. Although a detailed look at the contributing factors as well as the health and performance-related detrimental effects of insufficient sleep are out of the scope of this chapter, it is important to point out that domains of athletic performance (e.g., speed and endurance), neurocognitive function (e.g., attention and memory), and physical health (e.g., illness and injury risk, and weight maintenance) have all been shown to be negatively affected by insufficient sleep or

M. Singh (✉)
Department of Sleep Medicine, Thomas Roth Sleep Disorders Center, Henry Ford Health System, Detroit, MI, USA
e-mail: msingh2@hfhs.org

M. Workings
Department of Family Medicine, Henry Ford Health System, Detroit, MI, USA
e-mail: MWORKIN1@hfhs.org

C. Drake · T. Roth
Department of Sleep Medicine, Henry Ford Health System, Detroit, MI, USA
e-mail: CDRAKE1@HFHS.ORG; Troth1@HFHS.ORG

© Springer Nature Switzerland AG 2021
D. J. Engel, D. M. Phelan (eds.), *Sports Cardiology*,
https://doi.org/10.1007/978-3-030-69384-8_17

experimentally modeled sleep restriction [144]. Healthy adults are notoriously poor at self-assessing the magnitude of the presence and impact of sleep loss, underscoring the need for increased awareness of the importance of sleep among both elite athletes and practitioners managing their care. Education about the benefits of sleep and recovery, therefore are integral to helping athletes make the right choices about their sleep habits and environment.

Obstructive Sleep Apnea in Athletes

Obstructive sleep apnea (OSA) is a sleep disorder characterized by loud snoring, apneic episodes (cessation or reduced airflow), and arousals from sleep to open the airway (sleep fragmentation) [1]. The prevalence of OSA defined at an apnea-hypopnea index (AHI) ≥ 5 is estimated to be ~22% (range, 9–37%) in men and ~17% (range, 4–50%) in women in the USA [2]. Population-based epidemiologic studies have consistently shown that OSA affects primarily middle to older age adults, but may be present in the young adult especially those with certain risk factors including elevated body mass index (BMI) and enlarged neck sizes [3]. Thus, athletes with these physical traits have a higher prevalence of OSA particularly those in collision sports such as rugby and American football [4–7]. Sleep apnea is associated with numerous health problems, including cardiovascular disease (CVD), diabetes, and stroke [8, 9]. A causal role for sleep apnea in the pathogenesis of cardiometabolic disorders is supported by evidence that apnea and intermittent nocturnal hypoxemia augment sympathetic activation and contribute to the development of hypertension, endothelial dysfunction, and dyslipidemia [10]. Thus, identifying and treating sleep apnea is important for overall athlete health.

Despite the association of higher BMI and sleep apnea, there are a limited number of studies assessing the prevalence of apnea in high BMI athletes. Sleep apnea came into focus for the National Football League (NFL), when a 1994 study by the Centers for Disease Control and Prevention found that retired NFL linemen had a 52% higher rate of cardiovascular mortality than the general population and were three times more likely than other position players to die of heart disease [11]. It was speculated that a higher BMI among linemen was responsible for this increased cardiovascular mortality; however, most of the established cardiovascular risk factors were not assessed in this study. Given the link between sleep apnea, hypertension, and cardiovascular disease [12], a subsequent study was done in 257 retired NFL players that confirmed that linemen were more likely to have apnea (61% vs. 46%), hypertension (44.1 vs 34.0%, $p = 0.1$), and obesity (83% vs. 52%) than other position players [13].

George et al. evaluated 302 players from eight professional football teams in the NFL with specific sleep-related questionnaires and sleep laboratory assessment (polysomnography; PSG). The study estimated that 14% of NFL players had apnea [6].

Similarly, a Finnish study of professional ice hockey players found that 13% of the 107 athletes had OSA [14]. In a recent study aimed to determine the prevalence of sleep disorders in a team of 25 elite rugby union players (Australian) using in-laboratory PSG and sleep questionnaires, OSA was found to be present in 24% of players [15]. As the trend toward bigger collision sports players continues, unrecognized and untreated sleep apnea may affect not only the players' performance and productivity secondary to excessive sleepiness but also their future cardiovascular health [16]. As noted from NFL recruitment surveys, average NFL lineman weigh over 300 lbs; and this is now the norm compared with 3 decades ago (300 players in 2017 weighed over 300 lbs compared to only 10 players in 1986). A recent review of OSA among NFL players emphasized the unprecedented need for further studies on the health of NFL linemen, fueled by the unmeasured dangers of NFL athletes increasing neck size, weight, and BMI [17]. Indeed, a study exploring the mortality risk in recent NFL players showed that those with the highest playing-time BMI exhibited elevated cardiovascular mortality risk [39]. In addition to American football, other athletes like bodybuilders, sumo and professional wrestlers, etc., who have high BMI's and large necks are likely to exhibit higher rates of OSA, but epidemiological studies in these cohorts have yet to be performed.

Although limited, studies have also begun to evaluate the presence and consequences of sleep apnea in student-athletes. Iso et al. investigated 47 male freshman athletes on a rugby football team in Japan; 18 (43%) of the subjects evaluated met criteria for sleep apnea [18]. Additionally, the athletes with sleep apnea exhibited a significantly lower minimum oxygen saturation, and significantly higher oxygen desaturation index and elevated heart rate, compared to the athletes without apnea. Given that sleep apnea can be arrhythmogenic and is associated with increased risk of sudden cardiac death, [19, 20], it is critical to study the impact of undiagnosed and untreated sleep apnea on the cardiovascular health of young athletes, including student athletes.

In the past few years, there have been stories in the media of MLB players being diagnosed with sleep apnea, often after they have for years complained about symptoms of fatigue and tiredness. Typically, their BMI's are less than 30 and while they do not physically resemble NFL linemen, it is important to know that a substantial proportion of patients with apnea are not obese. Grey et al. reviewed data from 163 consecutive in-lab diagnostic sleep studies for participants referred to an academic teaching-hospital sleep clinic for suspected apnea and found that 25% of the participants with a diagnosis of OSA had a body mass index (BMI) within the normal range (BMI < 25 kg/m^2) and 54% had a BMI < 30 kg/m^2 [21]. Additionally, they found that nonobese OSA patients were more challenging to treat and less adherent and compliant with CPAP therapy. It is also important to point out that nearly a third of professional baseball players are of Hispanic/Latino origin, a population with a high prevalence of undiagnosed apnea [22]. The strong association of OSA with diabetes and hypertension, independent of obesity, is an additional factor highlighting the need for increased screening for sleep disorders in professional athletes [22].

Finally, many players in professional basketball have come forward in the media to share their stories related to sleep apnea, with the aim of increased recognition of this debilitating disorder in professional athletes. In contrast, few well-known players in professional hockey or soccer leagues have shared their OSA diagnosis, and there are minimal studies looking at sleep apnea in female athletes. Given the lack of good epidemiological studies looking at rates of apnea or treatment in these cohorts, sleep apnea is often not on the team physician's radar when evaluating tired athletes. It is however, important for team physicians to keep sleep apnea in their differential, especially when the presenting complaints include snoring, tiredness, and fatigue (even in the absence of obesity). Anatomical factors, such as small craniofacial structures, can lead to a crowded upper airway and increased upper airway collapsibility in certain nonobese patients with OSA [23]. Additionally, in approximately 70% of all patients with OSA, there is an increased propensity for awakening in response to respiratory stimuli (low respiratory arousal threshold), unstable ventilatory control (high loop gain), and ineffective upper-airway dilator muscles during sleep that can cause apnea, and thus an anatomical cause may not be present [24, 25].

All athletes who report daytime fatigue/sleepiness or snoring, gasping, snorting, or interruptions in breathing while sleeping should be asked about and examined for other features of OSA. These include awakening with a dry mouth or sore throat, moodiness or irritability, lack of concentration, memory impairment, decreased libido and impotence, nocturia, and gastroesophageal reflux disease (GERD) [26–28]. This information is useful for determining which patients to refer for further sleep evaluation.

The physical exam is frequently normal, except for a BMI >30 kg/m^2, a large neck >17 in., and a crowded oropharyngeal airway [29]. Due to lack of sensitivity and specificity of clinical signs and symptoms to effectively rule in or out sleep apnea [30], a variety of clinical questionnaires have been utilized using common signs and symptoms of OSA that are easily obtained and interpreted in the primary care setting [31]. While the diagnostic accuracy of self-report tools is limited, they have value in screening for OSA in symptomatic patients in high-risk settings (e.g., preoperative evaluation, high-risk populations). Such questionnaires have not been adequately tested as screening tools in athletes who may present with only snoring or fatigue. The Athlete Sleep Screening Questionnaire (ASSQ), a screening tool that was developed to detect clinically significant sleep disturbances and daytime dysfunction in athletes, uses the presence of loud snoring or choking or gasping to trigger a referral for further sleep apnea evaluation [32, 33].

Once apnea is suspected, objective diagnostic testing is necessary for the diagnosis. The American Academy of Sleep Medicine clinical practice guideline advocates this be performed in conjunction with a comprehensive sleep evaluation and adequate follow-up [34].

In clinical settings, recommendation for patients who are suspected of having mild sleep apnea (i.e., fewer signs and symptoms) is an in-lab polysomnographic sleep evaluation rather than an unattended in-home portable apnea test [34]. For patients with a high likelihood of moderate or severe uncomplicated sleep apnea (many presenting signs and symptoms), home testing is appropriate. However, the type of sleep evaluation utilized is largely influenced by third-party payers who tend to approve less expensive home testing over a more thorough in-lab evaluation. In the author's (MS) extensive experience working with professional athletes, in-lab testing approval is typically not an issue for payers covering professional league players. Student-athletes on the other hand, do not fall into this category.

Once diagnosed, the goals of therapy are to normalize the apnea-hypopnea index and oxyhemoglobin levels and improve alertness. In the athlete, the additional potential benefit of treating sleep apnea can include significant improvement in athletic performance. Although often reported anecdotally, a significant improvement in the average handicap index of golfers has been demonstrated following treatment of OSA with PAP therapy [35]. First-line therapy according to clinical practice guidelines for management of sleep apnea is positive airway pressure therapy [36–38]. In some cases where athletes prefer not to use positive airway pressure (i.e., CPAP mask) or are unable to tolerate it, oral appliances or upper airway surgery may be a more acceptable and better tolerated option. As athletes often travel to compete, positive airway pressure devices that are more travel friendly help with compliance as does involving the team travel department in having distilled water available to use for device humidifiers. Another point to remember is that surgical options often have to wait till the season is over and PAP may be needed in the interim. The overall message would be that the bar for getting tested for sleep apnea should be low and treatment helps address not just long-term health risk but also alertness and performance in the athlete.

Insomnia and Insomnia Complaints in Athletes

Insomnia disorder requires a report of a sleep initiation or sleep maintenance problem, despite adequate opportunities and circumstances to sleep, and daytime consequences associated with disturbed sleep (International Classification of Sleep Disorders, ICSD [40]). Insomnia is the most common sleep disorder in the USA with prevalence rates estimated between 15% and 24% among adults, and additionally at any point, 30% of adults have some symptoms of disturbed sleep [41]. Hyperarousal is a key component in the etiology of insomnia with overactive neurobiological and psychological systems contributing to difficult sleeping [42]. This hyperarousal in association with sleep-incompatible behaviors, sleep preoccupation, and excessive focus on sleep difficulties plays a role in the development and persistence of insomnia [43–45]. Additionally, there is evidence that certain personality traits associated with perfectionism can contribute as well [46]. For athletes, pre-competition anxiety and stress about performance may be a key component of this hyperarousal [47–49].

Sleep disturbance complaints prior to competition have been studied in athletes. In a survey study, the Competitive Sport and Sleep questionnaire and the Pittsburgh Sleep Quality Index were given to 283 elite Australian athletes. 64.0% of athletes indicated worse sleep on at least one occasion in the nights prior to an important competition over the past 12 months. 82.1% reported the main sleep problem was falling asleep. 83.5% attributed this problem to rumination about the competition and 43.8% reported nervousness [48]. In another study, 632 German athletes were surveyed and 65.8% of athletes reported experiencing poor sleep, with nervousness and rumination about the competition identified as causing significant problems falling asleep [47]. Additionally, athletes often report poor or no sleep after competition. Ten elite male rugby players were monitored over a twelve-night period for sleep duration and efficiency. There was a statistically significant difference in sleep duration on nights following a game compared to nongame nights, with players sleeping less on game nights, and going to sleep later on game nights [50]. In another study, 20 elite rugby players wore wrist activity monitors to objectively monitor sleep after an evening super rugby game. Compared to the nights leading up to the game, on the night after the game, players went to bed 3 h later (23:08 ± 66 min vs 02:11 ± 114 min; $p < 0.001$) and had 1:30 hour:min less sleep (5:54 ± 2:59 vs 8:02 ± 1:24 hour:min; $p < 0.05$) and four players did not sleep after the game [51]. There are multiple factors that can directly contribute to hyperarousal in athletes after competition, including increased circulating levels of cortisol, increased sympathetic hyperactivity, elevated core body temperature, caffeine use, increased exposure to light, and muscle pain [51–56]. In contrast, for pre-competition poor sleep, the main culprit appears to be anxiety or thoughts about competition itself.

Insomnia complaints have been studied in student-athletes as well. Hall et al. [57] surveyed 8683 student-athletes as part of the National College Health Assessment of US college/university students from 2011 to 2014. Prevalence for "sleep-difficulty" was 20%, insomnia was 22%, and tiredness was 61% [57]. Additionally, insomnia and daytime tiredness were associated with poorer academic performance. In the same group, researchers found that insomnia and daytime tiredness among student-athletes both independently predict risky/dangerous behavior and poor decision-making when drinking alcohol. Alternatively, risky behavior may also lead to poor self-care and worse sleep thus leading to a vicious cycle of exacerbation of sleep difficulties [58]. Student-athletes are unique in that they are balancing academics with athletics and thus are often overscheduled and frequently travel to compete. These conditions can lead to more vulnerability to sleep issues as compared to nonathlete students and should be assessed for and addressed early to prevent development of more chronic sleep problems.

Given all the pathways to hyperarousal and poor sleep in athletes, it is surprising that the prevalence of insomnia/disturbed sleep is not well explored. Lucida reported that 4% of Italian Olympic athletes met diagnostic criteria for insomnia using the Sleep Disorders Questionnaire [59, 60]. Schaal et al. reported a 6-month prevalence of insomnia symptoms of 22% in a sample of elite French athletes [61]. A recent study used questionnaires and home-based PSGs in 107 ice hockey players and reported a prevalence rate of disturbed sleep of 12% [14]. In the author's experience (MS), treating professional athletes, insomnia among this population is a frequent and clinically significant problem that can impact not only physical but mental health.

In the past decade, a number of observational studies have demonstrated an association between insomnia and incident cardiovascular disease (CVD) morbidity and mortality, including hypertension (HTN), coronary heart disease (CHD), and heart failure (HF) [146]. Although the pathogenesis underlying this relationship between insomnia and CVD is not fully understood, there are multiple mechanisms including dysregulation of the hypothalamic-pituitary (HPA) axis, sympathetic hyperactivity, increased systemic inflammation, and increased athero-genesis that are implicated.

It is also important to point out that insomnia frequently coexists with psychiatric disorders such as depression and anxiety [62]. Additionally, treating insomnia improves depression and anxiety symptoms, and treating anxiety/depression improves insomnia [63, 141–143]. Insomnia is also very common among patients with substance-use disorders and may be a risk factor for relapse [64]. In fact, patients who do not receive treatment for insomnia frequently seek over-the-counter remedies and have an increased risk of substance abuse. It is also important to explore the role of central nervous system stimulants such as caffeine, methylphenidate, amphetamines, etc., in contributing to insomnia complaints. Athletes who are diagnosed with ADHD will often take their stimulant medication just prior to game start-times to "help focus while playing". When game kick-off is in the evening, these medications contribute to the inability to fall asleep. Finally, in a recent study, insomnia was associated with increased sports-related concussion risk (RR = 3.13, 95% CI: 1.320e7.424, p = 0.015) [65]. In this study done in 190 NCAA division 1 athletes, moderate-to-severe insomnia more than tripled the athletes' risk of concussion. Team doctors should be cognizant of this relationship.

As reports of difficulty sleeping may be presenting symptoms for other sleep disorders such as sleep apnea, restless legs syndrome, and circadian rhythm disorders, these need to be ruled out during any medical evaluation. Patients with insomnia report increased fatigue, sleepiness, confusion, tension, and anxiety [66], and this results in a decreased quality of life and in athletes. Symptoms of insomnia and mental health disorders may result in degraded performance, thus identification and management in this cohort is important.

In clinical practice, subjective screening questionnaires can help identify insomnia [67–69]. While these questionnaires and scales may be appropriate for general or clinical populations, they lack specific questions that are tailored toward the sleep challenges faced by athletes. The ASSQ was designed to provide clinical screening with cutoff scores associated with the specific clinical interventions to manage sleep disorders and can be used to identify athletes who need insomnia workup and treatment [32, 33]. Additionally, the Athlete Sleep Behavior Questionnaire (ASBQ) is an 18-item survey that includes questions on sleeping behavior and habits thought to be common areas of concern for elite athletes and was designed as a practical tool to identify areas where improvements in sleep behavior could be made [70].

Once diagnosed, management of insomnia requires a stepwise approach, beginning with attempts to eliminate or at least minimize contributing factors that interfere with optimal sleep. Unfortunately, some of the contributing factors for athletes, including the effect of long-haul travel and high-intensity training [71], cannot not be eliminated. In addition, apart from the anxiety about competition and performance that athletes may have themselves, they may face further psychosocial stress about performance expectations from coaches, family, and competitors [72]. Thus, athletes may have unique thoughts and feelings that can influence behaviors, and cognitive-behavior therapy for insomnia (CBT-I) can help address these. In clinical practice, non-pharmacological sleep interventions including CBT-I, sleep hygiene education, and relaxation/mindfulness are first-line therapies [73, 74]. Overall, utilization of behavioral techniques can better help athletes learn the principles of sleep health, providing a more long-term solution to chronic sleep difficulties. In the author's (MS) experience working with professional athletes, these may be best initiated during the off-season due to time constraints. Athletes can then learn the principles and use them as needed during the season. Additionally, CBT-I approaches may not be readily available due to the limited number of providers, and other (digital CBT-I) approaches may be necessary.

Hypnotic medications may be utilized if non-pharmacological interventions are unsuccessful [73, 74]. However, pharmacological intervention may be best initiated during the off-season due to the risk of adverse events and the potential negative impact on daytime performance. In clinical practice, insomnia medications span multiple classes that can be categorized based on their mechanism of action or indication; and the choice of which to use is individualized based on a variety of factors, including patient age and comorbidities, type of insomnia complaint, side effect profiles, cost, and clinician and patient preference [75]. Although little is known about the epidemiology of prescribed and over-the-counter sleep medication use within professional sport, among student-athletes, 3% of NCAA collegiate athletes report nonprescription sleep aid use, and 18.7% of NCAA collegiate athletes report prescription sleep aid use [76].

For athletes, the two main circumstances that sleep medication may be used would be for those diagnosed with insomnia and to manage jet lag (chronobiological use-discussed in the next section). However, anecdotal evidence suggests that sleep medication use is frequent in athletes, both physician-prescribed/approved and otherwise, to combat pre/post-competition or post-training arousal (for its sedative action). Four main concerns are worth emphasizing here. Firstly, next day (or upon awakening) adverse effects of certain sleep medications on psychomotor performance have been reported [77]. However, the residual effects of such medication administered the evening before competition/training and their influence on subsequent athletic performance (i.e., the next day) is relatively unknown. Second, the "appropriateness" of using sleep medication to obtain the performance enhancement of improved sleep has been questioned [145]. Indeed, Olympic champions have openly been placed into drug rehabilitation due to dependence on sleep medication, and Australia recently banning all sleep medication use by their athletes selected for Rio 2016, advancing their previous ban for certain hypnotic medications employed only 3 weeks prior to London 2012. It, therefore, behooves team physicians to be acutely aware of and compliant with medical regulations in each of their sports and geographical locations [78] as these regulations are in a state of flux. One minor infraction can elicit severe consequences that can have a far-reaching impact, putting even more emphasis on the need for greater access to behavioral treatment options, including digital CBT-I which is widely available [141]. Thirdly, the potential for adverse events when used with other drugs (e.g., alcohol) need to be considered [79]. Finally, it is paramount for team physicians to be cognizant of the health-related concerns of sleep medication use (dependency, car accidents) [80, 81].

Circadian Rhythm Disorders in Athletes

Circadian sleep-wake rhythm disorders all involve a problem in the timing of when a person sleeps and is awake and in general three criteria must be met [40], a disrupted sleep-wake pattern, thought to be due to misalignment or malfunction of the circadian timing system; a complaint of difficulty sleeping, excessive sleepiness, or both; and suboptimal performance in an important area of functioning (e.g., occupation, education, social life, mental or physical health). The epidemiology of circadian rhythm disorders in athletes is largely unknown. However, circadian physiology modulates health and performance of athletes in multiple ways. Importantly, misalignment of the endogenous circadian timing system and sleep/wake and behavioral cycles may play a role in the onset and development of CVD and treatments aimed at mitigating circadian disruption may diminish CV risk [147].

First, a short primer on the circadian system: the *intrinsic circadian timekeeping* system modulates many physiological systems, and also actively drives *wakefulness* during the habitual waking day, helping to offset the progressive increase in sleepiness from the sleep homeostatic system, which accumulates sleep pressure across extended wakefulness [83–85]. At night, a properly aligned circadian system *increases sleep drive* at night, particularly in the latter half of the night once the homeostatic drive has been dissipated, helping to maintain sleep consolidation until normal wake-up time [86]. Additionally, *chronotype i*s a genetically determined trait that modifies each individual's preference to be most active in the morning (morning-larks), middle of the day (neither-type), or in the evening (evening-owls) [87]. Thus, sleep behavior may consequently vary depending on the athlete's chronotype and the time of day an athlete is required to train/compete [88]. For example, "night owls" who prefer to go to bed later and sleep in, may not be able to fall asleep earlier at the recommended time and may have to wake up early to train, which will cut their sleep duration. Such athletes may present with insomnia complaints when they try to fall asleep during the "forbidden zone for sleep" – the early evening period when it can be difficult (if not impossible) for them to initiate and maintain sleep [89]. In contrast, "morning larks" who prefer to go to bed early and wake up early, may need to go to bed later due to evening games and still wake up early, resulting in reduced sleep duration and excessive daytime sleepiness. As daily training/competition schedules with accompanying bedtimes are normally planned for the entire training group/team regardless of individual distinctions, planning individualized schedules based on athletes' preferred sleep schedules may be an effective measure to restore good sleep, but their practical applicability may be limited [90, 91]. In the author's experience working with athletes, this theoretical framework for sleep optimization is typically stymied by the rigid schedules that athletic teams have, that may have been in place for years.

Social jet lag is defined by the discrepancy between circadian and social clocks, which is measured as the difference in hours in midpoint of sleep between work days and free days – and this results in irregular sleep-wake patterns including significant sleep-wake timing discrepancies between workdays and free days [92]. Although, variability is a characteristic component of sleep-wake behavior [92], regularly heightened levels of inconsistency in sleep are considered unfavorable and thought to disrupt the synchrony of circadian rhythms, subsequently influencing sleep duration/quality, overall health, and performance [93, 94]. In the case of both professional and student athletes, training as well as competition schedules are prone to inducing inconsistency in sleep-wake timing among athletes. Student athletes are exposed to the common practice of early morning training and workouts, alternating with a tendency toward later times for falling asleep and waking up later on rest days, contributing to social jet lag and frequent performance impairing fatigue/sleepiness. Given the association of social jet lag with poor health, worse mood, and increased sleepiness/fatigue, it is critical to realign athletes' academic and training schedules to facilitate sleep and alert wakefulness. Alternatively, there are viable techniques to realign the sleep-wake schedule to accommodate irregular training schedules. Importantly, athletes who play mostly night/evening games can be compared to shift workers who must perform at night and thus experience difficulty with sleep or wakefulness at times that are imposed by shifts running counter to the environmental light–dark cycle [95, 96]. This is exemplified in MLB, where day games may alternate with night games resulting in a >3 h earlier wake up time on some mornings versus others. Similarly, in the NFL, the morning wake-up times on game days, for an evening game on the weekend may vary significantly from the wake-up times in the week leading up to the game when training schedules may start as early as 6 am. For most of the professional leagues where night/evening games prevail, frequent travel and family/social obligations further reduce sleep quality and quantity.

Rapid air travel across several time zones exposes the traveler to a shift in his/her internal biological clock. The result is a transient desynchronization of the circadian rhythm, called jet lag, lasting until the rhythm is realigned to the new environmental conditions [97]. Athletes often travel to compete, and competition may be proximal to travel time, thus not leaving enough time for resynchronization to the local time zone. Thus, athletes/support teams may develop symptoms of jet lag, including insomnia when they are supposed to sleep at the new time zone, sleepiness when they are supposed to be awake, fatigue, and reduced motivation. Traveling East tends to have a greater detrimental effect on sleep than traveling West [98–101]. Additionally, frequent traveling within the same time zone can also cause reduced sleep and the resulting travel fatigue can accumulate over the course of a season [102].

Finally, the influence of training/competition time is crucial to consider. Circadian rhythms regulate key physiological processes involved in athletic performance and thus can determine specific times at which peak performance is likely to occur based on intrinsic circadian factors [103–106]. In fact, studies done in multiple sports have shown peak performance in the late afternoon, with a nadir at roughly 3 AM, based on circadian factors [107, 108]. Thus, for teams that cross time zones to compete at various times of the day, some game timings may be disadvantageous for peak performance. In a study reviewing past 40 years of evening and daytime NFL games between west coast and east coast US teams, WC teams were found to have a consistent and major advantage in outcomes as compared to EC teams (above and beyond predicted outcomes) when playing evening games [109]. In another study, looking at 20 years of MLB data, authors observed that jet-lag effects on performance were largely evident after eastward travel with very limited effects after westward travel [110].

Typically, athletes with circadian rhythm sleep disorders present with disturbed sleep or excessive sleepiness. The key to the diagnosis is the recognition of the underlying abnormal sleep-wake patterns. Sleep diaries and/or actigraphs are critical in making the diagnosis as they provide reliable information regarding the timing sleep and wakefulness across several nights/day allowing patterns of sleep disturbance to be more readily identified.

Once diagnosed in clinical practice, the primary goal of treatment is to realign the circadian timing of sleep and wake with the desired or required sleep-wake period [111]. Appropriately timed melatonin, light therapy, and manipulations of bedtimes and rise times are important tools that help with realignment [112]. Jet lag management has both behavioral and pharmacological components. For short stop-overs, it is recommended to preserve the timing of sleep without modifying the circadian system. For longer trips, behavioral strategies before, during, and after the flight may advance or delay the sleep–wake cycle to help hasten realignment to the destination time zone [112]. A comprehensive plan taking into account flight timings, time zones crossed, length of stay, and timing of competition can be developed for both team and individual athletes. Recommended treatments include using timed bright light exposure, wake-promoting agents, hypnotics, and chronobiotics (i.e., melatonin and melatonin agonist) that shift internal rhythms can alleviate the symptoms of jet lag and hasten adaptation to the destination time zone and subsequently improved performance [113].

A short primer on melatonin is worth reviewing. Melatonin is intimately involved in the body's circadian regulation of sleep and essentially is a "darkness hormone" and not a "sleep hormone"; its secretion signals the length of the night with the ability to increase sleep propensity in humans (but not in nocturnal species, where it increases activity) [113, 114]. Thus, its endogenous role is to reinforce night-time physiology. It has both hypnotic (sleep-inducing) and phase-shifting (chronobiotic) properties, which in theory are ideal for jet-lag intervention, but to exploit both requires careful timing together with complete control of light exposure [115, 116].

The American Academy of Sleep Medicine recommends melatonin for jet lag and the doses of 0.5–5 mg were similarly effective; with higher doses being more effective at inducing sleep. Thus, when used correctly, melatonin can help with circadian phase advancement (falling asleep earlier) when taken in the early evening (eastward travel) and phase delay (falling asleep later) when taken in the very late evening or morning (westward travel) [117]. Exogenous melatonin is marketed as "benign" as well as a "natural" sleep aid, and this can be an issue as athletes will often buy it from health-food stores and use it indiscriminately for "any sleep" complaints. This can be problematic as melatonin product quality is a concern (including adulteration with other sedatives). Secondly, when used for phase shifting, if the dose is inappropriately timed relative to the individual's circadian timing or light exposure, it can lead to no, or even deleterious effects [118, 119]. The authors recommend it only be used with expert supervision.

Restless Legs Syndrome and Other Miscellaneous Sleep Disorders in Athletes

There are a few other sleep disorders that may be relevant to athletes. Restless legs syndrome (RLS) is a sleep-related movement disorder characterized by unpleasant or uncomfortable feeling in the lower limbs, accompanied by the urge to move that occurs during periods of inactivity, particularly in the evenings, and is transiently relieved by movement [40]. During sleep, most patients with RLS have characteristic limb movements called periodic limb movements of sleep (PLMS), which may or may not be associated with arousal from sleep. Although there are anecdotal reports suggesting that exercise or/and physical activity could worsen symptoms of motor restlessness during sleep, the prevalence of RLS in athletes is unknown. One study surveyed 60 marathon runners and reported an RLS prevalence rate of 13% [120]. Another recent study done in 107 professional ice hockey players reported a prevalence rate of RLS/PLMs of 4% [14]. There have been some reports looking at the role of high-intensity exercise sessions resulting in poor sleep; however, the results have not been consistent [121–123].

It is also important for team clinicians to know that insomnia can occur when sleeping at altitudes above 2000 m in the initial days after exposure that can be attributed to arousals caused by the hyper ventilatory response to arterial desaturation and sympathetic hyperactivity [124–126]. Often, the solution is a slow ascent with ample time to acclimate prior to training/competition [127]. In some cases, management with positive pressure devices and medications may become necessary [128, 129].

Finally, insomnia and poor sleep can be risk factors for injuries and concussions [65, 132, 133]. There is also ample evidence indicating that self-reported sleep disruption, daytime sleepiness, and fatigue are consequences of sports-related concussions [134–140]. This bidirectional relationship needs to be parsed further to help us understand if and how sleep issues after concussions contribute to further concussions and if treating the sleep issues would help in injury/concussion prevention and improvement. Thus is becomes important that screening and managing sleep disorders becomes an essential element of the athlete work up. Table 17.1 lists some of the screening tools used to identify sleep issues in the general clinical population versus those clinically validated to be used in athletes. Figure 17.1 shows an outline of how these screening tools might be used with athletes.

Table 17.1 Sleep assessment and evaluation: tools for providers

For Primary care providers	For Athlete health care providers
Epworth Sleepiness Scale (ESS) STOP BANG Sleep Screening Questionnaire (STOP BANG) Insomnia Severity Index (ISI) Pittsburgh Sleep Quality Index (PSQI) Global Sleep Assessment Questionnaire (GSAQ)	Athlete Sleep Screening Questionnaire (ASSQ)[a] Athlete Sleep Behavior Questionnaire (ASBQ)[b]

[a]Clinically validated to identify athletes that need further sleep assessment
[b]A valid and reliable tool for identifying maladaptive sleep practices in elite athletes
ESS 30, STOPBANG 30, ISI 68, PSQI- 67, ASSQ- 34, ASBQ 70

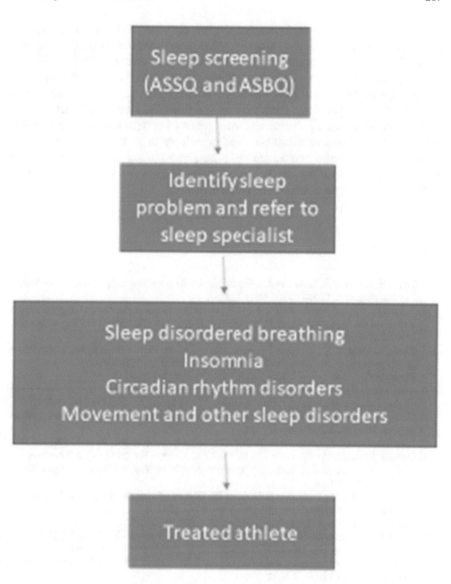

Fig. 17.1 Flow chart for screening and managing sleep issues for Athlete health care providers

Conclusions

Although optimizing sleep as a goal to optimal performance is gaining traction among athletes and coaches, sleep health in the athletic population may often be ignored. Certain populations of athletes may be at increased risk for sleep problems such as OSA, insomnia, and circadian rhythm disorders. This chapter presents a broad overview of the common sleep disorders in athletes, outlining epidemiology, presenting clinical symptoms as well as screening tools that would help in evaluation, diagnosis, and treatment. Since multiple sports-related factors including training and competition schedules, travel, sleep in hotels, etc., interact with athlete physiology and psychology, there may be variable effects on athlete sleep which require individualized assessment and management. For most sleep disorders, referral to sleep clinicians with expertise and experience in athlete issues would best serve the athlete. Proper assessment and management of sleep disorders in athletes is critical given prevailing trends and will help address downstream health risks with the added benefit of improving performance.

References

1. Patil SP, Schneider H, Schwartz AR, Smith PL. Adult obstructive sleep apnea: pathophysiology and diagnosis. Chest. 2007;132(1):325–37.
2. Franklin KA, Lindberg E. Obstructive sleep apnea is a common disorder in the population-a review on the epidemiology of sleep apnea. J Thorac Dis. 2015;7(8):1311–22. https://doi.org/10.3978/j.issn.2072-1439.2015.06.11.
3. Young T, Peppard PE, Gottlieb DJ. Epidemiology of obstructive sleep apnea: a population health perspective. Am J Respir Crit Care Med. 2002;165(9):1217–39.
4. Emsellem HA, Murtagh KE. Clin Sports Med. 2005;24(2):329–41. x
5. Swinbourne R, Gill N, Vaile J, Smart D. Prevalence of poor sleep quality, sleepiness and obstructive sleep apnoea risk factors in athletes. Eur J Sport Sci. 2016 Oct;16(7):850–8.
6. George CF, Kab V, Kab P, Villa JJ, Levy AM. Sleep and breathing in professional football players. Sleep Med. 2003;4(4):317–25.
7. Rice TB, Dunn RE, Lincoln AE, Tucker AM, Vogel RA, Heyer RA, Yates AP, Wilson PW, Pellmen EJ, Allen TW, Newman AB, Strollo PJ Jr, National Football League Subcommittee on Cardiovascular Health. Sleep-disordered breathing in the National Football League. Sleep. 2010;33(6):819–24.
8. Punjabi NM, Shahar E, Redline S, Gottlieb DJ, Givelber R, Resnick HE, Sleep Heart Health Study Investigators. Am sleep-disordered breathing, glucose intolerance, and insulin resistance: the Sleep Heart Health Study. J Epidemiol. 2004;160(6):521–30.
9. Gottlieb DJ, Yenokyan G, Newman AB, O'Connor GT, Punjabi NM, Quan SF, Redline S, Resnick HE, Tong EK, Diener-West M, Shahar E. Prospective study of obstructive sleep apnea and incident coronary heart disease and heart failure: the sleep heart health study. Circulation. 2010;122(4):352–60.
10. Butt M, Dwivedi G, Khair O, Lip GY. Obstructive sleep apnea and cardiovascular disease. Int J Cardiol. 2010;139(1):7–16.
11. Baron SRR. Health hazard evaluation report, National Football League players mortality study. Report No. HETA 88-085 1994 Centers for Disease Control and Prevention, National Institute for Occupational Safety and Health Atlanta, GA.
12. Somers VK, White DP, Amin R, et al. Sleep apnea and cardiovascular disease: an American Heart Association/American College of Cardiology Foundation scientific statement from the American Heart Association Council for High Blood Pressure Research Professional Education Committee, Council on Clinical Cardiology, Stroke Council, and Council on Cardiovascular Nursing. J Am Coll Cardiol. 2008;52:686–717.
13. Albuquerque FN, Kuniyoshi FH, Calvin AD, et al. Sleep-disordered breathing, hypertension, and obesity in retired National Football League players. J Am Coll Cardiol. 2010;56(17):1432–3.

14. Tuomilehto H, Vuorinen V-P, Penttilä E, Kivimäki M, Vuorenmaa M, Venojärvi M, Pihlajamäki J. Sleep of professional athletes: underexploited potential to improve health and performance. J Sports Sci. 2016;35(7):1–7.

15. Dunican IC, Walsh J, Higgins CC, Jones MJ, Maddison K, Caldwell JA, David H, Eastwood PR. Prevalence of sleep disorders and sleep problems in an elite super rugby union team. J Sports Sci. 2019;37(8):950–7.

16. Abernethy WB, Choo JK, Hutter AM Jr. Echocardiographic characteristics of professional football players. J Am Coll Cardiol. 2003;41(2):280–4.

17. Rogers AJ, Xia K, Soe K, et al. Obstructive sleep apnea among players in the national football league: a scoping review. J Sleep Disord Ther. 2017;6(5):278. https://doi.org/10.4172/2167-0277.1000278.

18. Iso Y, Kitai H, Kyuno E, Tsunoda F, Nishinaka N, Funato M, Nishimura E, Akihiro S, Tanuma H, Yonechi T, Geshi E, Sambe T, Suzuki H. Prevalence and significance of sleep disordered breathing in adolescent athletes. ERJ Open Res. 2019;5(1):00029-2019.

19. Rossi VA, Stradling JR, Kohler M. Effects of obstructive sleep apnoea on heart rhythm. Eur Respir J. 2013;41:1439–51.

20. Gami AS, Olson EJ, Shen WK, et al. Obstructive sleep apnea and the risk of sudden cardiac death: a longitudinal study of 10,701 adults. J Am Coll Cardiol. 2013;62:610–6.

21. Gray EL, McKenzie DK, Eckert DJ. Obstructive sleep apnea without obesity is common and difficult to treat: evidence for a distinct pathophysiological phenotype. J Clin Sleep Med. 2017;13(1):81–8. Published 2017 Jan 15. https://doi.org/10.5664/jcsm.6394.

22. Redline S, Sotres-Alvarez D, Loredo J, et al. Sleep-disordered breathing in Hispanic/Latino individuals of diverse backgrounds. The Hispanic Community Health Study/Study of Latinos. Am J Respir Crit Care Med. 2014;189(3):335–44. https://doi.org/10.1164/rccm.201309-1735OC.

23. Lam B, Ip MS, Tench E, Ryan CF. Craniofacial profile in Asian and white subjects with obstructive sleep apnoea. Thorax. 2005;60(6):504–10.

24. Eckert DJ, White DP, Jordan AS, Malhotra A, Wellman A. Defining phenotypic causes of obstructive sleep apnea. Identification of novel therapeutic targets. Am J Respir Crit Care Med. 2013;188(8):996–1004.

25. Owens RL, Edwards BA, Eckert DJ, Jordan AS, Sands SA, Malhotra A, White DP, Loring SH, Butler JP, Wellman A. An integrative model of physiological traits can be used to predict obstructive sleep apnea and response to non positive airway pressure therapy. Sleep. 2015;38(6):961–70.

26. Wallace A, Bucks RS. Memory and obstructive sleep apnea: a meta-analysis. Sleep. 2013;36(2):203.

27. Margel D, Shochat T, Getzler O, Livne PM, Pillar G. Continuous positive airway pressure reduces nocturia in patients with obstructive sleep apnea. Urology. 2006;67(5):974.

28. Gilani S, Quan SF, Pynnonen MA, Shin JJ. Obstructive sleep apnea and gastroesophageal reflux: a multivariate population-level analysis. Otolaryngol Head Neck Surg. 2016;154(2):390–5.

29. Epstein LJ, Kristo D, Strollo PJ Jr, Friedman N, Malhotra A, Patil J. Clinical guideline for the evaluation, management and long-term care of obstructive sleep apnea in adults. Clin Sleep Med. 2009;5(3):263.

30. Myers KA, Mrkobrada M, Simel DL. Does this patient have obstructive sleep apnea?: The Rational Clinical Examination systematic review. JAMA. 2013;310(7):731–41.

31. Jonas DE, Amick HR, Feltner C, Weber RP, Arvanitis M, Stine A, Lux L, Harris RP. Screening for obstructive sleep apnea in adults: evidence report and systematic review for the US preventive services task force. JAMA. 2017;317(4):415.

32. Samuels C, James L, Lawson D, Meeuwisse W. The Athlete Sleep Screening Questionnaire: a new tool for assessing and managing sleep in elite athletes. Br J Sports Med. 2016;50(7):418–22. https://doi.org/10.1136/bjsports-2014-094332.

33. Bender AM, Lawson D, Werthner P, Samuels CH. The clinical validation of the athlete sleep screening questionnaire: an instrument to identify athletes that need further sleep assess-

ment. Sports Med Open. 2018;4(1):23. Published 2018 Jun 4. https://doi.org/10.1186/s40798-018-0140-5.

34. Kapur VK, Auckley DH, Chowdhuri S, Kuhlmann DC, Mehra R, Ramar K, Harrod CG. Clinical practice guideline for diagnostic testing for adult obstructive sleep apnea: an American Academy of Sleep Medicine Clinical Practice Guideline. J Clin Sleep Med. 2017;13(3):479. Epub 2017 Mar 15

35. Benton ML, Friedman NS. Treatment of obstructive sleep apnea syndrome with nasal positive airway pressure improves golf performance. J Clin Sleep Med. 2013;9(12):1237–42.

36. Qaseem A, Holty JE, Owens DK, Dallas P, Starkey M, Shekelle P, Clinical Guidelines Committee of the American College of Physicians. Management of obstructive sleep apnea in adults: a clinical practice guideline from the American College of Physicians. Ann Intern Med. 2013;159(7):471.

37. Strohl KP, Brown DB, Collop N, George C, Grunstein R, Han F, Kline L, Malhotra A, Pack A, Phillips B, Rodenstein D, Schwab R, Weaver T, Wilson K, ATS Ad Hoc Committee on Sleep Apnea, Sleepiness, and Driving Risk in Noncommercial Drivers. An official American Thoracic Society Clinical Practice Guideline: sleep apnea, sleepiness, and driving risk in noncommercial drivers. An update of a 1994 statement. Am J Respir Crit Care Med. 2013 Jun;187(11):1259–66.

38. Patil SP, Ayappa IA, Caples SM, Kimoff RJ, Patel SR, Harrod CG. Treatment of adult obstructive sleep apnea with positive airway pressure: an American Academy of Sleep Medicine Systematic Review, Meta-Analysis, and GRADE Assessment. J Clin Sleep Med. 2019;15(2):301. Epub 2019 Feb 15

39. Lincoln AE, Vogel RA, Allen TW, Dunn RE, Alexander K, Kaufman ND, Tucker AM. Risk and causes of death among former national football league players (1986–2012). Med Sci Sports Exerc. 2018;50(3):486–93.

40. American Academy of Sleep Medicine. International classification of sleep disorders. 3rd ed. Darien: American Academy of Sleep Medicine; 2014.

41. Roth T, Coulouvrat C, Hajak G, Lakoma MD, Sampson NA, Shahly V, Shillington AC, Stephenson JJ, Walsh JK, Kessler RC. Prevalence and perceived health associated with insomnia based on DSM-IV-TR; International Statistical Classification of Diseases and Related Health Problems, Tenth Revision; and Research Diagnostic Criteria/International Classification of Sleep Disorders, Second Edition criteria: results from the America Insomnia Survey. Biol Psychiatry. 2011;69(6):592–600.

42. Kalmbach DA, Cuamatzi-Castelan AS, Tonnu CV, et al. Hyperarousal and sleep reactivity in insomnia: current insights. Nat Sci Sleep. 2018;10:193–201. Published 2018 July 17. https://doi.org/10.2147/NSS.S138823.

43. Espie CA, Broomfield NM, MacMahon KM, et al. The attention-intention-effort pathway in the development of psychophysiologic insomnia: a theoretical review. Sleep Med Rev. 2006;10(4):215–45.

44. Barclay NL, Ellis JG. Sleep-related attentional bias in poor versus good sleepers is independent of affective valence. J Sleep Res. 2013;22(4):414–21.

45. Jasnsson-Frojmark M, Bermas M, Kjellen A. Attentional bias in insomnia: the dot-probe task with pictorial stimuli depicting daytime fatigue/malaise. Cognit Ther Res. 2013;37(3):534–46.

46. van de Laar M, Verbeek I, Pevernagie D, et al. The role of personality traits in insomnia. Sleep Med Rev. 2010;14(1):61–8.

47. Erlacher D, Ehrenspiel F, Adegbesan O, et al. Sleep habits in German athletes before important competitions or games. J Sports Sci. 2011;29(8):859–66.

48. Juliff LE, Halson SL, Peiffer JJ. Understanding sleep disturbance in athletes prior to important competitions. J Sci Med Sport. 2015;18(1):13–8.

49. Ehrlenspiel F, Erlacher D, Ziegler M. Changes in subjective sleep quality before a competition and their relation to competitive anxiety. Behav Sleep Med. 2016;2:1–14.

50. Eagles A, Mclellan C, Hing W, Carloss N, Lovell D. Changes in sleep quantity and efficiency in professional rugby union players during home based training and match-play. J Sports Med Phys Fitness. 2014;

51. Dunican IC, Higgins CC, Jones MJ, Clarke MW, Murray K, Dawson B, Caldwell JA, Halson SL, Eastwood PR. Caffeine use in a Super Rugby game and its relationship to post-game sleep. Eur J Sport Sci. 2018;18(4):513–23.
52. O'Donnell S, Bird S, Jacobson G, et al. Sleep and stress hormone responses to training and competition in elite female athletes. Eur J Sport Sci. 2018;18:1–8.
53. Chennaoui M, Bougard C, Drogou C, et al. Stress biomarkers, mood states, and sleep during a major competition: success and failure athlete's profile of high-level swimmers. Front Physiol. 2016;7:94.
54. Kivlighan KT, Granger DA. Salivary alpha-amylase response to competition: relation to gender, previous experience, and attitudes. Psychoneuroendocrinology. 2006;31:703–14.
55. Veale JP, Pearce AJ. Physiological responses of elite junior Australian rules footballers during match-play. J Sports Sci Med. 2009;8:314–9.
56. Bonnet MH, Arand DL. Hyperarousal and insomnia: state of the science. Sleep Med Rev. 2010;14:9–15.
57. Hall K, Poling A, Athey P, Alfonso-Miller J, Gehrels MA, Grandner. Sleep difficulties associated with academic performance in student athletes. Sleep. 2017;40(suppl_1):A449.
58. Till K, Athey A, Chakravorty S, Killgore WD, Alfonso-Miller P, Gehrels J, Grandner MA. Insomnia and daytime tiredness in student athletes associated with risky behaviors and poor decision making when under the influence of alcohol. Sleep. 2017;40(suppl_1): A422–3.
59. Lucidi F, Lombardo C, Russo M, et al. Sleep complaints in Italian Olympic and recreational athletes. J Clin Sport Psychol. 2007;1:121–9.
60. Violani C, Devoto A, Lucidi F, Lombardo C, et al. Validity of a short insomnia questionnaire: the SDQ. Brain Res Bull. 2004;63(5):415–21.
61. Schaal K, Tafflet M, Nassif H, et al. Psychological balance in high level athletes: sex-based differences and sport-specific patterns. PLoS One. 2011;6(5):e19007.
62. Alvaro PK, Roberts RM, Harris JK. A systematic review assessing bidirectionality between sleep disturbances, anxiety, and depression. Sleep. 2013;36(7):1059.
63. Kalmbach DA, Cheng P, Arnedt JT, Anderson JR, Roth T, Fellman-Couture C, et al. Treating insomnia improves depression, maladaptive thinking, and hyperarousal in postmenopausal women: comparing cognitive-behavioral therapy for insomnia (CBTI), sleep restriction therapy, and sleep hygiene education. Sleep Med. 2019;55:124–34.
64. Brower KJ, Aldrich MS, Robinson EA, Zucker RA, Greden JF. Inomnia, self-medication, and relapse to alcoholism. Am J Psychiatry. 2001;158(3):399.
65. Raikes A, Athey A, Alfonso-Miller P, Killgore W, Grandner M. 0928 Self-reported insomnia and daytime sleepiness are better predictors of concussion risk than prior concussion history. Sleep. 2019;42:A373. https://doi.org/10.1093/sleep/zsz067.926.
66. Bonnet MH, Arand DL. Consequences of insomnia. Sleep Med Clin. 2006;1:351.
67. Buysse DJ, Reynolds CF, Monk TH, et al. The Pittsburgh sleep quality index: a new instrument for psychiatric practice and research. Psychiatry Res. 1989;28:193–213.
68. Bastien C, Vallières A, Morin CM. Validation of the Insomnia Severity Index as an outcome measure for insomnia research. Sleep Med. 2001;2:297–307.
69. Mastin DF, Bryson J, Corwyn R. Assessment of sleep hygiene using the Sleep Hygiene Index. J Behav Med. 2006;29(3):223–7.
70. Driller MW, Mah CD, Halson SL. Development of the athlete sleep behavior questionnaire: a tool for identifying maladaptive sleep practices in elite athletes. Sleep Sci. 2018;11(1):37–44.
71. Gupta L, Morgan K, Gilchrist S. Does Elite Sport Degrade Sleep Quality? A systematic review. Sports Med. 2017;47(7):1317–33.
72. Ommundsen Y, Roberts GC, Lemyre PN, Miller BW. Parental and coach support or pressure on psychosocial outcomes of pediatric athletes in soccer. Clin J Sport Med. 2006;16(6):522–6.
73. Qaseem A, Kansagara D, Forciea MA, Cooke M, Denberg TD, Clinical Guidelines Committee of the American College of Physicians. Management of chronic insomnia disorder in adults: a clinical practice guideline from the American College of Physicians. Ann Intern Med. 2016;165(2):125. Epub 2016 May 3

74. Brasure M, Fuchs E, MacDonald R, Nelson VA, Koffel E, Olson CM, Khawaja IS, Diem S, Carlyle M, Wilt TJ, Ouellette J, Butler M, Kane RL. Psychological and behavioral interventions for managing insomnia disorder: an evidence report for a clinical practice guideline by the American College of Physicians. Ann Intern Med. 2016;165(2):113–24. Epub 2016 May 03

75. Bertisch SM, Herzig SJ, Winkelman JW, Buettner C. National use of prescription medications for insomnia: NHANES 1999-2010. Sleep. 2014;37(2):343.

76. NCAA. National Study of Substance Use Habits of College Student Athletes, 2018.

77. Paul MA, Gray G, Kenny G, Pigeau RA. Impact of melatonin, zaleplon, zopiclone, and temazepam on psychomotor performance. Aviat Space Environ Med. 2003;74(12):1263–70.

78. NFLPA Drug Policies; Major League Baseball Joint Drug Prevention and Treatment Program; NBA Collective Bargaining Agreement; NHL Collective Bargaining Agreement; World Anti-Doping Agency's (WADA) Prohibited List.

79. https://pubs.niaaa.nih.gov/publications/arh23-1/40-54.pdf

80. Weaver MF. Prescription Sedative Misuse and Abuse. Yale J Biol Med. 2015;88(3):247–56. Published 3 Sept 2015.

81. Hansen RN, Boudreau DM, Ebel BE, Grossman DC, Sullivan SD. Sedative hypnotic medication use and the risk of motor vehicle crash. Am J Public Health. 2015;105(8):e64–9.

82. Aschoff J. Human circadian rhythms in activity, body temperature and other functions. Life Sci Space Res. 1967;5:159–73.

83. Wyatt JK, Ritz-De Cecco A, Czeisler CA, Dijk DJ. Circadian temperature and melatonin rhythms, sleep, and neurobehavioral function in humans living on a 20-h day. Am J Phys. 1999;277(4 Pt 2):R1152–63.

84. Dijk DJ, Czeisler CA. Paradoxical timing of the circadian rhythm of sleep propensity serves to consolidate sleep and wakefulness in humans. Neurosci Lett. 1994;166(1):63–8.

85. Wyatt JK. Chronobiology. In: Sheldon SH, Ferber R, Kryger MH, Gozal D, editors. Principles and practice of pediatric sleep medicine. 2nd ed. Philadelphia: Elsevier; 2014. p. 25.

86. Barclay NL, Watson NF, Buchwald D, Goldberg J. Moderation of genetic and environmental influences on diurnal preference by age in adult twins. Chronobiol Int. 2014;31(2):222–31.

87. Vitale JA, Bonato M, Galasso L, La Torre A, Merati G, Montaruli A, Roveda E, Carandente F. Sleep quality and high intensity interval training at two different times of day: a crossover study on the influence of the chronotype in male collegiate soccer players. Chronobiol Int. 2017;34(2):260–8.

88. Lavie P. Ultrashort sleep-waking schedule. III. 'Gates' and 'forbidden zones' for sleep. Electroencephalogr Clin Neurophysiol. 1986;63(5):414–25.

89. Samuels C. Sleep, recovery, and performance: the new frontier in high-performance athletics. Neurol Clin. 2008;26(1):169–80. ix–x

90. Scheer FA, Hu K, Evoniuk H, et al. Impact of the human circadian system, exercise, and their interaction on cardiovascular function. Proc Natl Acad Sci U S A. 2010;107:20541–6.

91. Rutters F, Lemmens SG, Adam TC, Bremmer MA, Elders PJ, Nijpels G, Dekker JM. Is social jetlag associated with an adverse endocrine, behavioral, and cardiovascular risk profile? J Biol Rhythm. 2014;29(5):377–83.

92. Bei B, Wiley JF, Trinder J, Manber R. Beyond the mean: a systematic review on the correlates of daily intraindividual variability of sleep/wake patterns. Sleep Med Rev. 2016;28:108–24.

93. Forbush S, Fisseha E, Gallagher R, Hale L, Malone S, Patterson F, Branas C, Barrett M, Killgore WD, Gehrels J, Alfonso-Miller Grandner MA. Sociodemographics, poor overall health, cardiovascular disease, depression, fatigue, and daytime sleepiness associated with social jetlag independent of sleep duration and insomnia. 2019;Sleep 40 (suppl_1):A396–A397.

94. Chennaoui M, Bougard C, Drogou C, Langrume C, Miller C, Gomez-Merino D, Vergnoux F. Stress biomarkers, mood states, and sleep during a major competition: "success" and "failure" Athlete's profile of high-level swimmers. Front Physiol. 2016;7:94.

95. Pilcher JJ, Lambert BJ, Huffcutt AI. Differential effects of permanent and rotating shifts on self-report sleep length: a meta-analytic review. Sleep. 2000;23(2):155–63.

96. Drake CL, Roehrs T, Richardson G, Walsh JK, Roth T. Shift work sleep disorder: prevalence and consequences beyond that of symptomatic day workers. Sleep. 2004;27(8):1453–62.

97. Manfredini R, Manfredini F, Fersini C, et al. Circadian rhythms, athletic performance, and jet lag. Br J Sports Med. 1998;32:101–6.

98. Kölling S, Treff G, Winkert K, et al. The effect of westward travel across five time zones on sleep and subjective jet-lag ratings in athletes before and during the 2015's World Rowing Junior Championships. J Sports Sci. 2017;35(22):2240–8.

99. Lastella M, Roach GD, Halson SL, et al. The effects of transmeridian travel and altitude on sleep: preparation for football competition. J Sports Sci Med. 2014;13:718.

100. Roach GD, Schmidt WF, Aughey RJ, et al. The sleep of elite athletes at sea level and high altitude: a comparison of sea-level natives and high-altitude natives (ISA3600). Br J Sports Med. 2013;47(Suppl 1):i114–20.

101. Fowler PM, Knez W, Crowcroft S, et al. Greater effect of east versus west travel on jet lag, sleep, and team sport performance. Med Sci Sports Exerc. 2017;49:2548–61.

102. Samuels CH. Jet lag and travel fatigue: a comprehensive management plan for sport medicine physicians and high-performance support teams. Clin J Sport Med. 2012 May;22(3):268–73.

103. Gauthier A, Davenne D, Martin A, Cometti G, Van Hoecke J. Diurnal rhythm of the muscular performance of elbow flexors during isometric contractions. Chronobiol Int. 1996;13:135–46.

104. Chtourou H, Souissi N. The effect of training at a specific time of day: a review. J Strength Cond Res. 2012;26:1984–2005.

105. Souissi N, Gauthier A, Sesboüé B, Larue J, Davenne D. Effects of regular training at the same time of day on diurnal fluctuations in muscular performance. J Sports Sci. 2002;20:929–37.

106. Drust B, Waterhouse J, Atkinson G, Edwards B, Reilly T. Circadian rhythms in sports performance: an update. Chronobiol Int. 2005;22:21–40.

107. Kline CE, Durstine JL, Davis JM, Moore TA, Devlin TM, Zielinski MR, Youngstedt SD. Circadian variation in swim performance. J Appl Physiol. 2007;102:641–9.

108. Atkinson G, Peacock O, Gibson ASC, Tucker R. Distribution of power output during cycling: impact and mechanisms. Sports Med. 2007;37:647–67.

109. Smith RS, Efron B, Mah CD, Malhotra A. The impact of circadian misalignment on athletic performance in professional football players. Sleep. 2013;36(12):1999–2001.

110. Song A, Severini T, Allada R. Jet lag and Major League Baseball. Proc Natl Acad Sci. 2017;114(6):1407–12. https://doi.org/10.1073/pnas.1608847114.

111. Auger RR, Burgess HJ, Emens JS, Deriy LV, Thomas SM, Sharkey KM, Clinical Practice Guideline for the Treatment of Intrinsic Circadian Rhythm Sleep-Wake Disorders: Advanced Sleep-Wake Phase Disorder (ASWPD), Delayed Sleep-Wake Phase Disorder (DSWPD), Non-24-Hour Sleep-Wake Rhythm Disorder (N24SWD), and Irregular Sleep-Wake Rhythm Disorder (ISWRD). An update for 2015: an American Academy of Sleep Medicine Clinical Practice Guideline. J Clin Sleep Med. 2015;11(10):1199. Epub 2015 Oct 15

112. Reilly T, Maskell P. Effects of altering the sleep-wake cycle in human circadian rhythms and motor performance. In: Proceedings of the first IOC World Congress on Sport Science. Colorado Springs: US Olympic Committee; 1989. p. 106.

113. Arendt J. Approaches to the pharmacological management of jet lag. Drugs. 2018;78(14):1419–31. https://doi.org/10.1007/s40265-018-0973-8.

114. Dijk DJ, Shanahan TL, Duffy JF, Ronda JM, Czeisler CA. Variation of electroencephalographic activity during non-rapid eye movement and rapid eye movement sleep with phase of circadian melatonin rhythm in humans. J Physiol. 1997;505(Pt 3):851–8.

115. Paul MA, Gray GW, Lieberman HR, Love RJ, Miller JC, Trouborst M, Arendt J. Phase advance with separate and combined melatonin and light treatment. Psychopharmacology. 2011;214(2):515–23.

116. Rajaratnam SM, Dijk DJ, Middleton B, Stone BM, Arendt J. Melatonin phase-shifts human circadian rhythms with no evidence of changes in the duration of endogenous melatonin secretion or the 24-hour production of reproductive hormones. J Clin Endocrinol Metab. 2003;88(9):4303–9.

117. Lewy AJ, Bauer VK, Ahmed S, Thomas KH, Cutler NL, Singer CM, Moffit MT, Sack RL. The human phase response curve (PRC) to melatonin is about 12 hours out of phase with the PRC to light. Chronobiol Int. 1998;15(1):71–83.
118. Forbes-Robertson S, Dudley E, Vadgama P, Cook C, Drawer S, Kilduff L. Circadian disruption and remedial interventions: effects and interventions for jet lag for athletic peak performance. Sports Med. 2012;42(3):185–208.
119. Atkinson G, Buckley P, Edwards B, Reilly T, Waterhouse. Are there hangover-effects on physical performance when melatonin is ingested by athletes before nocturnal sleep? J Int J Sports Med. 2001;22(3):232–4.
120. Fagundes SB, Fagundes DJ, Luna AA, et al. Prevalence of restless legs syndrome in runners. Sleep Med. 2012;13(6):771.
121. Brand S, Gerber M, Beck J, Hatzinger M, Pühse U, Holsboer-Trachsler E. High exercise levels are related to favorable sleep patterns and psychological functioning in adolescents: a comparison of athletes and controls. J Adolesc Health. 2010;46(2):133–41.
122. Killer SC, Svendsen IS, Jeukendrup AE, Gleeson M. Evidence of disturbed sleep and mood state in well-trained athletes during short-term intensified training with and without a high carbohydrate nutritional intervention. J Sports Sci. 2017;35(14):1402–10.
123. Kölling S, Wiewelhove T, Raeder C, Endler S, Ferrauti A, Meyer T, Kellmann M. Sleep monitoring of a six-day microcycle in strength and high-intensity training. Eur J Sport Sci. 2016 Aug;16(5):507–15.
124. Johnson PL, Edwards N, Burgess KR, et al. Sleep architecture changes during a trek from 1400 to 5000 m in the Nepal Himalaya. J Sleep Res. 2010;19:148–56.
125. Salvaggio A, Insalaco G, Marrone O, et al. Effects of high-altitude periodic breathing on sleep and arterial oxyhaemoglobin saturation. Eur Respir J. 1998;12:408–13.
126. Lastella M, Roach GD, Halson SL, Gore CJ, Garvican-Lewis LA, Sargent C. The effects of transmeridian travel and altitude on sleep: preparation for football competition. J Sports Sci Med. 2014;13:718–20.
127. Tang XG, Zhang JH, Gao XB, et al. Sleep quality changes in insomniacs and non-insomniacs after acute altitude exposure and its relationship with acute mountain sickness. Neuropsychiatr Dis Treat. 2014;10:1423–32. https://doi.org/10.2147/NDT.S67218.
128. Luks AM, Swenson ER, Bärtsch P. Acute high-altitude sickness. Eur Respir Rev. 2017;26(143):160096.
129. Mohsenin V. Common high altitudes illnesses a primer for healthcare provider. Br J Med Med Res. 2015;7(12):1017–25. https://doi.org/10.9734/BJMMR/2015/17501.
130. Halson SL. Sports Med. 2014;44(Suppl 1):13. https://doi.org/10.1007/s40279-014-0147-0.
131. Mah CD, Mah KE, Kezirian EJ, Dement WC. The effects of sleep extension on the athletic performance of collegiate basketball players. Sleep. 2011;34(7):943–50. Published 2011 Jul 1. https://doi.org/10.5665/SLEEP.1132.
132. Milewski MD, Skaggs DL, Bishop GA, et al. Chronic lack of sleep is associated with increased sports injuries in adolescent athletes. J Pediatr Orthop. 2014;34(2):129.
133. von Rosen P, Frohm A, Kottorp A, et al. Too little sleep and an unhealthy diet could increase the risk of sustaining a new injury in adolescent elite athletes. Scand J Med Sci Sports. 2017;27(11):1364e71.
134. Gosselin N, Duclos C. Insomnia following a mild traumatic brain injury: a missing piece to the work disability puzzle? Sleep Med. 2016;20:155e6.
135. Ouellet M-C, Beaulieu-Bonneau S, Morin CM. Insomnia in patients with traumatic brain injury: frequency, characteristics, and risk factors. J Head Trauma Rehabil. 2006;21(3):199e212.
136. Allan AC, Edmed SL, Sullivan KA, et al. Actigraphically measured sleep-wake behavior after mild traumatic brain injury: a case-control study. J Head Trauma Rehabil. 2017;32(2):E35.
137. Hoffman NL, O'Connor PJ, Schmidt MD, et al. Differences in sleep between concussed and nonconcussed college students: a matched caseecontrol study. Sleep. 2019;42(2) https://doi.org/10.1093/sleep/zsy222.
138. Raikes AC, Satterfield BC, Killgore WDS. Evidence of actigraphic and subjective sleep disruption following mild traumatic brain injury. Sleep Med. 2019;54:62e9.

139. Sufrinko AM, Howie EK, Elbin RJ, et al. A preliminary investigation of accelerometer-derived sleep and physical activity following sport-related concussion. J Head Trauma Rehabil. 2018;33(5):E64–74.
140. Raikes AC, Schaefer SY. Sleep quantity and quality during acute concussion: a pilot study. Sleep. 2016;39(12):2141e7.
141. Cheng P, Luik AI, Fellman-Couture C, Peterson E, Joseph CL, Tallent G, Tran KM, Ahmedani BK, Roehrs T, Roth T, Drake CL. Efficacy of digital CBT for insomnia to reduce depression across demographic groups: a randomized trial. Psychol Med. 2019;49(3):491–500. https://doi.org/10.1017/S0033291718001113.
142. Cheng P, Tallent G, Luik A, Peterson E, Tran K, Ahmedani B, Adler D, Roth T, Drake C. 0372 Digital cognitive behavioral therapy for insomnia reduces incident depression at one-year follow-up. Sleep. 2018;41:A142. Now accepted paper is SLEEP (2019).
143. Mason EC, Harvey AG. Insomnia before and after treatment for anxiety and depression. J Affect Disord. 2014;168:415–21.
144. Simpson NS, Gibbs EL, Matheson GO. Optimizing sleep to maximize performance: implications and recommendations for elite athletes. Scand J Med Sci Sports. 2017;27:266–74.
145. Taylor L, Chrismas BC, Dascombe B, Chamari K, Fowler PM. Sleep medication and athletic performance – the evidence for practitioners and future research directions. Front Physiol. 2016;7:83. https://doi.org/10.3389/fphys.2016.00083.
146. Javaheri S, Redline S. Insomnia and risk of cardiovascular disease. Chest. 2017;152(2):435–44. https://doi.org/10.1016/j.chest.2017.01.026.
147. Chellappa SL, Vujovic N, Williams JS, Scheer FAJL. Impact of circadian disruption on cardiovascular function and disease. Trends Endocrinol Metab. 2019;30(10):767–79. https://doi.org/10.1016/j.tem.2019.07.008.

Chapter 18
Chest Pain and Dyspnea

David C. Peritz and John J. Ryan

Introduction

Shortness of breath and chest pain, both associated and not associated with exercise, are common complaints among athletes. The causes of such are myriad (Table 18.1) with considerable overlap between the two symptoms. Indeed, even differentiating between the two symptoms can be challenging. As with most clinical concerns, a detailed history, and physical exam are paramount for determining the presence of life-threatening problems and for establishing the optimum diagnostic strategy, treatment, and management plan. In this chapter, we will describe the common conditions that cause dyspnea and chest pain in athletes and provide an algorithm and guidance as to the workup and evaluation.

Dyspnea

The evaluation of dyspnea in athletes can require extensive testing (Fig. 18.1). Both highly trained and amateur athletes commonly complain of shortness of breath during exercise despite there being no identifiable pathology. Poor exercise capacity should be ruled out with a thorough history of an athlete's training habits. Perceived shortness of breath related to limitations in functional capacity is often related to

D. C. Peritz (✉)
Heart and Vascular Center, Dartmouth Hitchcock Medical Center, Lebanon, NH, USA

Geisel School of Medicine, Lebanon, NH, USA
e-mail: david.c.peritz@hitchcock.org

J. J. Ryan
Division of Cardiovascular Medicine, Department of Internal Medicine, University of Utah, Salt Lake City, UT, USA
e-mail: john.ryan@hsc.utah.edu

© Springer Nature Switzerland AG 2021
D. J. Engel, D. M. Phelan (eds.), *Sports Cardiology*,
https://doi.org/10.1007/978-3-030-69384-8_18

Table 18.1 Etiologies of dyspnea and chest pain in athletes

Causes of dyspnea and chest pain			Recommended testing	Key findings
Cardiac	Structural	Valvular disease	Echocardiogram, cardiac MRI	Abnormal Echocardiogram
		Myocardial/pericardial	ECG, cMRI, echocardiogram	Diffuse ST elevation on ECG Gadolinium enhancement on cMRI
		Cardiomyopathy	Echocardiogram	
		Cardiac mass	Echocardiogram, cMRI	
	Electrical	Atrial fibrillation	ECG, remote ECG monitoring	Irregularly irregular rhythm
		Premature contractions	Remote monitoring, exercise stress test	
		Tachycardia		
		Bradycardia		
	Coronary	Ischemia	Stress testing, coronary CT, troponin	ST changes associated with stress Abnormal perfusion imaging
		Anomalous coronary artery	Coronary CT	Abnormal origin or path of coronary arteries
Pulmonary	Airway	Exercise-induced bronchoconstriction	Spirometry with bronchoprovocation Eucapnic voluntary hyperpnea	Symptoms early with exercise remain long after cessation Drop in FEV_1 of >20% with EVH or > 10% with exercise
		Pneumonia		
		Exercise-induced laryngeal obstruction	Continuous laryngeal endoscopy during exercise	Stridor Narrowing of vocal chords with both inspiration Inspiratory flattening of slow-volume loop
	Vascular	Pulmonary embolism	CT angiography Ventilation/perfusion scan	Lung perfusion defects on imaging
		Pulmonary arterial hypertension	Echocardiogram Right heart catheterization	Mean pulmonary artery pressure > 20 mmHg
	Extrinsic	Pleural effusion	CXR, chest CT	
		Pneumothorax	Auscultation, CXR	Absent breath sounds Tracheal deviation

Musculoskeletal		*Fractured rib*		
		Sternoclavicular joint/sternum		
		Costochondritis		
		Deconditioning	Exercise stress test, cardiopulmonary stress test	Low ventilatory threshold relative to peak VO_2 High chronotropic index Low-indexed VO_2
		Myopathy		
		Thyroid disease	TSH	Resting tachy/bradycardia
Other	Vascular	*Aortic dissection*		
	GI	*GERD*		
	Psychological	*Anxiety/depression*		
		Hyperventilation		

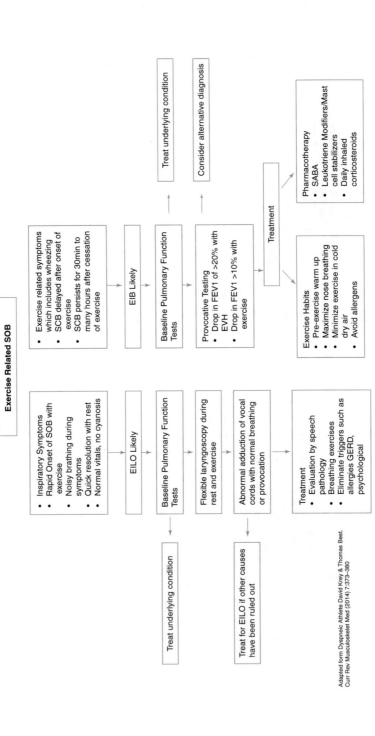

Fig. 18.1 Evaluation of Exercise-induced Shortness of Breath. EIB: exercise-induced bronchospasm; EILO: exercise-induced laryngeal obstruction; FEV1: forced expiratory volume; SABA: short acting β-agonists; SOB: shortness of breath. Adapted from David Krey & Thomas Best. *Curr Rev Musculoskelet Med* (2014) 7:373–380

changes in training and coaching expectations, such as moving from high school to college, changes in environment (different temperature or altitude, indoors versus outdoor training) or return to exercise after a period of deconditioning. While evaluating any changes in training behavior, it is important to ask about changes in weather or altitude of the training location as well as participation in unfamiliar exercises. A physician must also consider overtraining as a cause of symptomatic dyspnea [1]. In addition to a detailed exercise history, if a cardiac etiology is suspected, an electrocardiogram and echocardiogram should be part of the initial steps. A cardiopulmonary exercise testing (CPET) can be highly valuable in the assessment of inappropriate dyspnea, especially if initial testing remains inconclusive. In fact, CPET studies have shown that deconditioning is the identifiable cause of 23–67% of adolescents complaining of exercise-associated dyspnea [2]. Features that suggest deconditioning are a normal absolute peak VO_2 but a low-indexed VO_2 and O2 pulse. In addition, one might see a low ventilatory threshold relative to peak VO2 and high chronotropic index [3]. CPET information, however, may often not tell the whole story, especially without a baseline study to compare to. Many endurance athletes will have high maximum oxygen uptake (VO_2 max) values but still experience a perceived drop in performance. Without a prior VO_2 test to compare, it can be challenging to pick up subtle changes. This becomes even more difficult in nonendurance athletes whose VO_2 max would be closer to the normal range. While CPET testing is highly useful in the evaluation of a symptomatic athlete, a detailed guide to interpretation of CPET is beyond the scope of this chapter.

Exercise-Induced Bronchoconstriction

The prevalence of exercise-induced bronchoconstriction (EIB) is estimated to be between 10 and 50% within the athletic population and represents a major cause of morbidity [4]. It occurs in both asthmatic and nonasthmatic individuals and can affect athletes at any fitness level. EIB is frequently misdiagnosed because diagnosis is made based on symptoms which tend to be nonspecific. Unfortunately, it is common for a physician caring for an athlete to prescribe a trial a bronchodilators without baseline testing. As such, there are many athletes who use prescription bronchodilators but continue to have unresolved symptoms [5]. In the athletic population, it is prudent for physicians to provide a thorough initial evaluation as more serious diseases may masquerade as simply unresponsive EIB.

EIB is by definition an acute transient airway narrowing provoked by exercise. While the physiology is not entirely understood, leading hypotheses suggest that the bronchial mucosa becomes dry through increased ventilation and/or airway cooling. This, in turn, leads to inflammation and narrowing of the airway [6, 7]. During times of exercise, the high volume of exchanged and often cool air overwhelms the body's warming and humidifying mechanisms allowing for cold air to reach and irritate the distal bronchial tree. Given the proposed pathophysiology, it should not be surprising that this phenomenon is seen more often in outdoor and cold weather sports [8].

This reaction can also be triggered by other aerosolized irritants such as chemicals from a swimming pool [9] or automobile exhaust [10].

In addition to dyspnea, symptoms of EIB can consist of wheezing, cough, and chest tightness. Symptoms often start within 5–10 minutes of the initiation of exercise and may remain for 30 minutes after exercise is stopped. These two characteristics can often help differentiate EIB from exercise-induced laryngeal obstruction (EILO), which will be discussed subsequently.

Exercise-induced asthma (EIA) can also cause SOB. There tends to be significant symptom overlap between EIA and EIB. In fact, 80–90% of patients with EIA will also have EIB [11]. In addition, 10–40% of those with allergic rhinitis will also have EIB [12]. Unlike EIB, athletes with EIA may have chronic airway inflammation and symptoms of shortness of breath or wheezing at rest that become exacerbated with activity [13]. It is important to note, however, that there are asthmatics who only have symptoms with exercise and would need PFTs to further delineate.

Initial evaluation should begin with spirometry. Athletes with EIB will often normal spirometry at rest and should therefore undergo spirometry with bronchoprovocation. A dry air exercise challenge test which rests on the supposition that inherent to EIB is a dehydration of the respiratory tree and can often reveal restrictive physiology not noted at rest [14]. Similar in its effect on the airway, eucapnic voluntary hyperpnea (EVH) is another provocative test which is currently the gold standard for diagnosing EIB in athletes [15]. A drop in FEV1 of >20% with EVH is diagnostic of EIB [16]. Through hyperpnea with a dry gas, the test can mimic the effect that exercise has on the airway system. In addition to being used as a means of establishing response to treatment, EVH is also preferred in those who do not regularly exercise but have symptoms with activity [17, 18]. Lastly, the International Olympic Committee (IOC) requires EVH testing for documenting EIB in athletes [19]. In locations where EVH testing is not available, treadmill exercise testing in a pulmonary laboratory will suffice. In this method, the goal is an 8- to 12-minute test at 80–90% of max heart rate. A decrease in FEV1 of 10% or greater immediately following exercise as compared to pre-exercise is diagnostic of EIB [20]. Again, it is important to reiterate that if symptoms persist but testing has been negative alternative diagnoses much be considered.

Management for EIB should target symptom control both with medications and adjusting environmental allergen exposure whenever possible. There is reasonable evidence to support encouraging graduated pre-exercise warm-up, in addition encouraging nose breathing or breathing through scarf to warm/humidify air during cold weather sports [21]. While it is not recommended, it is not uncommon for physicians to initiate evaluation with a trial of short acting β-agonist such as albuterol [22]. The first-line medical therapy should be an inhaled Short-Acting β-agonist (SABA) used either in response to EIB symptoms or prior to exercise. If used prior to exercise, it is recommend that an athlete take 2 puffs, 15–30 minutes prior to activity [23]. Daily use of SABA can lead to tolerance, so frequent use should be avoided whenever possible. If symptoms persist to a point where daily medication is needed, it is first important for the prescriber to confirm that the inhaler is being used properly as this is a common and correctable error [24]. Once this is confirmed, a combination of inhaled corticosteroids and bronchodilators should be prescribed. Leukotriene modifiers are most effective when taken 2 hours prior to exercise and are recommended over long-acting β-agonists (LABA) [25, 26].

Exercise-Induced Laryngeal Obstruction

Exercise-induced laryngeal obstruction (EILO), previously referred to as vocal cord dysfunction (VCD), is another common cause of exercise-induced dyspnea in the athlete. With an average time to diagnosis of 4.5 years, it is also believed to be underdiagnosed [27, 28]. EILO is a more appropriate classification of the problem rather than vocal cord dysfunction because there is not necessarily a permanent alteration of the vocal cords, but instead it is characterized by abnormal closure at a supraglottic or glottis level of the larynx. This occurs only during inspiration and leads to intermittent narrowing of the airway [29]. This narrowing leads to restrictive airflow into the lungs and a sensation of SOB. This feeling is not present without exercise. There is a fair amount of overlap with EIB as up to 30% of patients with EILO also have EIB [30]. Both diseases present with shortness of breath and cough associated with exercise, but unlike EIB, the symptoms of EILO often rapidly resolve with cessation of exercise [31, 32]. Patients with EILO may also complain of more inspiratory symptoms rather than expiratory and in some cases demonstrate audible stridor or voice changes [33]. EILO is present in 5% of the athletic population, and following an evaluation by a pulmonologist, an estimated 35–70% of athletes referred for dyspnea on exertion were diagnosed with EILO [34]. It also appears to be more prevalent in athletes participating in outdoor sports as compared to indoor as well as more common in females and adolescents [35].

The diagnosis begins with a thorough history and physical involving the timing of symptoms. Symptoms from EIB tend to be slower onset and worst at 5–20 minutes after exercise. On the other hand, the symptoms of EILO are of rapid onset during exercise and resolve within 5 minutes of activity cessation (Fig. 18.1).

Despite these subtle differences, the diagnosis often requires pulmonary function testing as a thorough history is often not enough to differentiate EILO from EIB. Pulmonary function tests may show a reduction in both FEV1 and FVC. This is, however, not a very sensitive test; there is minimal difference between those with and without EILO at baseline. A decrease in FEV1 with methacholine challenge is suggestive of EIB, but it is worth noting that methacholine can act as an irritant and is known to provoke EILO as well [36].One notable characteristic of EILO during pulmonary function testing is that the expiratory loop of the flow-volume loop is typically normal, whereas the inspiratory loop is flattened. This pattern is most likely seen during symptomatic episodes [37]. The gold standard is continuous laryngeal endoscopy during exercise (CLE). While cumbersome, the exercise component is essential as symptoms often resolve quickly with rest. EILO is present if the vocal cords show narrowing with both inspiration and expiration, while patient has stridor or dyspnea [38]. EILO is more prevalent around supraglottic level as compared to glottis [39].

Much of the information we rely on for management is derived from treatment of VCD which is present at rest. This poses significant challenges in designing treatment protocols, but assessment and management by a speech and language pathologist continue to be of the utmost importance. Diaphragmatic breathing control exercises and laryngeal exercises under guidance of a speech pathologist have been shown to be up to 95% effective [40]. In addition, there are case reports of other strategies to managed EILO including supraglottic surgical intervention to strengthen vocal folds, biofeedback, psychotherapy, and hypnosis [41, 42]. It is important to treat any underlying conditions and help athletes to identify and eliminate triggers which may affect the vocal cords such as allergies, gastroesophageal reflux and psychological triggers such as anxiety [43].

Other Causes of Dyspnea

Structural Heart Disease

Identification of valvular heart disease usually occurs through identification of a murmur during a routine physical examination or preparticipation evaluation or when an athlete presents with exertional symptoms. Valvular heart disease can be divided into degenerative disease which usually affects those in their sixth decade onward and congenital disease which is often discovered at a much younger age. Congenital valvular disease affects 1–2% of individuals who pursue athletic endeavors [44]. Evaluation should begin with a detailed physical exam which includes blood pressures in both arms and one leg to rule out coarctation of the aorta. In addition, in most athletes with either an abnormal cardiac exam or unexplained dyspnea, an electrocardiogram and echocardiogram should be performed. This should screen for valvular disease as well as ventricular/atrial septal defects or patent ductus arteriosus. There are no large prospective studies evaluating the progression of valvular disease in athletes; thus, consensus guidelines have been created using data from the nonathletic population. Please see Chap. 6 for a detailed discussion on valvular disease in the athlete. In general, athletes should be monitored regularly with echocardiogram as well as exercise stress testing to evaluate progression. Athletes with symptoms should refrain from competitive sports but maintain an active lifestyle which should include 20–30 minutes of moderate cardiovascular exercise below their symptom threshold at least 5 times each week [45].

Those with bicuspid aortic valve should be screened for aortic enlargement. Those with bicuspid valve and aortic enlargement should be seen by a cardiologist trained in adult congenital disease in conjunction with the sports cardiology team to determine what, if any additional genetic testing should be done to look for connective tissue disease. Sports participation limitations in this group are based on aortic size as well as bicuspid aortic valve function [46]. Please refer to the chapter on exercise recommendations in congenital heart disease for a more detailed discussion and recommendations for athletes.

Anemia

Acute or chronic anemia should be within the differential for an athlete who presents with shortness of breath but without specific signs of airway disease. As an essential player in the delivery of oxygen to exercising muscles, a decrease in hemoglobin level may lead to compensatory mechanisms such as tachycardia or tachypnea [47]. Profound fatigue is also a common presenting complaint. These symptoms frequently mimic those caused by airway disease and can lead to a decrease in performance. Iron deficiency, which if left untreated can lead to anemia, is present in about 3% of athletes though may be more common in long distance runners [48]. The causes of anemia are broad, but within the athletic population, it is most commonly due to menstrual loss, gastrointestinal bleeding, or hemolysis due to repetitive impact of foot strikes during running/marching [49]. Diagnosis should begin with physical exam looking for generalized or conjunctival pallor. Laboratory studies should include a complete blood count (CBC) as well as iron studies (Ferritin, Transferrin, and total iron binding capacity). Treatment is dictated by addressing any identifiable cause of anemia and oral iron supplementation.

Pulmonary Embolism

Pulmonary embolism (PE) is a life-threatening cause of dyspnea in the athlete that was previously felt to be uncommon. The incidence in children and adolescents is particularly low (53/100,000) though there are an increasing number of case reports describing deep vein thrombosis (DVTs) and PE in otherwise healthy adult athletes [50, 51]. Unfortunately, the traditional algorithms often used when suspecting PE in the nonathletic population perform inadequately when applied to athletes. In fact, in a recent review of previously published case reports, the *Wells Score* performs strikingly poorly in the endurance athlete subpopulation [52]. Diagnosis still relies on a combination of clinical assessment, D-dimer measurement, lower extremity ultrasound, and computed tomography scan (CT). In addition to the potential life-threatening nature of the disease, thromboembolism can have a significant impact on an athlete's career with the average professional athlete losing 6.7 months of play after the diagnosis and treatment is made [53]. Moreover, there are also care reports of subjective loss of performance following total resolution of initial symptoms of PE [54].

Pneumothorax

While uncommon, primary spontaneous pneumothorax (PSP) is a serious condition which should be considered in any athlete presenting with pleuritic chest pain. Pneumothorax should be divided into traumatic or spontaneous. PSP is defined as a nontraumatic pneumothorax in the absence of prior lung disease. While most often occuring as a complication from rib fracture, traumatic pneumothorax should be suspected in athletes with difficulty breathing after a collision involving the chest, abdomen, or even flank [55]. Athletes may present in a delayed fashion and have trouble associating a specific trauma as the inciting event for symptoms. Though a rare event, PSP has been reported in numerous sports including weightlifting, SCUBA diving and running [56]. Typical presenting symptoms include pleuritic chest pain, dyspnea, and tachycardia. In severe cases, one may see asymmetric chest wall expansion, diminished breath sounds, deviation of trachea from midline and shifted cardiac apical impulse [57]. Initial decompression of a tension pneumothorax may be necessary in patients presenting with tenuous vital signs. In cases of less dramatic presentation, in addition to thorough lung auscultation, a chest x-ray is often necessary for diagnosis. Treatment depends on the size of the pneumothorax. In patients with their initial episode of PSP who are clinically stable and the pneumothorax is less than 3 cm, supplemental oxygen and observation typically are appropriate [58]. Those with large and symptomatic pneumothorax may require aspiration or chest tube placement [59]. The estimated recurrence rate of PSP is significant (23–50% over a 5 year period); thus, patient should be educated as to the elevated risk [60].Serial monitoring with x-rays to determine resolution should be done in 2–4 weeks. Return to play guidelines remains unclear though it is generally felt that athletes with either spontaneous or traumatic pneumothorax can return to their sport once symptoms resolve [61].

Chest Wall Abnormalities

Pectus excavatum is a common congenital deformity affecting 1:300 births. It is more common in males than females with a ratio of about 4:1 [62]. The deformity is characterized by an inward depression of the sternum relative to the ribcage and often worsens during late adolescence and early adulthood corresponding with deteriorating symptoms [63]. Exercise limitation is at least partially due to impaired augmentation of cardiac preload with exercise and restrictive pulmonary physiology with a reduction in total lung capacity [64]. The Haller Index or Pectus Severity Score is calculated using tomographic imaging, usually CT chest, and correlates well with reduction in exercise capacity [65]. CPET is usually required to define the cause and extent of cardiopulmonary limitation with severe limitations often mandating surgical intervention with the goal of alleviating mechanical obstruction and improving exercise capacity [66].

Scoliosis or curvature of the spine is relatively common in the general population with a prevalence ranging from 0.3–15% [67] and, like pectus excavatum, can cause restrictive lung physiology. In severe cases, there may be lung hypoplasia [68]. Breathing patterns in scoliosis tend to be altered as well with patients often demonstrating tachypnea and shallow breathing while relying heavily on accessory muscles [69]. These changes are often exacerbated during exercise where reduced respiratory system compliance, increased work of breathing, and blunted respiratory drive lead to lower performance [70]. Like patients with pectus excavatum, definitive treatment frequently involves consultation with orthopedic surgery.

Infectious Diseases

Infectious diseases including pneumonia, bronchitis, and systemic viral illnesses can cause shortness of breath in the athlete. Athletes tend to present with other more nonspecific complaints such as fatigue, muscle soreness, and upper respiratory symptoms. Upper respiratory illness (URI) is the common among athletes accounting for 35–65% of noninjury-related medical presentations. There remains an ongoing debate among exercise immunologists as to whether exhaustive exercise itself is immunosuppressive and accounts for the observed high incidence of URI or whether this is more likely related to other lifestyle issues that may increase exposure to infection (travel to competition, crowds at sporting events) or cause immunosuppression (poor sleep, anxiety, poor nutrition) [71].

Chest Pain

In the USA, chest pain affects nearly 70 million patients and accounts for almost 5% of all emergency room evaluations [72]. In athletes, the incidence is thought to be about 15/1000 participants, but that figure is likely an underestimate [73]. During initial evaluation of an athlete with chest pain, a physician's chief concern is to determine whether the pain is cardiac in nature and thus places the athlete at risk for sudden cardiac death (SCD). Although the vast majority of chest pain symptoms in both young and old athletes are noncardiac, the risk of cardiac disease increases with age [74]. Assessment should begin with a thorough history and physical exam as a significant proportion of noncardiac causes of chest pain can be delineated by a careful history and exam (Fig. 18.2). On symptom review, there are several high yield questions for predicting coronary disease which include the presence of exertional pain or radiation of pain to the arms or shoulder [75]. Lightheadedness during exercise along with palpitations or syncope may suggest arrhythmia. Positional pleuritic pain following a recent viral illness may suggest pericarditis. On the other hand, pain with palpation, certain movements, or pain at night while lying supine may shift the differential toward noncardiac causes.

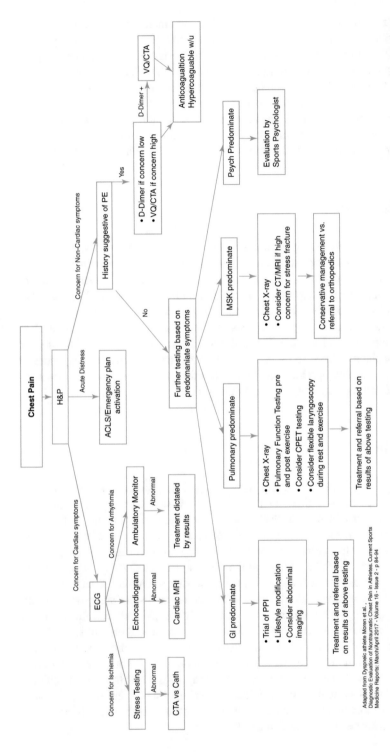

Adapted from Dyspnic athlete Moran et al.,
Diagnostic Evaluation of Nontraumatic Chest Pain in Athletes. Current Sports
Medicine Reports: March/April 2017 - Volume 16 - Issue 2 - p 84-94

Fig. 18.2 Evaluation of Chest Pain. PE: pulmonary embolism; VQ: ventilation perfusion scan; CTA: Computed tomography with angiography; MSK: Musculoskeletal; MRI: magnetic resonance imaging; CPET: cardiopulmonary exercise testing; ECG: electrocardiogram; GI: gastrointestinal; PPI: proton-pump inhibitor. Adapted from Moran et al. Diagnostic Evaluation of Nontraumatic Chest Pain in Athletes. *Current Sports Medicine Reports*: March/April 2017—Volume 16—Issue 2, p 84–94

A complete family history is also essential, especially as it relates to SCD or unexplained death. Any unexplained death in a family member under 50 years of age should increase a clinician's suspicion for genetic causes of chest pain such as hypertrophic cardiomyopathy (HCM), arrhythmogenic right ventricular cardiomyopathy (ARVC), or a connective tissue disorder. Lastly, a detailed history of medications (both prescribed and nonprescribed), supplements and illicit drug use should be gathered. Drugs which activate the sympathetic nervous system, including those for attention deficit disorder, can cause palpitations and chest pain [76].

Cardiac

Coronary Disease

Regular exercise is associated with a reduced morbidity and mortality from coronary artery disease (CAD); however, exercise should not be perceived as a panacea against the development of CAD. Autopsy results suggest that atherosclerotic disease is the most common cause of sudden cardiac death in the athlete over 35 years of age [77]. The exercise paradox highlights that while vigorous exercise increases the likelihood of short-term cardiac events by a factor of 5–7, habitual exercises are at lower overall risk compared to sedentary controls [78]. While it may seem counterintuitive, recent studies have suggested a higher burden of coronary artery calcium in long-term endurance athletes, though the clinic impact of this remains uncertain [79]. In any athlete over the age of 35 presenting with chest pain, specifically "warm-up" angina, a thorough evaluation for CAD is warranted. Workup should include a maximal exertion stress test. This may require an adjustment of the standard Bruce protocol for those of very high fitness. In those with a normal stress test and low cardiac risk profile, further testing can be avoided. In those with borderline or abnormal stress tests, CT angiogram can be helpful in confirming the extent of CAD and guiding further intervention [80]. Management should focus on aggressive risk factor modification and intervention when necessary. Statin-related muscle fatigue may be more common in the athletic population, but treatment with lipid lowering agents should remain a priority. Data on PCSK9 inhibitors in the athletic population are currently lacking but may present a helpful alternative to statin therapy.

Presenting often with both chest pain and pre-syncope, anomalous aortic origin of the coronary artery is a potentially life-threatening diagnosis. Occurring in 0.1–0.7% of the population, anomalous coronary arteries (ACA) can follow several different patterns, the most concerning of which involves the left coronary artery passing between the aorta and pulmonary artery (interarterial) and within the wall of the aorta (intramural) [81, 82]. Autopsy reports from collegiate athletes in the USA identified interarterial coronary artery anomalies as the second leading cause of sudden cardiac death [83]. SCD risk is difficult to determine but remains significantly higher in those with interarterial course of the left coronary artery (6.3%) as compared to the RCA (0.2%) [84]. Ischemia-induced malignant arrhythmias are related to vessel compression which is compounded by acute take-off angle and slit like orifice of the affected coronary artery as it runs within the wall of the aorta [85]. Diagnosis can often be made with echocardiography. If there is suspicion of an ACA, the athlete must be restricted from activity until further evaluation is made often in the form of cardiac computed tomography angiography (CCTA) or cardiac magnetic resonance imaging (cMRI). Stress testing is useful in determining whether there is inducible ischemia. All athletes with a left from right anomaly running an interarterial course should undergo surgery irrespective of symptoms or ischemia. Surgery is also recommended for those with a right from left anomaly running an interarterial course in the presence of symptoms or ischemia; in the absence of symptoms or demonstrable ischemia, competitive sports may be permitted after extensive shared decision making [86].

Myocarditis

Myocarditis is a nonischemic inflammatory process which affects the myocardium. The inflammation often leads to chest pain, myocardial dysfunction, and increased risk for arrhythmias [87]. The causes of myocarditis are often related to infectious etiologies, autoimmune, or toxic insults, with viral myocarditis being the most common. Clinical presentation can vary from mild chest pain or exertional dyspnea to decompensated heart failure and cardiogenic shock [88]. Initial evaluation should start with a detailed history including questions about recent illnesses, particularly viral symptoms as well as drug use. ECG findings are variable and include ST elevation or depression, conduction disturbances, and sustained arrhythmias. Transthoracic echocardiography will often show a decreased ejection fraction with/without wall motion abnormalities [89]. While the gold standard remains endomyocardial biopsy, the clinical use of this invasive procedure has waned due to the risks of complications and its limited sensitivity due to patchiness of the inflammation. Thus, cardiac MRI with demonstration of delayed gadolinium enhancement (DGE) in conjunction with elevated cardiac enzymes as well as clinical history of viral prodrome and chest pain is the more common method of diagnosis [90].

Myocarditis is a risk factor for SCD, an effect that appears to be compounded by exercise. In several SCD studies in those 40 years of age or younger, autopsy data demonstrated that myocarditis accounted for approximately 10% of the cases. Of those, about one-quarter of them were associated with exercise [91]. In the athletic population, once the diagnosis of myocarditis has been established, the chief concern is when is it safe to return to play. Currently, guidelines in the USA and Europe suggest that patient should refrain from exercise, while ongoing inflammation is present even in the face of normal LV function. Prior to returning to play, the patient should undergo exercise ECG, Holter monitor, echocardiogram, and biomarker testing to demonstrate resolution of inflammation and absence of arrhythmias. This should be done some time between 3 and 6 months after initial episode [92].The role of serial cMRI to monitor for scar formation and aid in risk stratification is unclear though there is strong evidence to suggest that presence of DGE portends a higher risk for malignant arrhythmias [93]. While data remain sparse and guidelines are not yet established, each of the major cardiology associations has developed return-to-play recommendations for those diagnosed with the novel Coronavirus disease 2019 (COVID-19) [94]. Early observations suggest COVID-19 can have a significant impact on the heart though myocarditis reports are scarce. We expect these recommendations for athletes with a history of COVID-19 to evolve as more is learned about the disease and the long-term sequelae. Understanding the virus's specific effects on the myocardium remains an area of significant research.

Pericarditis

Acute pericarditis is the most common of the pericardial diseases with an incidence of about 27.7 cases per 100,000 people each year [95]. In addition, acute pericarditis is identified in approximated 5% of emergency room visits for chest pain and about 0.1% of hospital admissions [96]. In the western world, the most common etiology is viral [97], while in the developing world, the most common cause remains tuberculosis [98]. Many patients will have a prodromal viral illness but present with abrupt onset characteristic precordial chest pain which worsens when lying flat or deep inspiration but improves with sitting and leaning forward. Radiation of pain to the trapezius ridge is considered pathognomonic [99]. ECG changes can vary but often show diffuse concave ST segment elevation with PR depression though in some cases only PR depression is present [100]. Cardiac exam may demonstrate a pericardial friction rub and tachycardia. In the case of a large pericardial effusion, an examiner may also note elevation in jugular venous pressure, muffled heart sounds and hypotension (Beck's Triad) suggestive of tamponade physiology. The diagnosis is based on the presence of at least two of the following signs and symptoms: chest pain consistent with pericarditis, a larger than trivial pericardial effusion, a pericardial friction rub or a characteristic ECG as described above. It is important to emphasize that friction rubs and ECG changes may be transient. Thus, repeating both may be necessary during the evaluation of a symptomatic patient. The use of steroids is limited to chronic or recurrent cases and should be avoided whenever possible [101].

Current recommendations state that competitive, high-intensity sports should be avoided until there is no longer any evidence of disease [102]. This includes resolution of symptoms, normalization of inflammatory markers and absence of pericardial effusion. These recommendations are based on the supposition that heavy physical activity may increase circulation of inflammatory markers and therefore increase the risk, development of pericardial effusion, refractory pericarditis, or progression to myocarditis. This evolution to myocarditis would then put the athlete at greater risk of SCD [103]. For recreational athletes, it may be reasonable to continue low-intensity exercise until symptoms resolve.

Aorta Dissection

Spontaneous aortic dissection is a rare but serious cause of death in the athlete most commonly associated with heavy weightlifting or other highly static exercises [104]. This is particularly important for those with identified connective tissue diseases who are at greater risk for aortic root dilation and possible rupture. Studies reporting larger aortic root dimensions in athletes as compared to controls are not longitudinal in nature and therefore cannot be used to determine if these minor differences are clinically relevant in those without genetic connective tissue disorders [105]. Efforts are underway to better understand normal aortic dimensions in larger professional athletes specifically American Football and Basketball players with the hopes better being able to screen those at higher risk for rupture [106, 107]. For a more in-depth discussion on this topic, please refer to Chap. 15.

Palpitations

Symptomatic variations in heart rhythm are usually benign [108]. However, because cardiac arrhythmia is often the trigger leading to SCD, any complaint of irregular rhythm or inappropriate tachycardia warrants further evaluation. Evaluation should involve a 12 lead ECG, as well as a detailed history and physical. Echocardiogram to rule out structural abnormalities is appropriate in most cases. If the resting ECG is normal, it becomes critical to try and capture symptomatic episodes using wearable rhythm monitors. Over the last few years, this task has become more easily achieved given the prevalence of smartphone-enabled monitors as well as long-term implantable recorders [109]. If the symptoms occur with exercise, exercise stress testing is indicated to eliciting symptoms and arrhythmia. If an abnormal rhythm is documented, treatment can be dictated based on the abnormality.

Gastrointestinal Causes

Gastroesophageal reflux (GERD) is common during exercise with the prevalence estimated to be as high as 50%. The exact mechanism by which GERD occurs during exercise is unknown, but it is believed to be in part due to decreased gastrointestinal blood flow and delayed gastric emptying as well as increased intra-abdominal pressure [110]. Food intake immediately prior to exercise as well as high-intensity exercise appears to be risk factors. Inquiring about use of nonsteroidal anti-inflammatory drug use as well as anorexic behaviors is important [111]. Patients often present with retrosternal burning or throat discomfort in addition to shortness of breath. GERD may also exacerbate symptoms of asthma. Treatment with activity modifications including reduction in high-intensity exercise, smaller meals with a longer delay prior to exercise and proton-pump inhibitors should be attempted prior to invasive diagnostics. If symptoms do not resolve, it is reasonable to consider endoscopy [112].

Chest Wall Pain

Musculoskeletal chest pain can occur in the ribs, sternum, or articulation of these structures. While more obvious causes include chest wall trauma or muscle strain, overuse injuries such as stress fractures have been reported in several sports. There is an increased risk associated with amenorrhea and low bone density. Stress fracture of the first rib more commonly occurs in sports with repetitive overhead movement and is likely due to a point of relative weakness where the subclavian artery passes underneath the first rib [113]. Patients usually present with a dull aching pain. Physical exam may reveal tenderness to palpation over the affected area. Radiographs are often negative in detecting stress fractures of the first rib; thus, if clinical suspicion is high, CT or MRI may be needed [114]. In the case of first rib stress fractures, treatment is conservative and involves biomechanical and strength training. A gradual return to overhead activity should be dictated by pain. Stress fractures of other ribs tend to involve ribs 4–8 and are associated primarily with rowing with one study reporting occurrence in 8–16% of elite rowers [115]. Treatment again involves rest, analgesia, and strengthening, but recovery tends to be more rapid and return to full training is often possible in 8–10 weeks [116].

Slipping rib syndrome often goes under-recognized and can be caused by repetitive trunk motion in sports such as running or swimming. It is felt to be caused by the sliding of floating ribs (8–12) under the adjacent ribs causing irritation of nerve cartilage and surrounding muscle [117]. Patients typically present with a sharp stabbing pain in the lower chest or back during activity followed by dull pain at rest that may last up to a few days. Pain can also be elicited by pressure over the ribs or by hooking one's fingers under the ribs and pulling anteriorly which causes a clicking sensation [118]. Imaging does not aid in the diagnosis. Treatment options include rest and reassurance although there are reports of anterior rib excision in some severe cases [119].

Costochondritis is commonly diagnosed in the general population as the cause of atypical chest pain. Though prevalence in the athlete is not well defined, one study reported that 30% of all patients who presented to the hospital with atypical symptoms were diagnosed with costochondritis [120]. Costochondritis most often occurs in the 2–5th costal cartilages and should be suspected in an athlete with dull anterior chest tenderness which does involve erythema or swelling which would be indicative of Tietze's Syndrome [121]. While there are reports of elevations in inflammatory markers as well as abnormalities on x-ray, CT or bone scan workup typically does not require imaging or laboratory testing. Treatment should focus on analgesia, reassurance, and rest [122].

Psychiatric

Psychogenic causes of chest pain are more commonly seen in children and adolescents. One study suggested that approximately 20% of chest pain in adolescents was due to hyperventilation or anxiety [123]. This should be a diagnosis of exclusion and involves a careful history including a discussion of life stressors or other associated symptoms.

Conclusion

Both chest pain and dyspnea are common presenting symptoms in athletes of all ages. While the vast majority of causes are benign, it is imperative that the managing physician keep a wide differential in mind. Noncardiac etiologies are far more prevalent in younger athletes who complain of chest pain, whereas in older athletes, cardiac concerns should be higher on the differential. In athletes of all ages presenting for evaluation of shortness of breath, the most common airway-related causes are EIB and EIA. Workup should focus on a detailed history and physical. Further testing, if any is required, should be dictated by the results of the initial evaluation as well as pretest probabilities based on the age of the athlete. While it remains a priority to limit the amount of time lost from sport, treating physicians should be prepared to hold an athlete with high-risk symptoms out of activity until workup is complete.

Acknowledgments Dr. Ryan and his research are supported by funding from The Reagan Corporation, The Gordon Family, and The Cushman Family.

References

1. Kreher JB, Schwartz JB. Overtraining syndrome: a practical guide. Sports Health. 2012;4:128–38.
2. Mahut B, Fuchs-Climent D, Plantier L, et al. Cross-sectional assessment of exertional dyspnea in otherwise healthy children. Pediatr Pulmonol. 2014;49:772–81.
3. LeClerc K. Cardiopulmonary exercise testing: a contemporary and versatile clinical tool. Cleve Clin J Med. 2017 Feb;84(2):161–8.
4. Parsons JP, Mastronarde JG. Exercise-induced bronchoconstriction in athletes. Chest. 2005;128:3966.

5. Smoliga JM, Weiss P, Rundell KW. Exercise induced bronchoconstriction in adults: evidence based diagnosis and management. BMJ. 2016;352:h6951.
6. Storms WW, Joyner DM. Update on exercise-induced asthma: a report of the Olympic exercise asthma summit conference. Phys Sports Med. 1997;25:45–55.
7. Anderson SD. Single dose agents in the prevention of exercise induced asthma: a descriptive review. Treat Respir Med. 2004;3:365–79.
8. Wilber RL, et al. Incidence of exercise-induced bronchospasm in Olympic winter sport athletes. Med Sci Sports Exerc. 2000;32:732–7.
9. Bougault V, Boulet LP. Airway dysfunction in swimmers. Br J Sports Med. 2012;46:402–6.
10. Price OJ, Ansley L, Menzies-Gow A, Cullinan P, Hull JH. Airway dysfunction in elite athletes - an occupational lung disease? Allergy. 2013;68:1343–52.
11. Feinstein RA, LaRussa J, Wang-Dohlman A, Bartolucci AA. Screening adolescent athletes for exercise-induced asthma. Clin J Sport Med. 1996;6:119–23.
12. Gotshall RW. Exercise-induced bronchoconstriction. Drugs. 2002;62:1725–39.
13. Jaworski CA. "Pulmonary". ACSM's sports medicine, a comprehensive review. In: O'Connor F. Wolters Kluwer Health. Lippincott Williams & Wilkins; 2013, p. 248–255.
14. Rundell KW, Wilber RL, Szmedra L, et al. Exercise-induced asthma screening of elite athletes: field vs laboratory exercise challenge. Med Sci Sports Exerc. 2000;32:309–16.
15. Hull JH, Ansley L, Price OJ, Dickinson JW, Bonini M. Eucapnic voluntary hyperpnea: gold standard for diagnosing exercise-induced bronchoconstriction in athletes? Sports Med. 2016;46(8):1083–93.
16. Holzer K, Anderson SD, Douglass J, et al. Exercise in elite summer athletes: challenges for diagnosis. J Allergy Clin Immunol. 2002;110:374–80.
17. Brannan JD, Koskela H. Anderson SD monitoring asthma therapy using indirect bronchial provocation tests. Clin Respir J. 2007;1(1):3–15.
18. Holley AB, Cohee B, Walter RJ, Shah AA, King CS, Roop S. Eucapnic voluntary hyperventilation is superior to methacholine challenge testing for detecting airway hyper-reactivity in nonathletes. J Asthma. 2012;49:614–9.
19. Fitch KD, Sue-Chu M, Anderson SD, Boulet LP, Hancox RJ, McKenzie DC, et al. Asthma and the elite athlete: summary of the International Olympic Committee's consensus conference, Lausanne, Switzerland, January 22–24, 2008. J Allergy Clin Immunol. 2008;122:254–60.
20. Hurwitz KM, Argyros GJ, Roach JM, et al. Interpretation of eucapnic voluntary hyperventilation in the diagnosis of asthma. Chest. 1995;108:1240–5.
21. Schachter EN, Lach E, Lee M, et al. The protective effect of a cold weather mask on exercised-induced asthma. Ann Allergy. 1981;46:12–6.
22. Brennan FH, Alent J, Ross MJ. Evaluating the athlete with suspected exercise-induced asthma or bronchospasm. Curr Sports Med Rep. Mar 2018;17(3):85–9.
23. Parsons JP, Hallstrand TS, Mastronarde JG, et al. An official American thoracic society clinical practice guideline: exercise induced bronchoconstriction. Am J Respir Crit Care Med. 2013;187:1016–27.
24. Harnett CM, Hunt EB, Bowen BR, et al. A study to assess inhaler technique and its potential impact on asthma control in patients attending an asthma clinic. J Asthma. 2014 May;51(4):440–5.
25. Philip G, Villaran C, Pearlman DS, et al. Protection against exercise-induced bronchoconstriction two hours after a single oral dose of montelukast. J Asthma. 2007;44:213–7.
26. Ferrari M, Segattini C, Zanon R, et al. Comparison of the protective effect of formoterol and of salmeterol against exercise-induced bronchospasm when given immediately before a cycloergometric test. Respiration. 2002;69:509–12.
27. Patel NJ, Jorgensen C, Kuhn J, et al. Concurrent laryngeal abnormalities in patients with paradoxical vocal fold dysfunction. Otolaryngol Head Neck Surg. 2004;130:686–9.
28. Cohen SM, Belluci E. Health utilization among patients with vocal cord dysfunction. Nurs Forum. 2011;46:177–85.
29. Christensen PM, Heimdal JH, Christopher KL, et al. ERS/ELS/ACCP 2013 international consensus conference nomenclature on inducible laryngeal obstructions. Eur Respir Rev. 2015;24:445–50.

30. Johansson H, Norlander K, Berglund L, et al. Prevalence of exercise-induced bronchocon-striction and exercise-induced laryngeal obstruction in a general adolescent population. Thorax. 2015;70:57–63.
31. Al-Alwan A, Kaminsky D. Vocal cord dysfunction in athletes: clinical presentation and review of the literature. Phys Sportsmed. 2012;40:22–7.
32. Nielsen EW, Hull JH, Backer V. High prevalence of exercise-induced laryngeal obstruction in athletes. Med Sci Sports Exerc. 2013;45:2030–5.
33. Marcinow AM, Thompson J, Chiang T, et al. Paradoxical vocal fold motion disorder in the elite athlete: experience at a large division I university. Laryngoscope. 2014;124:1425–30.
34. Hanks CD, Parsons J, Benninger C, et al. Etiology of dyspnea in elite and recreational ath-letes. Phys Sports Med. 2012;40:28–33.
35. Rundell KW, Spiering BA. Inspiratory stridor in elite athletes. Chest. 2003;123:468–74.
36. Morris MJ, Deal LE, Bean DR, et al. Vocal cord dysfunction in patients with exertional dys-pnea. Chest. 1999;116:1676–82.
37. Deckert J, Deckert L. Vocal cord dysfunction. Am Fam Physician. 2010;81(2):156–9.
38. Heimdal JH, Roskund OD, Halvorsen T, et al. Continuous laryngoscopic exercise test: a method for visualizing laryngeal dysfunction during exercise. Laryngoscope. 2006;116:52–7.
39. Røksund OD, Heimdal JH, Olofsson J, Maat RC, Halvorsen T. Larynx during exercise: the unexplored bottleneck of the airways. Eur Arch Otorhinolaryngol. 2015 Sep;272(9):2101–9.
40. Sullivan MD, Heywood BM, Beukelman DR. A treatment for vocal cord dysfunction in female athletes: an outcome study. Laryngoscope. 2001;111:1751–5.
41. Norlander K, Johansson H, Jansson C, et al. Surgical treatment is effective in severe cases of exercise-induced laryngeal obstruction: a follow-up study. Acta Otolaryngol. 2015;135:1152–9.
42. Powell DM, Karanfilov BI, Beechler KB, et al. Paradoxical vocal cord dysfunction in juve-niles. Arch Otolaryngol Head Neck Surg. 2000;126:29–34.
43. Kolnes LJ, Stensrud T. Exercise-induced laryngeal obstruction in athletes: contributory fac-tors and treatment implications. Physiother Theory Pract. 2018 May;14:1–12.
44. Nishimura RA, McGoon MD, Shub C, et al. Echocardiographically documented mitral-valve prolapse. Long-term follow-up of 237 patients. N Engl J Med. 1985;313:1305–9.
45. Gati S, Malhotra A, Sharma S. Exercise recommendations in patients with valvular heart disease. Heart. 2019;105:106–11.
46. Braverman AC, Harris KM, Kovacs RJ, Maron BJ. Eligibility and disqualification recom-mendations for competitive athletes with cardiovascular abnormalities: task force 7: aor-tic diseases, including Marfan syndrome: a scientific statement from the American Heart Association and American College of Cardiology. J Am Coll Cardiol. 2015;66(21):2398–405.
47. Shaskey DJ, Green GA. Sports haematology. Sports Med. 2000;29:27–38.
48. Zoller H, Vogel W. Iron supplementation in athletes – first do no harm. Nutrition. 2004;20:615–9.
49. Fazal AA, Whittemore MS, DeGeorge KC. Foot-strike haemolysis in an ultramarathon run-ner. BMJ Case Rep. 2017;13:2017.
50. Moffatt K, Silberberg PJ, Gnarra DJ. Pulmonary embolism in an adolescent soccer player: a case report. Med Sci Sports Exerc. 2007;39(6):899–902.
51. Sanz de la Garza M, Lopez A, Sitges M. Multiple pulmonary embolisms in a male marathon athlete: is intense endurance exercise a real thrombogenic risk? Scand J Med Sci Sports. 2017;27(5):563–6.
52. Zaleski AL, Taylor BA, Pescatello LS, Thompson PD, Denegar C. Performance of wells score to predict deep vein thrombosis and pulmonary embolism in endurance athletes. Phys Sportsmed. 2017;45(4):358–64.
53. Bishop M, Astolfi M, Padegimas E, DeLuca P, Hammoud S. Venous thromboembolism within professional American sport leagues. Orthop J Sports Med. 2017;5(12):2325967117745530.
54. Dumitrescu D, Gerhardt F, Viethen T, Schmidt M, Mayer E, Rosenkranz S. Case report: sub-jective loss of performance after pulmonary embolism in an athlete- beyond normal values. BMC Pulm Med. 2016;16:21.

55. David PF. Primary spontaneous pneumothorax in a track athlete. Clin J Sport Med. 2002;12(5):318–9.
56. Marnejon T, Sarac S, Cropp AJ. Spontaneous pneumothorax in weightlifters. J Sports Med Phys Fitness. 1995;35(2):124–6.
57. Partridge RA, Coley A, Bowie R, Woolard RH. Sports-related pneumothorax. Ann Emerg Med. 1997;30(4):539–41.
58. Kelly AM, Kerr D, Clooney M. Outcomes of emergency department patients treated for primary spontaneous pneumothorax. Chest. 2008;134(5):1033.
59. Janssen J, Cardillo G. Primary spontaneous pneumothorax: towards outpatient treatment and abandoning chest tube drainage. Respiration. 2011;82(2):201.
60. Baumann MH, Strange C, Heffner JE, et al. Management of spontaneous pneumothorax: an American College of Chest Physicians Delphi consensus statement. Chest. 2001;119(2):590.
61. Curtin SM, Tucker AM, Gens DR. Pneumothorax in sports: issues in recognition and follow-up care. Phys Sportsmed. 2000;28(8):23–32.
62. Nuss D, Obermeyer RJ, Kelly RE. Pectus excavatum from a pediatric surgeon's perspective. Ann Cardiothorac Surg. 2016;5(5):493–500.
63. Williams A, Crabbe D. Pectus deformities of the anterior chest wall. Paediatr Respir Rev. 2003;4:237–42.
64. Rowland T, Moriarty K, Banever G. Effect of pectus excavatum deformity on cardiorespiratory fitness in adolescent boys. Arch Pediatr Adolesc Med. 2005;159(11):1069–73.
65. Malek M, Fonkalsrud E, Cooper C. Ventilatory and cardiovascular responses to exercise in patients with pectus excavatum. Chest. 2003;124:870–82.
66. Obermeyer RJ, Cohen NS, Jaroszewski DE. The physiologic impact of pectus excavatum repair. Semin Pediatr Surg. 2018;27(3):127–32.
67. Tsiligiannis T, Grivas T. Pulmonary function in children with idiopathic scoliosis. Scoliosis. 2012;7(1):7.
68. McMaster MJ, Glasby MA, Singh H, Cunningham S. Lung function in congenital kyphosis and kyphoscoliosis. J Spinal Disord Tech. 2007;20(3):203–8.
69. Lisboa C, Moreno R, Fava M, Ferretti R, Cruz E. Inspiratory muscle function in patients with severe kyphoscoliosis. Am Rev Respir Dis. 1985;132(1):48–52.
70. Kearon C, Viviani GR, Kirkley A, Killian KJ. Factors determining pulmonary function in adolescent idiopathic thoracic scoliosis. Am Rev Respir Dis. 1993;148(2):288–94.
71. Simpson RJ, Campbell JP, Gleeson M, et al. Can exercise affect immune function to increase susceptibility to infection? Exerc Immunol Rev. 2020;26:8–22.
72. Achem SR. Noncardiac chest pain-treatment approaches. Gastroenterol Clin N Am. 2008;37:859–78.
73. Rowland TW. Evaluating cardiac symptoms in the athlete: is it safe to play? Clin J Spor Med. 2005;15:416–20.
74. Lee TH, Goldman L. Evaluation of the patient with acute chest pain. N Engl J Med. 2000;342:1187–95.
75. Goodacre S, Locker T, Morris F, Campbell S. How useful are clinical features in the diagnosis of acute, undifferentiated chest pain? Acad Emerg Med. 2002;9:203–8.
76. Wilens T, Prince J. Stimulants and sudden death: what is a physician to do? Pediatrics. 2006;118:1215–9.
77. Eckart R, Shry E, Burke A. Sudden death in young adults: an autopsy-based series of a population undergoing active surveillance. J Am Coll Cardiol. 2011;58(12):1254–61.
78. Parker MW, Thompson PD. Prog Cardiovasc Dis. 2012;54:416–22.
79. Merghani A, Maestrini V, Rosmini S. Prevalence of subclinical coronary artery disease in masters endurance athletes with a low atherosclerotic risk profile. Circulation. 2017;136(2):126–37.
80. Borjesson M, Delborg M, Niebauer J, et al. Recommendations for participation in leisure time or competitive sports in athletes-patients with coronary artery disease: a position statement from the Sports Cardiology Section of the European Association of Preventative Cardiology (EAPC). Eur Heart J. 2019;40(1):13–8.

81. Davis JA, Cecchin F, Jones TK, Portman MA. Major coronary artery anomalies in a pediatric population: incidence and clinical importance. J Am Coll Cardiol. 2001;37:593–7.
82. Basso C, Maron BJ, Corrado D, Thiene G. Clinical profile of congenital coronary artery anomalies with origin from the wrong aortic sinus leading to sudden death in young competitive athletes. J Am Coll Cardiol. 2000;35:1493–501.
83. Maron BJ, Haas TS, Murphy CJ, Ahluwalia A, Rutten-Ramos S. Incidence and causes of sudden death in U.S. College athletes. J Am Coll Cardiol. 2014;63:1636–43.
84. Brothers J, Carter C, McBride M, Spray T, Paridon S. Anomalous left coronary artery origin from the opposite sinus of valsalva: evidence of intermittent ischemia. J Thorac Cardiovasc Surg. 2010;140:e27–9.
85. Ali M, Hanley A, McFadden EP, Vaughan CJ. Coronary artery anomalies: a practical approach to diagnosis and management. Heart Asia. 2011;3(1):8–12.
86. Van Hare GF, Ackerman MJ, Evangelista JA, et al. Eligibility and disqualification recommendations for competitive athletes with cardiovascular abnormalities: task force 4: congenital heart disease: a scientific statement from the American Heart Association and American College of Cardiology. Circulation. 2015;132:e281–91.
87. Basso C, Carturan E, Corrado D, Thiene G. Myocarditis and dilated cardiomyopathy in athletes: diagnosis, management, and recommendations for sport activity. Cardiol Clin. 2007;25:423–9.
88. Woodruff JF. Viral myocarditis. A review. Am J Pathol. 1980;101:423–84.
89. Brennan FH, Stenzier B, Oriscello R. Diagnosis and management of myocarditis in athletes. Curr Sports Med Rep. 2003;2(2):65–71.
90. Aquaro GD, Perfetti M, Camastra G, et al. Cardiac MR with late gadolinium enhancement in acute myocarditis with preserved systolic function: ITAMY study. J Am Coll Cardiol. 2017;70:1977–87.
91. van der Werf C, van Langen IM, Wilde AA. Sudden death in the young: what do we know about it and how to prevent? Circ Arrhythm Electrophysiol. 2010;3:96–104.
92. Maron BJ, Zipes DP, Kovacs RJ. Eligibility and disqualification recommendations for competitive athletes with cardiovascular abnormalities: Task Force 3: Hypertrophic Cardiomyopathy, Arrhythmogenic Right Ventricular Cardiomyopathy and Other Cardiomyopathies, and myocarditis. Circulation. 2015;132:e237–80.
93. Zorzi A, Perazzolo Marra M, Rigato I, et al. Nonischemic left ventricular scar as a substrate of life-threatening ventricular arrhythmias and sudden cardiac death in competitive athletes. Circ Arrhythm Electrophysiol. 2016;9(7):e004229.
94. Phelan D, Kim JH, Chung EH. A game plan for the resumption of sport and exercise after coronavirus disease 2019 (COVID-19) infection. [published online ahead of print, 2020 May 13]. JAMA Cardiol. 2020; https://doi.org/10.1001/jamacardio.2020.2136.
95. Maisch B, Seferovic PM, Ristic AD, et al. Guidelines on the diagnosis and management of pericardial diseases executive summary; the task force on the diagnosis and management of pericardial diseases of the European Society of Cardiology. Eur Heart J. 2004;25:587–610.
96. LeWinter MM. Acute Pericarditis. N Engl J Med. 2014;371:2410–6.
97. Seidenberg PH, Haynes J. Pericarditis: diagnosis, management, and return to play. Curr Sports Med Rep. 2006;5(2):74Y9.
98. Sliwa K, Mocumbi AO. Forgotten cardiovascular diseases in Africa. Clin Res Cardiol. 2010;99:65–74.
99. Shabetai R. The pericardium. Norwell: Kluwer; 2003.
100. Seferovic PM, Ristic AD, Maksimovic R, et al. Pericardial syndromes: an update after the ESC guidelines 2004. Heart Fail Rev. 2013;18:255–66.
101. Imazio M, Brucato A, Trinchero R, Spodick D, Adlery Y. Colchicine for pericarditis: hype or hope? Eur Heart J. 2009;30:532–9.
102. Maron B, Zipes DP, Kovacs RJ. Eligibility and disqualification recommendations for competitive athletes with cardiovascular abnormalities: preamble, principles and general consid-

erations: a scientific statement from the American Heart Association and American College of Cardiology. J Am Coll Cardiol. 2015;66:2343–9.

103. Friman G, Wesslen L. Special feature for the Olympics: infections and exercise in high-performance athletes. Immunol Cell Biol. 2000;78:510–22.

104. Hatzaras I, Tranquilli M, Coady M, Barrett PM, Bible J, Elefteriades JA. Weight lifting and aortic dissection: more evidence for a connection. Cardiology. 2007;107(2):103–6.

105. Eijsvogels TMH, Fernandez AB, Thompson PD. Are there deleterious cardiac effects of acute and chronic endurance exercise? Physiol Rev. 2016;96(1):99–125.

106. Engel DJ, Schwartz A, Homma S. Athletic cardiac remodeling in US professional basketball players. JAMA Cardiol. 2016;1(1):80–7.

107. Gentry JL, Carruthers D, Joshi PH, et al. Ascending aortic dimensions in former National Football League athletes. Circ Cardiovasc Imaging. 2017;10(11):e006852.

108. Washington RL. Dysrhythmic heart disease. In: Goldberg B, editor. Sports and exercise for children with chronic health conditions. Champaign: Human Kinetics Publishers; 1995. p. 237–46.

109. Peritz DC, Howard A, Ciocca M, Chung EG. Smartphone ECG aids real time diagnosis of palpitation in the competitive college athlete. J Electrocardiol. 2015;48(5):896–9.

110. Jozkow P, Wasko-Czopnik D, Medras M, Paradowski L. Gastroesophageal reflux disease and physical activity. Sports Med. 2006;36(5):385Y91.

111. Collings KL, Pierce Pratt F, Rodriguez-Stanley S, et al. Esophageal reflux in conditioned runners, cyclists, and weightlifters. Med Sci Sports Exerc. 2003;35(5):730Y5.

112. Parmelee-Peters K, Moeller JL. Gastroesophageal reflux in athletes. Curr Sports Med Rep. 2004;3(2):107–11.

113. Coris EE, Higgins HW. First rib stress fractures in throwing athletes. Am J Sports Med. 2005;33(9):1400Y4.

114. Wild AT, Begly JP, Garzon-Muvdi J, Desai P, McFarland EG. First-rib stress fracture in a high-school lacrosse player: a case report and short clinical review. Sports Health. 2011;3(6):547–9.

115. McDonnell LK, Hume PA, Nolte V. Rib stress fractures among rowers: definition, epidemiology, mechanisms, risk factors and effectiveness of injury prevention strategies. Sports Med. 2011;41(11):883–901.

116. Gregory PL, Biswas AC, Batt ME. Musculoskeletal problems of the chest wall in athletes. Sports Med. 2002;32(4):235Y50.

117. Udermann BE, Cavanaugh DG, Gibson MH, et al. Slipping rib syndrome in a collegiate swimmer: a case report. J Athl Train. 2005;40(2):120Y2.

118. Khan N, Waseem S, Ullah S, Mehmood H. Slipping rib syndrome in a female adult with long-standing intractable upper abdominal pain. Case Rep Med. 2018;2018:7484560. Published online 2018 Jul 2.

119. Foley CM, Sugimoto D, Mooney DP, Meehan WP, Stracciolini A. Diagnosis and treatment of slipping rib syndrome. Clin J Sport Med. 2019;29(1):18–23.

120. Disla E, Rhim HR, Reddy A, et al. Costochondritis: a prospective analysis in an emergency department setting. Arch Int Med. 1994;154(21):2466–9.

121. Mendelson G, Mendelson H, Horowitz SF, et al. Can (99m)-technetium methylene diphosphonate bone scans objectively document costochondritis? Chest. 1997;111(6):1600–2.

122. Aspegren D, Hyde T, Miller M. Conservative treatment of a female collegiate volleyball player with costochondritis. J Manipulative Physiol Ther. 2007;30(4):321Y5.

123. Singh AM, McGregor RS. Differential diagnosis of chest symptoms in the athlete. Clin Rev Allergy Immunol. 2005;29(2):87Y96.

Chapter 19
The Evaluation of Palpitations and Dizziness in the Athlete

Brad Witbrodt and Jonathan H. Kim

Palpitations

Palpitations are best described as the gradual or sudden onset of the awareness of one's heartbeat [5]. Because of the profound subjectivity within this definition, athletes with palpitations may present to clinicians with a variety of symptoms that occur in a wide variety of clinical scenarios. For example, a sizable portion of cases will be identified during preparticipation sports screening exams, while others result from athletes seeking medical consultation due to symptomatic palpitations that occur during exercise [6]. Similar to the general population, the incidence of significant underlying cardiac disease varies with respect to risk factors for cardiac disease, with age representing the strongest predictor of risk [7, 8]. While also nonspecific, a personal history of cardiac disease or a family history of cardiac disease is also important risk factors that should be considered during the evaluation [4, 8]. Given the wide differential for palpitations in athletes, a *thorough* history and physical examination are the essential first step in directing the course of diagnosis and management.

History

A detailed history is critical in determining whether key descriptive variables are present that may be indicative of pathology. It is important to appreciate that the term "palpitations" may not be understood by all athletes or consistent with the athlete's interpretation of this nonspecific symptom. Practitioners should appreciate the variety of sensations that athletes may use to describe this symptom. As such,

B. Witbrodt · J. H. Kim (✉)
Emory Clinical Cardiovascular Research Institute, Atlanta, GA, USA
e-mail: Bradley.Witbrodt@bjc.org; jonathan.kim@emory.edu

© Springer Nature Switzerland AG 2021
D. J. Engel, D. M. Phelan (eds.), *Sports Cardiology*,
https://doi.org/10.1007/978-3-030-69384-8_19

321

we believe it is important to characterize palpitations using lay terms. Patients may indicate that they feel "skipping beats," "their heart beating out of their chest," "racing," "fluttering," or other nonspecific sensations in their chest. Occasionally, patients may describe odd sensations in their neck, throat, generalized weakness, or unease, all of which could be consistent with palpitations. In our practice, we question for the presence of palpitations followed by lay descriptions in order for the athlete to completely comprehend the line of questioning.

While obtaining the initial history, it is important to capture the athlete's general level of stress that coincide with symptoms. Understanding the athlete's level of concern is valuable when forming an initial treatment plan, particularly when the history supports etiologies that are more benign. For some athletes, the sensation of palpitations may be a simple annoyance, while for others, there may be significant lifestyle-limiting symptoms or an associated deterioration in athletic performance. These distinctions are important when determining best management approaches, as benign palpitations that typically require no medical treatment, such as nonincessant atrial (APC) or premature ventricular contractions (PVC), could still lead to significant functional limitations or performance issues for which further medical therapy could be considered.

The most critical aspect of the history is determining whether the palpitations are happening at rest or with exertion. The majority of malignant arrhythmias associated with sudden cardiac death occur during exertion [9]. Episodes of palpitations that lead to abrupt syncope during vigorous physical exertion (practice, training, competition) warrant an in-depth evaluation and immediate restriction of physical activity [4]. These palpitations that occur abruptly during exercise or out of proportion to the athlete's level of effort should be differentiated from palpitations that occur at rest. With exercise-induced palpitations, it is important to record the intensity of exertion associated with the onset of palpitations. It is also important to determine whether the palpitations are simple "skipped beats" versus potential sustained tachycardia. This distinction differentiates the presence of incident supraventricular tachycardia (SVT), including atrial fibrillation, atrioventricular nodal reentry tachycardia (AVNRT), atrioventricular reentrant tachycardia (AVRT), and ventricular tachycardia from normal ectopic APCs or PVCs. In addition, second-degree AV block Type I (Wenckebach) may present as nonpathologic palpitations in athletes (Table 19.1).

It is important to inquire about mechanisms of symptom termination or other factors associated with relief or cessation of palpitations. Common responses often include deep breathing while supine or vagal-type maneuvers (bearing down, cough, cold compress). Sustained palpitations that respond to vagal maneuvers typically indicate an AV nodal-dependent arrhythmia. Tachyarrhythmias that are not readily terminated using Valsalva typically indicate arrhythmias that are not completely AV node-dependent such as atrial tachycardia, atrial fibrillation, or ventricular arrhythmias. Other useful termination questions include whether the patient feels a "strong beat" after a short pause. This sensation may be indicative of a postrecovery pause in the setting of benign ectopy. Finally, supplement use, particularly energy supplements, and caffeine intake should be recorded.

Table 19.1 Common etiologies of palpitations

	Common Etiologies	Historical Key Features
Benign Ectopy	Atrial premature contractions Premature ventricular contractions Wenckebach conduction Ectopic atrial rhythms	Sensation of "skipped beats" Pauses with "strong beats" Usually no association with physical activity
Arrhythmias	Supraventricular tachycardia Atrial fibrillation Atrial tachycardia Atrioventricular nodal reentry tachycardia (AVNRT) Atrioventricular reentry tachycardia (AVRT)	Sudden onset and termination Irregularity Heart rate out of proportion to activity May be self-terminated by vagal maneuvers (AVNRT/AVRT)
	Ventricular tachycardia	More likely associated with underlying structural heart disease Suspect if there is a family history of sudden cardiac death or inherited channelopathy

Physical Exam

The physical exam should focus on excluding underlying structural heart disease. Cardiac auscultation should include assessment for the presence of murmurs, gallops, or rubs and for carotid bruits. Clinicians should utilize provocative maneuvers to exclude signs of dynamic left ventricular outflow tract obstruction as could be present in hypertrophic cardiomyopathy (HCM) [10]. Specific examples of provocative maneuvers include auscultation with and without Valsalva and auscultation with squatting and standing. With these maneuvers (Valsalva and immediate standing), there is a dynamic decrease in left ventricular preload, which can enhance murmurs of dynamic outflow tract obstruction [11]. Radial pulse should be checked to assess for the presence of ectopy. Finally, the American Heart Association (AHA) athlete preparticipation screening guidelines recommend assessment of simultaneous radial and femoral pulses [12, 13]. A significant delay in femoral pulses could indicate aortic coarctation, which accounts for 4–6 percent of all congenital heart defects [14].

Evaluation

Risk stratification is the primary directive when formulating a diagnostic and treatment plan for palpitations. Low-risk athletes, based on the findings of history, physical, and sometimes 12-lead electrocardiogram (ECG) may require little to no additional testing. However, any high-risk features require further investigation. Athletes with affirmative answers to the AHA 14-point athletic screen (Table 19.2) [13] and abnormal ECG findings based on International Consensus Criteria (Table 19.3) [15] warrant further evaluation that should include further cardiac

Table 19.2 American Heart Association 14-point athletic cardiovascular screening questionnaire

Personal History

1. Exertional chest pain/discomfort
2. Exertional syncope or near syncope
3. Excessive exertional and unexplained fatigue/fatigue associated with exercise
4. Prior recognition of a heart murmur
5. Elevated systemic blood pressure
6. Prior restriction from participation in sports
7. Prior testing for the heart ordered by a physician

Family history

8. Premature death sudden and unexpected before age of 50 years due to heart disease in one or more relatives
9. Disability from heart disease in a close relative <50 years old
10. Specific knowledge of certain cardiac conditions in family members: hypertrophic or dilated cardiomyopathy, long QT syndrome or other ion channelopathies, Marfan syndrome, or clinically important arrhythmias

Physical exam

11. Heart murmur—exam supine and standing or with Valsalva, specifically to identify murmurs of dynamic left ventricular outflow tract obstruction
12. Femoral pulses to exclude aortic coarctation
13. Physical stigmata of Marfan syndrome
14. Brachial artery blood pressure (sitting, preferably taken in both arms)

Adapted from Maron et al. [13]

Table 19.3 International Criteria for Electrocardiographic Interpretation in Athletes

Normal ECG Findings	Borderline ECG Findings[a]	Abnormal ECG Findings
Increased QRS voltage for LVH or RVH	Left axis deviation	Abnormal T wave inversions
Incomplete RBBB	Left atrial enlargement	ST segment depression
Early repolarization/ST segment elevation	Right axis deviation	Pathologic Q waves
ST elevation followed by T wave inversions in V1–V4 in black athletes	Right atrial enlargement	LBBB
T wave inversions in V1–V3 in ≤16 years old	Complete RBBB	QRS >140 ms
Sinus bradycardia or sinus arrhythmia		Epsilon wave
Ectopic atrial or junctional rhythm		Delta wave
1st degree AV block		QT interval prolongation
Mobitz Type 1, 2nd degree AV block (Wenckebach)		Brugada pattern
		Resting heart rate < 30 bpm
		PR interval > 400 ms
		Mobitz II or 3rd degree AV block
		≥2 PVCs per 10 sec tracing
		Any atrial or ventricular tachyarrhythmia

Adapted from Drezner et al. [15]

AV atrioventricular, *bpm* beats per minute, *LBBB* left bundle branch block, *LVH* left ventricular hypertrophy, *PVC* premature ventricular contraction, *RBBB* right bundle branch block, *RVH* right ventricular hypertrophy

[a]One borderline finding is normal; 2 borderline findings require further evaluation

imaging and assessment modalities such as echocardiogram, cardiac magnetic resonance imaging (CMR), stress testing, and extended heart rhythm monitoring. In clinical situations where no high-risk features are identified, ambulatory rhythm monitoring can still be considered to try to identify the etiology of the palpitations. In patients with symptomatic palpitations, prior data demonstrate that ambulatory Holter or cardiac event monitoring yields a diagnosis 33–35% and 72–80% of the time, respectively [16]. Ruling out the presence of structural cardiac disease is mandatory for athletes with high-risk features [9, 15]. A summary of our clinical approach to the evaluation of palpitations in the athlete is discussed later in this chapter (Fig. 19.1).

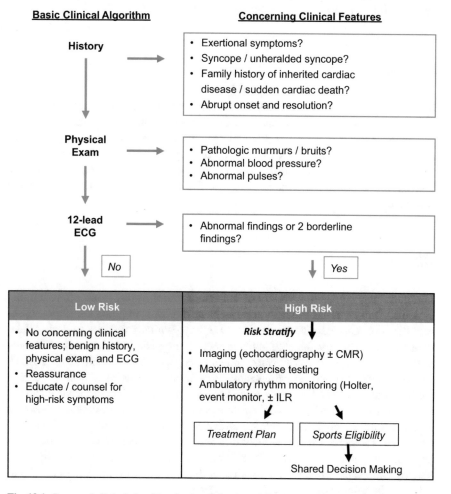

Basic Clinical Algorithm

History

Physical Exam

12-lead ECG

Concerning Clinical Features

- Exertional symptoms?
- Syncope / unheralded syncope?
- Family history of inherited cardiac disease / sudden cardiac death?
- Abrupt onset and resolution?

- Pathologic murmurs / bruits?
- Abnormal blood pressure?
- Abnormal pulses?

- Abnormal findings or 2 borderline findings?

No   *Yes*

Low Risk

- No concerning clinical features; benign history, physical exam, and ECG
- Reassurance
- Educate / counsel for high-risk symptoms

High Risk

Risk Stratify

- Imaging (echocardiography ± CMR)
- Maximum exercise testing
- Ambulatory rhythm monitoring (Holter, event monitor, ± ILR

Treatment Plan   *Sports Eligibility*

Shared Decision Making

Fig. 19.1 Proposed clinical algorithm for the evaluation of dizziness and palpitations in the athlete. CMR cardiac magnetic resonance imaging, ECG electrocardiogram, ILR implantable loop recorder

Prognosis

Palpitations that are nonsustained and occur only at rest are common and are usually benign in athletes [4]. Most benign resting palpitations are related to high resting vagal tone, common in highly conditioned athletes [7]. As previously described, common etiologies include APCs, PVCs, Wenckebach, ectopic atrial rhythms, and junctional rhythms (Table 19.1) [15]. In particular, PVCs have been shown to occur in 40–75% of healthy individuals during 24-hour Holter monitoring [17, 18]. Small studies among athletes have demonstrated that PVCs occur at a higher incidence in endurance athletes with 70% of endurance athletes versus 55% of nonathletes exhibiting ventricular ectopy and 25% of endurance athletes versus 5% of nonathletes exhibiting complex ventricular ectopy [19].

Dizziness

Similar to palpitations, dizziness is a relatively common symptom reported by athletes [20], but some experiences of dizziness can cause significant discomfort in athletes and prompt further medical evaluation. The differential diagnosis for dizziness is broad and requires detailed and specific historical questioning to direct the appropriate evaluation. As such, the approach to dizziness in athletes is heavily reliant on an accurate history as the most important first step in the evaluation.

History

Dizziness may equate to a variety of sensations that manifest from different organ systems. Thus, it is essential to accurately scrutinize symptoms and differentiate whether a primary cardiac workup is necessary. While definitions and classifications of dizziness vary, the commonly accepted categories based on history include *presyncope, vertigo, disequilibrium,* and *nonspecific dizziness* (Table 19.4) [20, 21]. Careful classification of symptoms into one of these categories is critical in focusing the physical exam and forming a more precise differential diagnosis. Most cardiac causes of dizziness will include symptoms consistent with presyncope, however symptoms of vertigo do not exclude cardiac etiologies [22]. A history and physical exam that is solely consistent with vertigo or disequilibrium should be triaged to the appropriate specialist for further care. Nonspecific dizziness may be the most challenging clinical presentation that requires in-depth questioning and a detailed physical exam in order to exclude cardiac etiologies.

Table 19.4 Common accepted categories of dizziness

	Historical Clues	Physical Exam Clues	Key Differential
Presyncope	Sensation and prodrome of near fainting (orthostasis) Prodrome of diaphoresis, nausea (vasovagal) Palpitations (arrhythmia)	Orthostatics: SBP decrease of 20 mmHg; DBP decrease of 10 mmHg; pulse increase of 30 bpm Pathologic murmurs	Orthostasis Cardiovascular etiologies: arrhythmias, valve disease, structural heart disease, vascular disease Autonomic dysfunction
Vertigo	Sensation of spinning Sensation of movement extraneous to the patient History of hearing loss	Nystagmus Positive Dix-Hallpike maneuver	BPPV Labyrinthitis Meniere's disease Vestibular neuritis Acoustic neuroma Migraines
Disequilibrium	Unsteadiness of gait Paresthesia or decreased sensation in lower extremities Symptoms are minimal or not present when sitting or supine	Decreased sensation in lower extremities Shuffling gait, positive Romberg sign, or poor balance	Diabetes TIA/CVA Parkinson's disease
Nonspecific Dizziness	Vague symptoms of mental "cloudiness," "heaviness," or other nonspecific descriptions	Normal neurologic exam Reproducibility with hyperventilation	Anxiety Depression Substance abuse Iatrogenic History of concussion Hyperventilation

BPPV benign paroxysmal positional vertigo, *CVA* cerebrovascular accident, *SBP* systolic blood pressure, *TIA* transient ischemic attack

Physical Exam

A comprehensive physical exam is required, in combination with the detailed history, for the athlete who reports symptoms of dizziness. Provocative maneuvers to assess for structural heart disease, as previously discussed, represent a necessary component of the exam. To accurately evaluate autonomic tone and postural hemodynamic responses, orthostatic blood pressures should be recorded [23]. A drop in systolic blood pressure of ≥20 mmHg or ≥10 mmHg for diastolic blood pressure within 3 minutes of standing up from a supine position is considered an orthostatic response [23]. Patients may demonstrate supine hypertension, which is a risk factor for autonomic dysfunction, with an increase in blood pressure of 30 mmHg from standing to supine generally accepted as abnormal [23]. The heart rate response to standing should additionally be documented to evaluate for positional tachycardia, in which an increase of 30 beats per minute over 10 minutes is classified as abnormal [23, 24].

A basic neurologic exam should include cranial nerve testing, assessment for gait abnormalities, and testing for cerebellar signs. The exam should also assess for the presence of tremors, focal weakness, or peripheral neuropathy. In patients with classic vertigo, a basic otolaryngology evaluation is necessary including otoscopic examination, assessment of extraocular movements, and evaluation for nystagmus utilizing the Dix-Hallpike maneuver [25].

Noncardiac Dizziness

The ability to differentiate symptoms of dizziness that may arise from a cardiac versus noncardiac origin is the most crucial aspect of the clinical history. Dizziness that occurs spontaneously at rest, or after a physical maneuver such as standing up, rolling over, or lying down, is more likely to be vertiginous in etiology. Dizziness that presents as vertigo will typically be described as feeling "off-balance" or as "spinning" akin to riding a roller coaster or merry-go-round. Etiologies are often due to underlying oculomotor or vestibular (inner ear) pathology or other neurologic conditions [26–29]. From a cardiovascular perspective, vertigo can represent the initial presenting sign of cerebrovascular disease such as transient ischemic attack, stroke, or carotid artery stenosis. Similar to vertigo, disequilibrium is primarily a disease of either the peripheral or the central nervous system that is best managed by neurology or otolaryngology specialists. However, disequilibrium can also be a manifestation of cerebrovascular or peripheral vascular disease because of the strong association with diabetes mellitus [26, 30–32]. Thus, within cases of noncardiac dizziness, there is opportunity to screen for underlying cardiovascular disease and initiate appropriate primary prevention when necessary [33].

In challenging cases, the history and physical includes signs and symptoms of both cardiac and noncardiac conditions. For example, athletes who experience classic vertigo may also endorse palpitations during symptomatic episodes. In these cases, treatment options may require a multidisciplinary approach. It remains critical in these scenarios to balance the concern for underlying cardiac disease with the likelihood of benign noncardiac etiologies. This overarching philosophy holds true for the evaluation of both dizziness and palpitations.

Cardiac Dizziness

The majority of cases of cardiogenic dizziness fall into the presyncope category (Table 19.5). The athlete will typically indicate that they are going to "faint" or "pass out," as opposed to experiencing vertigo or disequilibrium. In clear cases of presyncope, it is mandatory to determine if symptoms are occurring at rest, during exertion, or immediately following the termination of exercise. Exertional presyncope is pathologic until proven otherwise and requires a more detailed cardiac evaluation. Among athletes who present with presyncope or frank syncope, 39% are due

Table 19.5 Differentiating cardiac versus noncardiac dizziness by history and physical exam

	Cardiac Dizziness	Noncardiac Dizziness
History	Presyncope Vasovagal prodrome Associated with palpitations Associated with exertion History of prior cardiac disease	Vertigo/disequilibrium/atypical dizziness Associated with head movements or laying down History of prior neurological disease Hearing loss/tinnitus
Physical Exam	Pathologic murmurs Carotid bruits Abnormal pulses Orthostatic blood pressures Heart rate increase of >30 beats per minute with standing	Neuropathy Nystagmus Abnormal gait Hearing or visual acuity abnormalities Tremors/ataxia

to cardiovascular causes, while 36% have no identifiable etiology [34, 35]. Among cases with no known etiology, 30% are typically orthostatic in nature or reflex/autonomic mediated episodes [35]. Autonomic dysfunction, discussed in detail in the following section, is more common in older athletes but can also occur in younger athletes [36]. It is felt that elevated parasympathetic tone present among highly conditioned athletes increases the risk for neurogenic mediated episodes of presyncope/syncope observed in this population [37, 38]. Despite the significant anxiety and discomfort that vagal episodes incur, it is a benign condition and thus reassuring from the sports cardiology perspective [35].

Reflex (Vasovagal) Dizziness and Autonomic Dysfunction

Similar to vertigo, dizziness that stems from autonomic dysfunction may be positional in nature. When the history indicates that vasovagal origins of the patient's symptoms are most likely, it is reasonable to forgo further diagnostic testing [35].

Autonomic dysfunction encompasses a variety of different conditions that result in orthostasis, due to inappropriate pooling of blood in the lower extremities leading to a drop in cerebral blood flow, cerebral hypoperfusion, and corollary symptomatic dizziness [39]. There are three primary variants of autonomic dysfunction:

1. reflex or vasovagal episodes
2. postural tachycardia (POTS) syndrome
3. (rare) pure autonomic failure syndromes include multisystem atrophy seen almost exclusively in elderly patients [23].

Reflex or vasovagal dizziness (neurocardiogenic dizziness) is extremely common in the general population, including in athletes, and constitutes approximately 33% of all cases of dizziness [35, 40]. The underlying physiology of a vasovagal episode is the initiation of an autonomic reflex resulting from a sudden stimulus to the parasympathetic nervous system, leading to the abrupt onset of hypotension and bradycardia. This autonomic reflex can be triggered in a variety of ways including prolonged standing, the site of blood or other perceived disturbing visual stimuli, or profound emotional stressors [41, 42]. Although minimal data exist, it is thought that athletes may have a higher propensity for vasovagal reflex reactions due to the baseline increased resting parasympathetic tone inherently present in highly conditioned athletes [43–45]. Importantly, vasovagal reactions are typically diagnosed via history alone, with the classic presentation inclusive of a noticeable prodrome of diaphoresis, plus a feeling of generalized warmth and nausea accompanying the symptoms of presyncope. Upon resolution of the initial symptoms, it is common for postepisode generalized fatigue and/or malaise to persist for several minutes.

The POTS syndromes are generally described as mild, less severe forms of pure autonomic dysfunction with the hallmark presentation characterized by excessive increases in heart rate ($\geq$30 bpm) after 10 minutes of standing in the absence of an orthostatic drop in blood pressure [23]. POTS encompasses two known variants, peripheral and centrally mediated POTS [46]. Peripherally mediated POTS is thought to be related to failure of the peripheral vasculature to adequately maintain systemic vascular resistance in response to either sudden or prolonged changes in orthostatic stress. This lack of peripheral vascular tone leads to increased heart rate and cardiac contractility that can be felt as dizziness, fatigue, visual disturbance, or exercise intolerance [39, 47]. Centrally mediated POTS is associated with similar symptoms, but is caused by abnormal feedback to central baroreceptors [37–39, 47, 48]. It is noteworthy that patients with POTS tend to have *daily symptoms* as the underlying pathophysiology is inherently present at all times [39, 47]. POTS contrasts with reflex-mediated autonomic dysfunction in which patients typically describe long periods of quiescent symptoms. Some studies suggest that POTS may be an earlier presentation of more severe autonomic dysfunction and rare patients ($\leq$10%) may progress to pure autonomic failure [47].

Occasionally, the athlete's symptoms will be difficult to classify or significant functional debilitation will be present as part of the underlying history. In these cases, proceeding with a heads-up tilt table test may be considered for risk stratification and prognostication. In our opinion, the decision to obtain a tilt table test should be approached with caution as a negative tilt study does not necessarily exclude the presence of autonomic dysfunction. Moreover, the management of many of these conditions lacks robust, evidenced-based practice guidelines [40, 49]. Unique to sports cardiology, there may also be psychological undertones present in the athlete as part of the clinical presentation that may be exacerbated by repetitive and undue medical testing. In complex cases, we favor a multidisciplinary approach, which may include specialists in autonomic dysfunction, if clinically appropriate.

Exertional Cardiac Dizziness

Exertional dizziness in an athlete is a high-risk finding that warrants further evaluation to exclude underlying structural heart disease or a primary arrhythmic disorder [34, 50–54]. Despite the relative infrequency of primary inherited cardiac conditions, the increased risk of sudden cardiac death associated with these diseases

Table 19.6 Underlying cardiac etiologies associated with exertional dizziness and palpitations in athletes

Diseases of the Myocardium	
Myopericarditis	
Genetic cardiomyopathy (e.g., hypertrophic cardiomyopathy, arrhythmogenic right ventricular cardiomyopathy, dilated cardiomyopathy, noncompaction cardiomyopathy)	
Hypertensive heart disease	
Coronary Artery Anomalies	
Anomalous Aortic Origin of the Coronary Arteries	
Conduction System Abnormalities	
Atrial fibrillation	Ventricular tachycardia
Atrial flutter	Atrial premature contractions
Atrial tachycardia	
Other supraventricular tachycardia (e.g., AVNRT, AVRT)	Premature ventricular contractions
	2nd degree AV block Type 1 (Wenckebach)
	2nd degree AV block Type 2

AVNRT AV nodal reentrant tachycardia, *AVRT* AV reentry tachycardia

prioritizes identifying symptomatic athletes that harbor these conditions. In the evaluation of the athlete with exertional dizziness, there are three primary categories to consider diseases of the myocardium, coronary artery anomalies, and conduction system abnormalities (Table 19.6) [55, 56]. It is important to acknowledge that while manifestations of these diseases can be precipitated by strenuous activity, sometimes clinical presentations may be subtle. Exertional presyncope and unheralded syncope are always pathologic until proven otherwise and require a careful and thorough diagnostic approach.

Postexertional Dizziness

In general, dizziness that occurs postexertion, such as following the completion of a competitive endurance event, is less concerning and often related to peripheral vasodilation postexercise [57]. During dynamic exercise, arterial vasodilatation is present and systemic vascular resistance is reduced that allows shunting of oxygenated blood to exercising skeletal muscle [58]. Postexertional orthostatic episodes are common in endurance athletes and classically occur close to or immediately after the termination of prolonged exercise [50]. The mechanism underlying these episodes is related to the abrupt loss of skeletal muscle contraction (i.e., musculovenous pump) and decreased heart rate in an athlete whose peripheral vasculature remains vasodilated. This situational physiology leads to a drop in cerebral perfusion and presyncopal orthostasis [59]. These episodes can be exacerbated by dehydration, fatigue, and potentially environmental (i.e., hot and humid) conditions.

Diagnostic Approach to Palpitations and Dizziness in the Athlete

Our general approach toward palpitations and/or dizziness in athletes is described in this section. First, it is imperative to determine if the palpitations and/or dizziness are manifestations of a serious underlying cardiac condition and to differentiate low-risk versus high-risk athletes. This requires an in-depth history and physical exam in combination with appropriate and focused diagnostic testing. Second, recommendations for ongoing or cessation of athletic training need to be determined throughout the diagnostic evaluation. Finally, once the diagnosis is made, counseling, treatment, and, if applicable, shared decision making for return to play and sports eligibility represent the final steps. Figure 19.1 shows a proposed clinical algorithm for the evaluation of dizziness and palpitations in the athlete.

Low-Risk Athletes

Athletes deemed to have low-risk symptoms should be reassured with avoidance of further diagnostic testing. The athlete should be counseled that their symptoms are benign and not indicative of an underlying malignant cardiac issue. Patients in this low-risk category generally have the following characteristics:

1. no exercise-induced or "red-flag" symptoms
2. infrequent symptoms
3. absence of high-risk findings on ECG
4. normal physical exam.

Athletes in this low-risk category may report symptoms consistent with APCs, PVCs, vasovagal symptoms, and milder presentations of orthostasis or autonomic dysfunction. Patients with benign ectopy will generally notice symptoms occurring at rest. In addition, symptoms are not noticed or will dissipate completely during exercise. Similarly, patients with a classic history of vasovagal, postexertional, or orthostatic dizziness are typically diagnosed based on historical clues. Rarely, further in-depth evaluations may be necessary when the history is unclear, or when other high-risk findings are discovered that may or may not be related to the patient's presenting complaint. More commonly, it is appropriate to educate the athlete on red-flag symptoms to watch for that would trigger future concerns.

High-Risk Athletes

High-risk athletes are classified based on data gathered from the history and physical exam. These athletes will require further diagnostic testing. Decisions regarding ongoing   exercise/athletic   participation   during   the   evaluation   should   be individualized based on the initial concerns from the sports cardiologist. Even at this stage, embracing a shared decision-making approach may be appropriate, particularly for nonsanctioned recreational athletes. With shared decision making, the clinical judgment of the sports cardiologist in concert with the beliefs of the patient is both accounted for in prescribing physical activity levels during the diagnostic evaluation. Athletes with a clear family history of sudden cardiac death, unheralded syncope, or a documented ventricular arrhythmia should be considered high risk, and cessation of strenuous activity should be strongly recommended until the diagnostic evaluation has been completed.

It is important to assess specific historical features of symptoms in the athlete's presentation. For example, the characteristics of symptoms (such as prodrome or no prodrome), the timing of symptoms (rest, exercise, or both), and the presence of any exacerbating or relieving factors should be scrutinized. Palpitations that occur at maximum intensity (such as during high-intensity interval training or at the end of competitive racing) should impact the design of specific exercise protocols performed as part of the diagnostic evaluation. The AHA 14-point questionnaire provides a useful framework outlining key historical questions for athletes presenting with palpitations and/or dizziness (Table 19.2) [13]. High-risk athletes require additional testing beyond a detailed physical exam and 12-lead ECG. This evaluation usually includes, at minimum, imaging by transthoracic echocardiography (TTE) and ambulatory rhythm monitoring (Holter, event monitor, or mobile cardiac telemetry).

12-Lead ECG

There are numerous findings detected by 12-lead ECG that can indicate underlying structural cardiac pathology, arrhythmia, or an arrhythmia syndrome. As detailed in Table 19.3, normal athletic variants must also be recognized [15]. Specific to palpitations and/or dizziness, the presence of a delta wave or short PR interval is consistent with preexcitation (Wolff-Parkinson-White pattern) [60]. The corrected QT interval should be measured [15, 61, 62]. The presence of ectopy, either APCs or PVCs, should be noted. While single PVCs on a standard 12-lead ECG are not classified as pathologic, if ≥2 PVCs are detected on any standard 10-second ECG strip, this typically warrants further evaluation. With frequent PVCs, subsequent 24-hr Holter monitoring would be appropriate to determine the aggregate PVC burden. Finally, the presence of significant repolarization abnormalities, ST depressions, pathologic Q waves, or abnormal T wave inversions (2 or more contiguous leads) in young athletes elicits concern for a potential underlying genetic cardiomyopathy and warrants further evaluation.

Transthoracic Echocardiography (TTE)

TTE is a core cardiac diagnostic imaging test utilized in the evaluation of athletes given the information gleaned from the test, technical ease, portability, and cost-effectiveness [63]. Pertinent elements taken from TTE include differentiation of adaptations due to exercise-induced cardiac remodeling from cardiomyopathies and excluding significant valvular pathology [64, 65]. With congenital sonographers or with general sonographers appropriately trained, TTE can also exclude the presence of anomalous aortic origin of the coronary arteries (AAOCA) [66–69], which can potentially spare the need for coronary CT angiography (CTA) and intravenous contrast administration and radiation. CTA, however, remains the diagnostic test of choice if the suspicion for AAOCA is high on the differential [70]. Some studies have cited TTE as being a poor test for identifying coronary ostia, with 62% missing images [71], while other experienced labs have cited >90% reliability in identifying each of the primary coronary ostia [72]. In our practice, we utilize congenital TTE as our first-line imaging study and reserve CTA for cases in which the ostia cannot be readily identified by TTE.

Ambulatory Rhythm Monitoring

Ambulatory rhythm monitoring by Holter or event monitoring remains the gold standard methodology in the workup of symptomatic palpitations and/or dizziness with concern for underlying arrhythmias. There are pros and cons of the differing methodologies of remote cardiac rhythm monitoring, balancing the likelihood of identifying the rhythm abnormality while also minimizing patient inconvenience. In most cases, a 2- to 4 -week event monitor is best to increase yield, particularly if symptoms are occurring relatively frequently [16]. Moreover, most modern event monitors utilize a nonintrusive patch and are water-resistant. This is especially useful in the sports cardiology clinic as most athletes can wear the device and continue exercise training with the exception of water immersion sports. 24- to 48-hour Holter monitoring is best for quantifying the burden of arrhythmia or ectopy, or if symptoms are incessant in frequency. In certain high-risk patients, such as those in whom ventricular arrhythmias are suspected, mobile cardiac telemetry can be considered given the ability to notify physicians expeditiously if a malignant arrhythmia is detected [73].

Exercise Testing

Maximum exercise testing is necessary for risk stratification in athletes presenting with symptoms of palpitations or dizziness. In these cases, exercising with 12-lead ECG monitoring may elicit and identify arrhythmias that are triggered by exertion. As previously discussed, it is imperative to customize exercise protocols to ensure that the exercise intensity associated with symptoms is achieved and to ensure that the test concludes with volitional fatigue rather than basic heart rate thresholds. In circumstances where symptoms are provoked during sprint drills or intervals, we routinely proceed with start–stop intervals on the treadmill, rather than a gradual ramp protocol, in attempt to elicit symptoms.

While not mandatory as part of a sports cardiology practice, we find that the additional physiologic data obtained from cardiopulmonary exercise testing (CPET) are valuable in providing information regarding exercise performance. CPET includes respiratory gas exchange for measurement of peak oxygen uptake (VO_2) during exercise [74]. For those athletes in which a tailored exercise prescription is requested, data from CPET provide appropriate heart rate thresholds that can aid in this process [75, 76]. CPET can also exclude psychogenic etiologies of exercise-induced symptoms [74].

Additional Diagnostic Testing

Certain clinical situations necessitate the need for more expansive testing. Examples include situations where a final diagnosis requires further risk stratification and/or prognostication, or situations where high-risk features are present, but no definitive diagnosis is made after the initial evaluation. In cases of palpitations and/or dizziness, cardiac MRI (CMR) and invasive electrophysiologic (EP) studies may be employed as part of the clinical algorithm.

Cardiac MRI

CMR allows more detailed characterization of the myocardium and/or valvular apparatus beyond traditional cardiac imaging [77–79]. CMR also provides structural and hemodynamic assessments that can add to the clinical information obtained by the echocardiogram [77]. With the addition of IV gadolinium contrast, CMR can detect myocardial inflammation and scarring (delayed gadolinium enhancement), in cases of myocarditis, genetic cardiomyopathy (HCM and arrhythmogenic right ventricular cardiomyopathy), and coronary artery disease [80].

EP Studies and Implantable Monitors

Invasive EP testing allows for in-depth assessment of the electrical activity of the heart. While safe, it remains typically reserved in athletes for cases in which ablation would be indicated or cases in which arrhythmia (SVT) is highly likely, but elusive from the prior diagnostic workup [81, 82]. Athletes diagnosed with classic SVT are generally best managed by confirmatory testing with an EP study followed by ablation given the successful cure rate in experienced centers [83–85]. An early invasive strategy for SVT may be preferred by athletes because it provides a high likelihood of definitive treatment, while simultaneously avoiding medications and risk of side effects from antiarrhythmic and beta blocker therapy. Provocative testing for high-grade AV block and induction of ventricular arrhythmias in high-risk patients are other clinical scenarios in which an EP study may be indicated [86].

The use of implantable loop recorders (ILR) is increasing in frequency and becoming extremely helpful in cases where the etiology of dizziness, palpitations, or syncope remains elusive. These devices are small (USB sized) and are implanted under the skin in the left upper chest wall. The specific benefits of ILR in the diagnostic algorithm stem from the ability to perform continuous monitoring for an extended period, usually up to 3 years, without the need of any external apparatus [16, 87, 88]. In our practice, in cases of syncope or recurrent sustained/symptomatic palpitations in which the comprehensive evaluation is negative, we find use of ILR for ongoing ambulatory monitoring clinically useful, particularly when the athlete is allowed back to full sports participation.

Shared Decision Making

Within medicine, respecting core patient values in treatment decisions and proceeding with a shared decision-making approach has evolved as a fundamental tenet in clinical practice. Within sports cardiology, as it relates to sports participation for patients who harbor cardiovascular risk or disease, involving the athlete and other potential stakeholders in the decision-making process has become a point of emphasis. Athletes with cardiovascular disease are educated and counseled on the risks and benefits of ongoing exercise and sport participation [89]. The sports cardiologists' mandate is to provide as accurate and best possible risk assessment based on individualized diagnostic data and the scientific evidence available [4, 12, 90]. The athlete and other stakeholders are able to contribute their own core beliefs prior to making the best decisions for the athlete. This approach, the avoidance of physician paternalism and sole reliance on expert opinion, has garnered momentum in recent years [89, 91, 92]. In addition, there are new evidenced-based data demonstrating sports safety in previously deemed high-risk conditions [93–95]. The shared decision-making process relies heavily on education and close and frequent communications between all parties involved.

Conclusions

Palpitations and dizziness that present among athletes have numerous and often overlapping etiologies and the diagnostic pathways and treatment plans can be complex. An accurate and thorough history is essential and provides the key differentiating factors between low versus high-risk processes. The physical exam and 12-lead

ECG should be used to augment the history and guide the extent of the subsequent diagnostic evaluation. From an athletic standpoint, the primary objective of the sports cardiologist is to risk stratify, treat, and attempt to guide a safe return for the athlete back to training and competition. Similar to other arenas within sports cardiology, shared decision making between the treatment team and the athlete has become an integral aspect of any treatment plan provided to the athlete.

References

1. Pelliccia A, Culasso F, Di Paolo FM, et al. Prevalence of abnormal electrocardiograms in a large, unselected population undergoing pre-participation cardiovascular screening. Eur Heart J. 2007;28:2006–10.
2. Kroenke K, Arrington ME, Mangelsdorff AD. The prevalence of symptoms in medical outpatients and the adequacy of therapy. Arch Intern Med. 1990;150:1685–9.
3. Weber BE, Kapoor WN. Evaluation and outcomes of patients with palpitations. Am J Med. 1996;100:138–48.
4. Zipes DP, Garson A. 26th Bethesda conference: recommendations for determining eligibility for competition in athletes with cardiovascular abnormalities. Task force 6: arrhythmias. J Am Coll Cardiol. 1994;24:892–9.
5. Cooper JM. Palpitations. Circulation. 2005;112:e299–301.
6. Magnani JW, Wang N, Benjamin EJ, et al. Atrial fibrillation and declining physical performance in older adults: the health, aging and body composition study (health ABC). Circ Arrhythm Electrophysiol. 2016;9:e003525.
7. Lawless CE, Briner W. Palpitations in athletes. Sports Med. 2008;38:687–702.
8. Thavendiranathan P, Bagai A, Khoo C, Dorian P, Choudhry NK. Does this patient with palpitations have a cardiac arrhythmia? JAMA. 2009;302:2135–43.
9. Maron BJ. Sudden death in young athletes. N Engl J Med. 2003;349:1064–75.
10. Houston BA, Stevens GR. Hypertrophic cardiomyopathy: a review. Clin Med Insights Cardiol. 2014;8:53–65.
11. Magnani JW, Wang N, Benjamin EJ, et al. Atrial fibrillation and declining physical performance in older adults: the health, aging, and body composition study. Circ Arrhythm Electrophysiol. 2016;9:e003525.
12. Maron BJ, Araújo CG, Thompson PD, et al. Recommendations for preparticipation screening and the assessment of cardiovascular disease in masters athletes: an advisory for healthcare professionals from the working groups of the World Heart Federation, the International Federation of Sports Medicine, and the American Heart Association Committee on exercise, cardiac rehabilitation, and prevention. Circulation. 2001;103:327–34.
13. Maron BJ, Friedman RA, Kligfield P, et al. Assessment of the 12-Lead ECG as a screening test for detection of cardiovascular disease in healthy general populations of young people (12–25 years of age). Circulation. 2014;130:1303–34.
14. Hoffman JIE, Kaplan S. The incidence of congenital heart disease. J Am Coll Cardiol. 2002;39:1890–900.
15. Drezner JA, Sharma S, Baggish A, et al. International criteria for electrocardiographic interpretation in athletes: consensus statement. Br J Sports Med. 2017;51:704–31.
16. Hoefman E, Bindels PJE, van Weert HCPM. Efficacy of diagnostic tools for detecting cardiac arrhythmias: systematic literature search. Neth Heart J Mon J Neth Soc Cardiol Neth Heart Found. 2010;18:543–51.
17. Kennedy HL, Whitlock JA, Sprague MK, Kennedy LJ, Buckingham TA, Goldberg RJ. Long-term follow-up of asymptomatic healthy subjects with frequent and complex ventricular ectopy. N Engl J Med. 1985;312:193–7.

18. Lampert R. Evaluation and management of arrhythmia in the athletic patient. Prog Cardiovasc Dis. 2012;54:423–31.
19. Palatini P, Maraglino G, Sperti G, et al. Prevalence and possible mechanisms of ventricular arrhythmias in athletes. Am Heart J. 1985;110:560–7.
20. Sloane PD, Coeytaux RR, Beck RS, Dallara J. Dizziness: state of the science. Ann Intern Med. 2001;134:823–32.
21. Klenck CA. The dizzy athlete. Curr Sports Med Rep. 2007;6:25–31.
22. Newman-Toker DE, Dy FJ, Stanton VA, Zee DS, Calkins H, Robinson KA. How often is dizziness from primary cardiovascular disease true vertigo? A systematic review. J Gen Intern Med. 2008;23:2087–94.
23. Freeman R, Wieling W, Axelrod FB, et al. Consensus statement on the definition of orthostatic hypotension, neurally mediated syncope and the postural tachycardia syndrome. Clin Auton Res. 2011;21:69–72.
24. Plash WB, Diedrich A, Biaggioni I, et al. Diagnosing postural tachycardia syndrome: comparison of tilt test versus standing hemodynamics. Clin Sci. 2013;124:109–14.
25. Huh Y-E, Kim J-S. Bedside evaluation of dizzy patients. J Clin Neurol (Seoul, Korea). 2013;9:203–13.
26. Karatas M. Vascular vertigo: epidemiology and clinical syndromes. Neurologist. 2011;17:1–10.
27. Lempert T, Neuhauser H. Epidemiology of vertigo, migraine and vestibular migraine. J Neurol. 2009;256:333–8.
28. Neuhauser HK. Epidemiology of vertigo. Curr Opin Neurol. 2007;20:40–6.
29. Neuhauser HK. The epidemiology of dizziness and vertigo. Handb Clin Neurol. 2016;137:67–82.
30. D'Silva LJ, Lin J, Staecker H, Whitney SL, Kluding PM. Impact of diabetic complications on balance and falls: contribution of the vestibular system. Phys Ther. 2016;96:400–9.
31. Vinik AI, Maser RE, Mitchell BD, Freeman R. Diabetic autonomic neuropathy. Diabetes Care. 2003;26:1553–79.
32. Kim SK, Lee KJ, Hahm JR, et al. Clinical significance of the presence of autonomic and vestibular dysfunction in diabetic patients with peripheral neuropathy. Diabetes Metab J. 2012;36:64–9.
33. Arnett DK, Blumenthal RS, et al. 2019 ACC/AHA guideline on the primary prevention of cardiovascular disease. J Am Coll Cardiol. 2019;140:26–9.
34. Colivicchi F, Ammirati F, Santini M. Epidemiology and prognostic implications of syncope in young competing athletes. Eur Heart J. 2004;25:1749–53.
35. Soteriades ES, Evans JC, Larson MG, et al. Incidence and prognosis of syncope. N Engl J Med. 2002;347:878–85.
36. Shibao C, Grijalva CG, Raj SR, Biaggioni CII, Griffin MR. Orthostatic hypotension-related hospitalizations in the United States. Am J Med. 2007;120:975–80.
37. Calkins H, Seifert M, Morady F. Clinical presentation and long-term follow-up of athletes with exercise-induced vasodepressor syncope. Am Heart J. 1995;129:1159–64.
38. Levine BD, Lane LD, Buckey JC, Friedman DB, Blomqvist CG. Left ventricular pressure-volume and Frank-Starling relations in endurance athletes. Implications for orthostatic tolerance and exercise performance. Circulation. 1991;84:1016–23.
39. Grubb BP. Neurocardiogenic syncope and related disorders of orthostatic intolerance. Circulation. 2005;111:2997–3006.
40. Shen W-K, Sheldon Robert S, Benditt David G, et al. 2017 ACC/AHA/HRS guideline for the evaluation and management of patients with syncope: executive summary: a report of the American College of Cardiology/American Heart Association task force on clinical practice guidelines and the Heart Rhythm Society. Circulation. 2017;136:e25–59.
41. Kosinski D, Grubb BP, Temesy-Armos P. Pathophysiological aspects of neurocardiogenic syncope: current concepts and new perspectives. Pacing Clin Electrophysiol. 1995;18:716–24.
42. Mosqueda-Garcia R, Furlan R, Tank J, Fernandez-Violante R. The elusive pathophysiology of neurally mediated syncope. Circulation. 2000;102:2898–906.

43. Coote JH, White MJ. CrossTalk proposal: bradycardia in the trained athlete is attributable to high vagal tone. J Physiol. 2015;593:1745–7.
44. Kosinski D, Grubb B, Karas B, Frederick S. Exercise-induced neurocardiogenic syncope: clinical data, pathophysiological aspects, and potential role of tilt table testing. Europace Eur Pacing Arrhythm Card Electrophysiol J Work Groups Card Pacing Arrhythm Card Cell Electrophysiol Eur Soc Cardiol. 2000;2:77–82.
45. Sneddon JF, Scalia G, Ward DE, McKenna WJ, Camm AJ, Frenneaux MP. Exercise induced vasodepressor syncope. Br Heart J. 1994;71:554–7.
46. Sheldon RS, Grubb BP, Olshansky B, et al. 2015 heart rhythm society expert consensus statement on the diagnosis and treatment of postural tachycardia syndrome, inappropriate sinus tachycardia, and vasovagal syncope. Heart Rhythm. 2015;12:e41–63.
47. Grubb BP, Calkins H, Rowe PC. Postural tachycardia, orthostatic intolerance, and the chronic fatigue syndrome. In: Syncope: mechanisms and management. John Wiley & Sons, Ltd, Hoboken, NJ. 2007. p. 225–44.
48. Kanjwal Y, Kosinski D, Grubb BP. The postural orthostatic tachycardia syndrome: definitions, diagnosis, and management. Pacing Clin Electrophysiol. 2003;26:1747–57.
49. Sagristà-Sauleda J, Romero-Ferrer B, Moya A, Permanyer-Miralda G, Soler-Soler J. Variations in diagnostic yield of head-up tilt test and electrophysiology in groups of patients with syncope of unknown origin. Eur Heart J. 2001;22:857–65.
50. Holtzhausen LM, Noakes TD, Kroning B, de Klerk M, Roberts M, Emsley R. Clinical and biochemical characteristics of collapsed ultra-marathon runners. Med Sci Sports Exerc. 1994;26:1095–101.
51. Basso C, Maron BJ, Corrado D, Thiene G. Clinical profile of congenital coronary artery anomalies with origin from the wrong aortic sinus leading to sudden death in young competitive athletes. J Am Coll Cardiol. 2000;35:1493–501.
52. Hobbs JB, Peterson DR, Moss AJ, et al. Risk of aborted cardiac arrest or sudden cardiac death during adolescence in the long-QT syndrome. JAMA. 2006;296:1249–54.
53. Corrado D, Basso C, Thiene G, et al. Spectrum of clinicopathologic manifestations of arrhythmogenic right ventricular cardiomyopathy/dysplasia: a multicenter study. J Am Coll Cardiol. 1997;30:1512–20.
54. Maron BJ, Shirani J, Poliac LC, Mathenge R, Roberts WC, Mueller FO. Sudden death in young competitive athletes: clinical, demographic, and pathological profiles. JAMA. 1996;276:199–204.
55. Liberthson RR. Sudden death from cardiac causes in children and young adults. N Engl J Med. 1996;334:1039–44.
56. Shivanshu Madan MEHC, MD, FACC. The Syncopal Athlete American College of Cardiology; 2016.
57. O'Connor FG, Oriscello RG, Levine BD. Exercise-related syncope in the young athlete: reassurance, restriction or referral? Am Fam Physician. 1999;60:2001–8.
58. Warltier David C, editor, Campagna Jason A, Carter C. Clinical relevance of the Bezold–Jarisch reflex. Anesthesiology J Am Soc Anesthesiol 2003;98:1250–1260.
59. Casey DP, Joyner MJ. Local control of skeletal muscle blood flow during exercise: influence of available oxygen. J Appl Physiol (1985). 2011;111:1527–38.
60. Keating L, Morris FP, Brady WJ. Electrocardiographic features of Wolff-Parkinson-White syndrome. Emerg Med J. 2003;20:491–3.
61. Bazett HC. An analysis of the time relations of electrocardiograms. Heart. 1920;7:353–70.
62. Johnson JN, Ackerman MJ. QTc: how long is too long? Br J Sports Med. 2009;43:657–62.
63. American College of Cardiology Foundation Appropriate Use Criteria Task Force, American Society of E, American Heart A, et al. ACCF/ASE/AHA/ASNC/HFSA/HRS/SCAI/SCCM/SCCT/SCMR 2011 appropriate use criteria for echocardiography. A report of the American College of Cardiology Foundation Appropriate Use Criteria Task Force, American Society of Echocardiography, American Heart Association, American Society of Nuclear Cardiology, Heart Failure Society of America, Heart Rhythm Society, Society for Cardiovascular

Angiography and Interventions, Society of Critical Care Medicine, Society of Cardiovascular Computed Tomography, Society for Cardiovascular Magnetic Resonance American College of Chest Physicians. J Am Soc Echocardiogr Off Publ Am Soc Echocardiogr. 2011;24:229–67.

64. Grazioli G, Sanz M, Montserrat S, Vidal B, Sitges M. Echocardiography in the evaluation of athletes. F1000Research. 2015;4:151.

65. Weiner RB, Baggish AL. Exercise-induced cardiac remodeling. Prog Cardiovasc Dis. 2012;54:380–6.

66. Lytrivi ID, Wong AH, Ko HH, et al. Echocardiographic diagnosis of clinically silent congenital coronary artery anomalies. Int J Cardiol. 2008;126:386–93.

67. Cohen MS, Herlong RJ, Silverman NH. Echocardiographic imaging of anomalous origin of the coronary arteries. Cardiol Young. 2010;20:26–34.

68. Walsh R, Nielsen JC, Ko HH, et al. Imaging of congenital coronary artery anomalies. Pediatr Radiol. 2011;41:1526–35.

69. Frommelt PC, Berger S, Pelech AN, Bergstrom S, Williamson JG. Prospective identification of anomalous origin of left coronary artery from the right sinus of valsalva using transthoracic echocardiography: importance of color Doppler flow mapping. Pediatr Cardiol. 2001;22:327–32.

70. Stout KK, Daniels CJ, Aboulhosn JA, et al. 2018 AHA/ACC guideline for the management of adults with congenital heart disease: a report of the American College of Cardiology/American Heart Association task force on clinical practice guidelines. Circulation. 2019;139:e698–800.

71. Lorber R, Srivastava S, Wilder TJ, et al. Anomalous aortic origin of coronary arteries in the young: echocardiographic evaluation with surgical correlation. J Am Coll Cardiol Img. 2015;8:1239–49.

72. Hussain T, Mathur S, Peel SA, et al. Coronary artery size and origin imaging in children: a comparative study of MRI and trans-thoracic echocardiography. BMC Med Imaging. 2015;15:48.

73. Derkac WM, Finkelmeier JR, Horgan DJ, Hutchinson MD. Diagnostic yield of asymptomatic arrhythmias detected by mobile cardiac outpatient telemetry and autotrigger looping event cardiac monitors. J Cardiovasc Electrophysiol. 2017;28:1475–8.

74. Wasserman K. Principles of exercise testing and interpretation: including pathophysiology and clinical applications. Wolters Kluwer health/Lippincott Williams & Wilkins, Philadelphia, PA. 2012.

75. Hossack K, Hartwig R. Cardiac arrest associated with supervised cardiac rehabilitation. J Cardiac Rehabil. 1982;2:402–8.

76. Hauer K, Niebauer J, Weiss C, et al. Myocardial ischemia during physical exercise in patients with stable coronary artery disease: predictability and prevention. Int J Cardiol. 2000;75:179–86.

77. Shah S, Chryssos ED, Parker H. Magnetic resonance imaging: a wealth of cardiovascular information. Ochsner J. 2009;9:266–77.

78. American College of Cardiology Foundation Task Force on Expert Consensus D, Hundley WG, Bluemke DA, et al. ACCF/ACR/AHA/NASCI/SCMR 2010 expert consensus document on cardiovascular magnetic resonance: a report of the American College of Cardiology Foundation task force on expert consensus documents. J Am Coll Cardiol. 2010;55:2614–62.

79. von Knobelsdorff-Brenkenhoff F, Schulz-Menger J. Role of cardiovascular magnetic resonance in the guidelines of the European Society of Cardiology. J Cardiovasc Magn Reson. 2016;18:6.

80. Marcus FI, McKenna WJ, Sherrill D, et al. Diagnosis of arrhythmogenic right ventricular cardiomyopathy/dysplasia (ARVC/D). Circulation. 2010;121:1533–41.

81. Bhaskaran A, Chik W, Thomas S, Kovoor P, Thiagalingam A. A review of the safety aspects of radio frequency ablation. IJC Heart Vasc. 2015;8:147–53.

82. Horowitz LN, Kay HR, Kutalek SP, et al. Risks and complications of clinical cardiac electrophysiologic studies: a prospective analysis of 1,000 consecutive patients. J Am Coll Cardiol. 1987;9:1261–8.

83. Cheng CH, Sanders GD, Hlatky MA, et al. Cost-effectiveness of radiofrequency ablation for supraventricular tachycardia. Ann Intern Med. 2000;133:864–76.
84. Spector P, Reynolds MR, Calkins H, et al. Meta-analysis of ablation of atrial flutter and supraventricular tachycardia. Am J Cardiol. 2009;104:671–7.
85. Jackman WM, Beckman KJ, McClelland JH, et al. Treatment of supraventricular tachycardia due to atrioventricular nodal reentry by radiofrequency catheter ablation of slow-pathway conduction. N Engl J Med. 1992;327:313–8.
86. Katritsis DG, Josephson ME. Electrophysiological testing for the investigation of bradycardias. Arrhythmia Electrophysiol Rev. 2017;6:24–8.
87. Sreeram N, Gass M, Apitz C, et al. The diagnostic yield from implantable loop recorders in children and young adults. Clin Res Cardiol. 2008;97:327–33.
88. Zimetbaum P, Goldman A. Ambulatory arrhythmia monitoring choosing the right device. Circulation. 2010;122(16):1629–36.
89. Baggish AL, Ackerman MJ, Putukian M, Lampert R. Shared decision making for athletes with cardiovascular disease: practical considerations. Curr Sports Med Rep. 2019;18:76–81.
90. Maron BJ, Chaitman BR, Ackerman MJ, et al. Recommendations for physical activity and recreational sports participation for young patients with genetic cardiovascular diseases. Circulation. 2004;109:2807–16.
91. Baggish AL, Ackerman MJ, Lampert R. Competitive sport participation among athletes with heart disease: a call for a paradigm shift in decision making. Circulation. 2017;136:1569–71.
92. McNutt RA. Shared medical decision making: problems, process, progress. JAMA. 2004;292:2516–8.
93. Aziz PF, Sweeten T, Vogel RL, et al. Sports participation in genotype positive children with long QT syndrome. JACC Clin Electrophysiol. 2015;1:62–70.
94. Lampert R, Olshansky B, Heidbuchel H, et al. Safety of sports for athletes with implantable cardioverter-defibrillators. Circulation. 2013;127:2021–30.
95. Johnson JN, Ackerman MJ. Competitive sports participation in athletes with congenital long QT syndrome. JAMA. 2012;308:764–5.

Chapter 20
The Collapsed Athlete

Justine S. Ko and George Chiampas

Introduction

Sideline management involves the ability to assess an athlete's symptoms and sudden changes in health. Injuries can vary from musculoskeletal to cardiovascular to neurologic in nature. The collapsed athlete is defined as an athlete who experiences sudden loss of postural tone that results in the inability to continue with event participation [1]. Athletic collapse, while frequently benign, can result in significant harm to the athlete and therefore requires immediate medical attention. Overall, fatal events are rare. In the most recent 2017 Annual Report, the National Center for Catastrophic Sport Injury Research (NCCSIR) noted 862 nontraumatic catastrophic injuries since 1982, with 44 fatal injuries at the collegiate level over that time period [2].

With the progression of sports medicine and expansion of sideline management, the quick assessment and early intervention in the collapsed athlete has become a crucial component of athlete care. While there can be many causes for athletic collapse, there is a limited differential for severe and potentially life-threatening conditions that should guide initial diagnosis and management. These main causes include cardiac arrest, hyponatremia, exertional heat stroke, hypothermia, respiratory distress, hypoglycemia, trauma, and exertional sickling. The evaluation and management of each topic will be reviewed in this chapter.

J. S. Ko (✉)
Department of Emergency Medicine, Feinberg School of Medicine, Northwestern University, Chicago, IL, USA

G. Chiampas
Departments of Emergency Medicine and Orthopedic Surgery, Feinberg School of Medicine, Northwestern University, Chicago, IL, USA

© Springer Nature Switzerland AG 2021
D. J. Engel, D. M. Phelan (eds.), *Sports Cardiology*,
https://doi.org/10.1007/978-3-030-69384-8_20

343

Approach to the Collapsed Athlete

An algorithmic approach should be utilized in the collapsed athlete in the absence of obvious trauma. The following algorithm, used in the Chicago Marathon, can be used as a guide for the management of the collapsed athlete (Fig. 20.1) [3]. In the initial assessment, the patient's pulse should be palpated for no more than 10 seconds. If a palpable pulse is not obtained, sudden cardiac arrest is presumed. CPR and advanced cardiovascular life support (ACLS) should be initiated, with emphasis on hands-only CPR as described below. For the patient with a pulse, further workup and history is warranted to evaluate the patient.

The athlete's medical history, including diabetes, sickle cell trait, cardiac abnormalities, should be considered when differentiating possible causes. In a hemodynamically stable and awake patient, further historical pieces of information, including symptoms, prior history, and trauma, can be obtained from the patient to guide diagnosis. Witness accounts will also help with differentiating trauma, indirect causes of collapse, and seizure. If resources allow, a rectal temperature, cardiac monitoring, and early metabolic evaluation with point-of-care glucose and sodium levels should be obtained in an altered patient.

Cardiac Arrest

Sudden cardiac death is the most common cause of atraumatic deaths in athletes. While rare, with an estimated incidence of approximately 1:43,700 in collegiate athletes and 1:200,000 in high school athletes per academic year, this scenario is the most feared and should always be assessed for first [4]. A large proportion of these fatalities are linked to cardiac conditions, including arrythmias, congenital cardiac conditions such as hypertrophic cardiomyopathy, and atherosclerotic coronary artery disease. In the young athlete, the most common cause of sudden cardiac death has been linked to hypertrophic cardiomyopathy, which can predispose an athlete to ventricular dysrhythmias [5].

In the event of cardiac arrest, immediate CPR, automated external defibrillator (AED) application, and activation of emergency medical response teams should be done as soon as possible [6]. Early bystander resuscitation, access to AED, and early defibrillation have been shown to improve outcomes given the predisposition to ventricular dysrhythmias as described above [7, 8]. Recent CPR guidelines shifted their focus from A-B-C (Airway-Breathing-Circulation) to C-A-B (Circulation-Airway-Breathing). These recommendations were re-emphasized in the 2015 AHA Guidelines to highlight compression-only CPR, with adequate depth and rate of compressions, and the importance of limiting interruptions [9]. While there may be an innate desire to transport these patients immediately, it is important to perform on-site resuscitation and application of the AED to assess the patient's rhythm. Early CPR and defibrillation within 3–5 minutes of collapse has correlated with higher survival rates [10, 11]. Cardiac arrest as a cause of the collapsed athlete will be discussed in more detail in a later chapter.

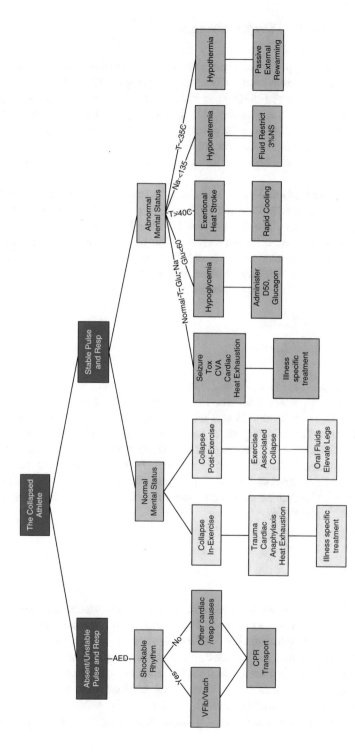

Fig. 20.1 The Collapsed Athlete Algorithm. This algorithm is used at the Chicago marathon for medical personnel training

Exercise-Associated Hyponatremia

Exercise-associated hyponatremia (EAH) is defined as a low serum sodium concentration, generally a sodium level <135 mmol/L, during or after exercise. EAH first came to the forefront in the 1980s after multiple reports surfaced in runners at the Comrades Marathon in South Africa [12]. In recent years, EAH has continued to interest medical personnel due to its potential for significant morbidity and mortality. The reported prevalence of this condition varies, likely due to underreporting in asymptomatic individuals; however, it has been cited to be as high as 50% in ultra-runners [13].

In a prospective study on Boston Marathon runners, risk factors for development of EAH included excessive fluid intake, longer race times, and significant weight gain during the race [14]. The cause of EAH is thought to be related to an increase in total body water caused by overconsumption of fluids by the athlete and an increase in vasopressin secretion [15–17]. The exact mechanism for vasopressin secretion in this setting is not well defined, but is thought to be related to inflammatory cytokines, and nonspecific stressors [15].

Presentation & Diagnosis

The presentation for exercise-associated hyponatremia varies significantly. Symptoms range from asymptomatic to seizures and severe encephalopathy. The majority of symptomatic athletes will present with complaints of headache, dizziness, or weakness [17]. Notably, these symptoms overlap with other common syndromes in athletes such as exertional heat exhaustion and dehydration. Prompt diagnosis with rapid sodium levels is optimal. In the Statement of the Third International Exercise-Associated Hyponatremia Consensus Development Conference, it was recommended that on-site evaluation of sodium levels be available if resources allow [16].

Treatment

Once EAH has been diagnosed with a serum sodium level, treatment involves fluid restriction in mild to moderate cases and hypertonic saline in more severe cases. In patients who are asymptomatic but with a serum sodium level <130 mmol/L, oral hypertonic solutions can be considered to prevent development of symptomatic hyponatremia [16]. In the absence of a sodium level in a collapsed and altered athlete, oral hypotonic hydration and intravenous administration of normal saline should be deferred as to avoid exacerbating symptoms of possible EAH. In the presence of seizure or severe mental status changes, hypertonic saline is recommended in the form of a 100 mL 3% hypertonic saline bolus. Importantly, the initial postrace serum sodium level may be significantly overestimated due to retained fluid in the gastrointestinal tract that has yet to be absorbed or a delayed effect of an elevated vasopressin level. As such, continued monitoring should be pursued, especially in a symptomatic patient [17].

Prevention

Given that EAH has been linked to overconsumption of fluids, prevention of this condition centers around athlete education. Education on drinking to thirst and the dangers of overdrinking has been shown to reduce the incidence of EAH [16]. Sodium-containing sports drinks, however, have not been shown to prevent EAH due to their low sodium content and hypotonicity [17]. Athletes should also be educated on the importance of monitoring their pre- and post-workout weights as a surrogate for fluid consumption. In general, athletes who gain weight after exercise are drinking too much. Athletes who lose greater than 2–3% of their body weight are drinking too little. Optimizing their fluid consumption during training months can improve performance and prevent EAH [15, 18].

Exertional Heat Stroke

Exertional heat stroke (EHS) is the most severe illness along the spectrum of exertional heat illnesses. It is the third leading cause of death in athletes [19]. EHS is generally associated with a core body temperature ≥ 40.5 °C and is caused by an increase in heat production or a decrease in heat loss [20, 21]. The human body regulates an elevated temperature based on four main mechanisms: radiation, convection, conduction, and vaporization. The most efficient of the four mechanisms is vaporization, which is seen with sweating and evaporation of the sweat at the skin surface [19, 22].

Multiple factors contribute to the rise in temperature in exertional heat stroke. During intense exercise, skeletal muscle use generates heat at significantly higher levels compared to rest. This heat is transferred through the blood and to the capillaries at the surface of the skin, where the blood is then cooled. During exercise, EHS occurs when regulatory heat dissipation via sweat and radiant heat loss can no longer match the heat production, and a resultant rise in temperature occurs. Environmental changes, such as an increase in humidity, can contribute to EHS by decreasing the heat gradient between the body and its surroundings and limiting evaporative heat [19]. Furthermore, decreased cardiac function and dehydration can also affect cooling, as it impedes the ability of the blood to be transported to the body surface [22].

Presentation & Diagnosis

Early symptoms of EHS can include dizziness, vomiting, and fatigue. More severe symptoms include altered mental status, loss of consciousness, and even seizures. Risk factors for development of clinically significant EHS include lack of heat acclimatization, hot and humid exercise environment, and poor physical fitness [23]. Morbidity associated with EHS has been linked to duration of hyperthermia rather than the degree of hyperthermia. As such, rapid diagnosis with a core (rectal) temperature and immediate on-site treatment is warranted [24].

Treatment

The mainstay of treatment for EHS is rapid cooling, which can be done through several methods such as conductive cooling via immersion or evaporative cooling via sprayed water and fanning. For EHS, cooling via immersion in an ice-water bath is the most effective and can decrease temperatures by nearly 1 °C/min. In the absence of an ice-water bath, conductive cooling via ice packs to the axilla, neck, and groin is a reasonable alternative. This can be facilitated by evaporative methods, which involves spraying the body with water and cooling with fanned air [25]. In a 2016 meta-analysis on cooling methods, cold water immersion (CWI) demonstrated faster cooling and lead to better outcomes compared to passive recovery. Based on the meta-analysis, a cold water temperature of ≤10 °C is recommended [26].

Timing of treatment in EHS is critical – reduction of temperature to <40 °C within 30 minutes has been shown to limit fatality rates to near zero [24]. In the recent consensus statement on prehospital EHS management, treatment with on-site cooling is recommended to ensure rapid temperature reduction and to decrease organ damage and morbidity from hyperthermia [27]. Once a patient is immersed, continuous core temperature monitoring should be performed and patients should be removed when the core temperature reaches 38–39 °C or ~102 °F to avoid hypothermia [25, 28].

Prevention

Given the environmental impact on the risk of developing EHS, prevention involves a keen awareness of the weather prior to partaking or starting events. The wet bulb globe temperature (WBGT) is an index that factors in ambient temperature, relative humidity, and radiant heat load from the sun. This index has been used by several event coordinators and associations to determine necessity for event modifications [29]. For instance, in the Bank of America Chicago Marathon, an event alert system (EAS) that was developed in 2008 with recommended WBGT cutoffs is utilized to warn medical personnel and participants regarding possible dangers (Table 20.1).

Table 20.1 Bank of America Chicago Marathon Event alert system

Alert level	Event conditions	Recommended actions	Temperature
Extreme	Event cancelled/ extreme and dangerous conditions	Participation stopped/ follow event official instruction	WBGT > 82˚F
High	Potentially dangerous conditions	Slow down/observe course changes/follow event official instruction/consider stopping	WBGT 73-82˚F
Moderate	Less than ideal conditions	Slow down/be prepared for worsening conditions	WBGT 65-73˚F
Low	Good conditions	Enjoy the event/be alert	WBGT 40-65°F

WBGT=Wet bulb globe temperature

WBGT **wet bulb globe temperature**

In the U.S. Soccer Recognize to Recover website (recognizetorecover.org), WBGT cutoffs are further separated based on geographic location. Higher WBGT cutoffs are allowed for warmer climates due to heat acclimatization by athletes. Overall, it is recommended that hydration breaks become longer and more frequent as the WBGT rises, with the consideration of shortening or even canceling events and practices when extreme conditions are present [30]. Importantly, medical directors and trainers should also factor in medical personnel, treatment resources, and prior event history into their event modification decisions [29, 31].

Hypothermia

In contrast to EHS, hypothermia is defined as a core temperature <35 °C and occurs when heat loss exceeds that of heat production [32]. Although a less common cause of athletic collapse, hypothermia must be considered, especially during colder weather conditions. Normally, in response to the cold, the body will try to preserve core body temperature by increasing metabolic heat production, which arises through involuntary shivering or increased voluntary activity. The body will also reduce heat loss by inducing peripheral vasoconstriction to preserve core body temperature and increase insulation provided by the body shell [32].

Hypothermia in an athlete usually involves excessive heat loss related to clothing that is wet. Water exposure, such as rain, sleet, snow, swimming, increases the risk for hypothermia as there is a higher amount of heat loss via convection [33]. Additional risk factors for hypothermia include age >60 years old, lower percentage body fat, and participation in shorter or lower intensity activities [32].

Table 20.2 Classification of hypothermia [33, 34]

	Core temperature	Symptoms	Shivering	Cardiac abnormalities	Field interventions
Mild hypothermia	32–35 °C	Behavior change, dysarthria, apathy	Present	Tachycardia	PER, warm PO fluids
Moderate hypothermia	28–32 °C	Dilated pupils, stupor	Decreased	Bradycardia, cardiac arrhythmias	PER, warm IV fluids
Severe hypothermia	<28 °C	Unconsciousness	Absent	Bradycardia, ventricular fibrillation	PER, warm IV fluids

PER = Passive external rewarming

Presentation and Diagnosis

Hypothermia presents with a range of symptoms, which often correlates with the athlete's core temperature. It is separated into three categories – mild, moderate, and severe hypothermia – as detailed in Table 20.2. In mild hypothermia, athletes will present with shivering and may become more aloof with behavioral changes. In moderate to severe hypothermia, the body's shivering response declines and the core temperature drops further. As temperatures fall below 32 °C, athletes experience more extensive CNS changes such as confusion, stupor, and loss of consciousness. Furthermore, severe bradycardia and cardiac arrhythmias can develop and the risk of cardiac arrest increases. As with EHS, diagnosis involves a core rectal temperature.

Treatment

Rapid warming is the mainstay of treatment for hypothermia and its associated sequelae. In contrast to EHS, which requires rapid onsite cooling, rewarming these patients may require equipment and techniques that are not available onsite. Transfer to a medical facility should be initiated as soon as possible. Extra care needs to be provided during transport as large movements can induce cardiac arrhythmias in a cold and irritable heart.

Passive external rewarming (PER) is the warming modality of choice for mild hypothermia. In these patients, any wet clothes should be removed first, the patient should be brought into a warm and dry environment, and warm blankets and heating packets should be applied. PER can increase core temperature by approximately 0.5 °C/h [35]. For moderate to severe hypothermia, active external rewarming is implemented. It requires a higher level of care at a medical facility and utilizes a Bair Hugger or external heating device to facilitate warming. More aggressive care with internal rewarming strategies should be considered for temperatures below

28 °C. Warm IV fluids at 4 °C can be infused. Additionally, more invasive extracorporeal rewarming with hemodialysis or extracorporeal membrane oxygenation (ECMO) can be utilized in severe cases [36, 37].

In the setting of cardiac arrest in a hypothermic patient, cardiac resuscitation should not cease until the patient has been fully rewarmed given the significant myocardial irritation that occurs with hypothermia. In a retrospective study in Norway, it was noted that patients with accidental hypothermia survived temperatures as low as 13.7 °C and required as long as nearly 7 hours of CPR during the rewarming process prior to return of spontaneous circulation [38].

Prevention

Prevention of hypothermia, similar to EHS, entails event modifications based on weather and environmental conditions. Similar to WBGT, the wind chill temperature (WCT) index can be used to assess risk for hypothermia and guide event modifications. This index factors in wind speed and temperature. The U.S. Soccer Recognize to Recover website recommends limiting skin exposure and providing frequent rewarming opportunities based on the WCT (Table 20.3) [30].

In cold weather, athletic clothing also plays a big role in preventing hypothermia and it is recommended that patients dress in layers. The bottom layer should be a thin, moisture-wicking material that allows moisture to move away from the skin and to the surface. This prevents conductive heat loss. The middle layer usually provides insulation via materials such as fleece, wool, and down. Finally, the outer layer should be wind/water-resistant, which allows moisture from the bottom layers to cross and evaporate [36].

Table 20.3 Hypothermia alert level

Alert level	WCT (F)	Event conditions	Recommended action
Black	<0	Extreme conditions[a]	Cancel or attempt to move activities indoors. Frostbite could occur
Red	1–15	High risk for cold-related illness[a]	Consider modifying activity to limit exposure and allow for more frequent chances to rewarm
Orange	16–24	Moderate risk for cold-related illness[a]	Provide additional protective clothing, cover as much exposed skin as practical, and provide opportunities and facilities for rewarming
Yellow	25–30	Less than ideal conditions[a]	Be aware of the potential for cold injury and notify appropriate personnel of the potential
Green	>30	Good conditions	Normal activities

[a]In wet environments with colder conditions, the following situations are accelerated. Use additional caution to recognize potential cold injuries. (NOTE: These WCT guidelines were adapted from the NATA position statement: Environmental Cold Injuries [39]
Used with permission from U.S. Soccer Recognize to Recover

Respiratory Distress (Anaphylaxis, Asthma)

While cardiac causes are the leading cause of sudden death in athletes, respiratory distress can also cause collapse. It is important to remember that athletes may have chronic medical problems, such as asthma and allergies, despite their overall active and healthy appearance. These problems can present themselves acutely during exercise and decrease an athlete's exercise tolerance. Furthermore, there are several exercise-associated respiratory conditions that providers should be familiar with when caring for athletes.

Anaphylaxis

Anaphylaxis is a severe hypersensitivity reaction that involves two or more organ systems. Fatal injuries from anaphylaxis are cited as 0.63–0.76 per million in adults [40]. It results from various stimulants, most commonly a food or drug allergy. Environmental exposures, such as bee stings or other insect bites, can also be a potential source. Patients present with lip swelling, tongue swelling, rash, shortness of breath, and/or gastrointestinal discomfort. Treatment of anaphylaxis requires prompt intramuscular epinephrine administration in conjunction with steroids and antihistamines.

Exercise-induced anaphylaxis (EIA) is when anaphylaxis occurs after physical exercise and is often associated with consumption of a food allergen around the time of exercise. The exact mechanism behind this phenomenon is not well known; however, it has been suggested that the redistribution of blood from the gut during exercise causes ingested allergens to activate mast cells and results in an anaphylactic reaction [41]. Treatment for EIA is similar to other anaphylactic reactions – intramuscular epinephrine injection.

Exercise-induced Bronchoconstriction and Asthma

Exercise-induced bronchoconstriction (EIB) and exercise-induced asthma are two disease processes in which there is transient narrowing of the airways during or after exercise. Exercise-induced asthma occurs in athletes with a history of asthma while exercise-induced bronchoconstriction occurs in patients with no prior diagnosis [42]. Incidence of EIB has been reported to be as high as 10% in the general population [43]. As with normal asthmatic patients, these athletes will present with wheezing, cough, and shortness of breath.

Risk factors for EIB include activities that require a higher minute ventilation, such as marathon running and soccer, and activities in colder, drier conditions. Compliance to medication in athletes with known asthma helps to prevent exercise-associated asthma. Athletes should be counseled on the importance of long-term control and the potential dangers of weather changes. Treatment involves inhaled beta-agonists for acute symptom management. Inhaled corticosteroids are the most effective for long-term prevention of EIB and can be used in conjunction with inhaled beta-agonists [42].

Exertional Sickling

Sickle cell trait (SCT) is a heterozygous condition in which individuals inherit one mutated sickle hemoglobin gene from one of their parents, resulting in the HgbAS genotype. Normal hemoglobin molecules are made of four subunits, each one containing an oxygen-carrying heme group and a globin molecule. In a normal hemoglobin molecule, there are two alpha subunits and two beta subunits. In sickle hemoglobin (HgbS), two mutated beta subunits are present, which causes polymerization of hemoglobin molecules at the cell membrane surface in the deoxygenated state. This change to the cell membrane surface causes the "sticky" nature of red blood cells in sickle cell disease patients that leads to vaso-occlusive events [44]. In sickle cell trait, one mutant beta subunit is present and leads to an approximate concentration of 40% HgbS in each red blood cell [45].

Sickle cell trait affects approximately 8% of the African American population and approximately 0.01–0.05% of the remaining population [46]. Individuals with SCT are generally asymptomatic; however, HgbAS can still sickle, especially in acidotic and hypoxic states. The dangers of exertional sickling in athletes with sickle cell trait surfaced after multiple deaths in college football athletes between 1974 and 2010. Many of these deaths occurred during periods with maximal physical exertion, such as during conditioning exercises [46].

Presentation & Diagnosis

Exercise provides the perfect storm for sickling in athletes with SCT – acidosis, hypoxia, and dehydration [47]. The vaso-occlusive events that develop under these circumstances lead to rhabdomyolysis, renal failure, and severe metabolic derangements that can ultimately result in death [46].

Diagnosis of exertional sickling requires a high clinical suspicion. Athletes can present with a wide range of symptoms. They usually present after several minutes of maximal exertion with muscle weakness and fatigue. The muscle pain and weakness come on very quickly, unlike the cramping associated with heat illness which may present over hours. In addition, the pain associated with exertional sickling is milder and athletes will complain of more weakness. Muscles in exertional sickling will also not appear to be tense and cramping, as the root cause occurs at the microvascular level and does not cause large contractures of the muscles [48].

Treatment & Prevention

After the death of a collegiate athlete in 2010, the National Collegiate Athletic Association (NCAA) implemented a mandatory genetic screening for sickle cell trait. In a 2012 policy impact analysis, it was estimated that this mandatory screening would prevent approximately seven collegiate athlete deaths over the course of a 10-year period [49]. Athletes, however, can still refuse to present documentation and choose to sign a waiver. As such, a high clinical suspicion should be present, even at the elite collegiate level. In athletes with known SCT, they should be coached to build endurance slowly and work at their own pace with frequent rests as needed [46]. These athletes should avoid participating in timed drills to avoid exceeding their tolerated pace.

Treatment of exertional sickling is mainly supportive with supplemental oxygen and cooling as needed. In suspected collapse from exertional sickling, the athlete should be transferred to a medical facility where the treatment of fulminant rhabdomyolysis with parental fluid resuscitation and more aggressive supportive care can be initiated [50].

Hypoglycemia

In any collapsed individual, hypoglycemia should be ruled out. Hypoglycemia is defined as a blood glucose level <60 mg/dL and should especially be considered in athletes with known diabetes mellitus. It can present with various symptoms, including headache, lightheadedness, sweating, and confusion. Prompt point-of-care glucose testing on the sideline is important for diagnosis; however, if onsite testing is not available, prophylactic treatment should be started. For athletes with mild hypoglycemia, oral glucose supplementation with juice, sugar, or other carbohydrates is preferred. In severe hypoglycemia, where the athlete may be altered, intravenous dextrose administration or intramuscular glucagon administration should be utilized [48]. Repeat serum glucose monitoring must be performed after treatment to ensure no refractory or rebound hypoglycemia. Additional observation and treatment may be needed if low blood glucose levels persist.

Athletes need to be counseled on the symptoms of hypoglycemia. In diabetic athletes, a developed care plan with their physician will help avoid exercise-associated hypoglycemia. Additionally, these athletes should eat carbohydrates before, during, and after activities and have frequent glucose monitoring [48].

Exercise-associated Collapse

Exercise-associated collapse (EAC) is defined as an athlete's inability to stand or walk due to lightheadedness or dizziness after exercise. It generally occurs immediately after exercise or a sudden halt in activity. The etiology of EAC is thought to be related to postural hypotension that results from the sudden reduction in the action of skeletal muscles. During exercise, skeletal muscle acts as "the second heart," pumping blood back to the heart from the vasodilated extremity vessels. When exercise ceases, there is a sudden decrease in venous return and pooling of the blood in the lower extremities as skeletal muscle contractions decrease. This, coupled with skin and muscle vasodilatation, causes a rapid reduction in preload, which then results in postural hypotension and collapse [51, 52]. Patients present with lightheadedness, dizziness, or syncope. Mental status is usually preserved, however, and patients tend to improve quickly. While EAC is the most common diagnosis in athletic collapse, it is a diagnosis of exclusion. Athletes should be evaluated for the life-threatening causes of collapse as described in the prior sections. A rectal temperature, point-of-care glucose, and rapid serum sodium are advised [51].

Treatment & Prevention

A patient with EAC should be laid down and their legs should be elevated to facilitate blood return to the heart and to increase preload. Furthermore, once other causes of collapse are excluded, oral or IV rehydration can be started. With oral rehydration, patients should drink to their thirst. Athletes are also advised to avoid abrupt cessation of activity to prevent EAC. For instance, in marathon runners, it is recommended that they continue walking after completion of the race to avoid the sudden drop in cardiac preload and collapse.

Seizures

Seizures should also be considered on the differential. They are defined as an abnormal firing of a group of neurons in the cerebral cortex [53]. There are many forms of seizures; however, the most common are generalized tonic-clonic seizures where there are rhythmic, repetitive motions of the body. This is associated with an altered state during and after the event [54]. Approximately 10% of the US population will experience at least one seizure in their lifetime. Most seizures are self-limiting, lasting 1–2 minutes. During the seizure, supportive care may be needed in the form of airway support, such as a jaw thrust or supplemental oxygen, as patients tend to hypoventilate during seizure activity. Patients should be positioned in a way to avoid self-harm and airway compromise [55].

Importantly, sudden cardiac arrest can lead to abnormal movements that can be mistaken for seizures. In a nontraumatic collapse of an athlete with no known history of seizures, prompt assessment for cardiac causes is necessary and initiation of CPR should be considered. Neuro-cardiogenic syncope (NCS) can also appear like seizures. The etiology of NCS is related to a transient loss of consciousness from cerebral hypoperfusion [56]. Unlike seizures, movements from NCS are usually associated with a prodrome, such as lightheadedness, and is associated with a rapid recovery and return to baseline.

If seizure activity persists, benzodiazepines are the mainstay of treatment. On the sideline, where IV access may not be available, intranasal or intramuscular benzodiazepine administration can be utilized [55]. Other causes of seizures must also be considered, including hypoglycemia and hyponatremia. Metabolic derangements, if present, should be corrected to help cease seizure activity.

Trauma

Traumatic causes of collapse also account for a significant portion of athletic collapse and even death. In a study of 1866 young athlete deaths from 1980 to 2006, an estimated 22% were related to traumatic causes, mainly from head or neck injuries [57]. In an athlete with collapse of unknown etiology, a provider should search for physical signs of trauma. If there is suspicion for trauma, the athlete should be stabilized on the field with cervical spine precautions [34]. Further management should follow Advanced Trauma Life Support (ATLS) guidelines.

Emergency Preparedness

With each of these causes, an important component to management lies in emergency action plans (EAPs) and preparedness with staff and emergency personnel. Studies have shown that an EAP, access to an AED, and early defibrillation increase survival rates [8]. Early defibrillation is key in cardiac arrest, with survival rates decreasing 7–10% with each minute of delay [10]. Emergency action plans help to organize and provide a unified approach among medical personnel at a large event. These plans enable a practiced response from onsite personnel to initiate early CPR, and activation of the EMS system. It is recommended that every institution or organization have a written EAP for a planned event. Key components to the plan include a communication system, training of personnel, adequate equipment and transportation, and a coordinated plan of action. The EAP should be reviewed and practiced with medical providers and trainers each year to limit uncertainty and confusion during actual events [58].

Summary

Management of sideline emergencies is a key component of athlete care. A collapsed athlete requires prompt assessment and diagnosis. Several conditions, as described above, can lead to collapse and result in significant morbidity and mortality if not addressed appropriately. Providers should be familiar with the life-threatening causes so that prompt treatment can be initiated when the need arises.

An algorithmic approach, as depicted in Fig. 20.1, can be used to guide initial diagnosis and management. When available, a core temperature, rapid serum glucose, and rapid serum sodium should be obtained. Finally, an established EAP and knowledge on the use and location of an AED can help facilitate an organized process in an otherwise chaotic situation.

References

 1. Blue JG, Pecci MA. The collapsed athlete. Orthop Clin North Am. 2002;33(3):471–8.
 2. Reports – National Center for Catastrophic Sport Injury Research [Internet]. [cited 2019 Sept 17]. Available from: https://nccsir.unc.edu/reports/.
 3. Chiampas G, Jaworski C. Preparing for the surge: perspectives on marathon medical preparedness. Curr Sports Med Rep. 2009;8(3):131–5.
 4. Harmon KG, Asif IM, David K, Drezner Jonathan A. Incidence of sudden cardiac death in national collegiate athletic association athletes. Circulation. 2011;123(15):1594–600.
 5. Wasfy MM, Hutter AM, Weiner RB. Sudden cardiac death in athletes. Methodist Debakey Cardiovasc J. 2016;12(2):76–80.
 6. Toresdahl B, Courson R, Börjesson M, Sharma S, Drezner J. Emergency cardiac care in the athletic setting: from schools to the Olympics. Br J Sports Med. 2012;46(Suppl 1):i85–9.
 7. Drezner JA, Toresdahl BG, Rao AL, Huszti E, Harmon KG. Outcomes from sudden cardiac arrest in US high schools: a 2-year prospective study from the National Registry for AED use in sports. Br J Sports Med. 2013;47(18):1179–83.
 8. Drezner JA, Rao AL, Justin H, Bloomingdale Megan K, Harmon Kimberly G. Effectiveness of emergency response planning for sudden cardiac arrest in United States high schools with automated external defibrillators. Circulation. 2009;120(6):518–25.
 9. Neumar RW, Shuster M, Callaway CW, Gent LM, Atkins DL, Bhanji F, et al. 2015 American Heart Association Guidelines Update for CPR and ECC: executive summary. Circulation. 2015;132(Suppl 2):S315–67.
10. Rao AL, Standaert CJ, Drezner JA, Herring SA. Expert opinion and controversies in musculoskeletal and sports medicine: preventing sudden cardiac death in young athletes. Arch Phys Med Rehabil. 2010;91(6):958–62.
11. Rothmier JD, Drezner JA. The role of automated external defibrillators in athletics. Sports Health. 2009;1(1):16–20.
12. Noakes TD, Speedy DB. Case proven: exercise associated hyponatraemia is due to overdrinking. So why did it take 20 years before the original evidence was accepted? Br J Sports Med. 2006;40(7):567–72.
13. Urso C, Brucculeri S, Caimi G. Physiopathological, epidemiological, clinical and therapeutic aspects of exercise-associated hyponatremia. J Clin Med. 2014;3(4):1258–75.
14. Almond CSD, Shin AY, Fortescue EB, Mannix RC, Wypij D, Binstadt BA, et al. Hyponatremia among runners in the Boston Marathon. N Engl J Med. 2005;352(15):1550–6.
15. Hew-Butler T, Loi V, Pani A, Rosner MH. Exercise-Associated Hyponatremia: 2017 Update. Front Med [Internet]. 3 Mar 2017 [cited 2019 Sept 19];4. Available from: https://www.ncbi.nlm.nih.gov/pmc/articles/PMC5334560/.
16. Hew-Butler T, Rosner M, Fowkes-Godek S, Dugas J, Hoffman M, Lewis D, et al. Statement of the third international exercise-associated hyponatremia consensus development conference, Carlsbad, California, 2015. Clin J Sport Med. 2015;25(4):303–20.
17. Rosner MH, Kirven J. Exercise-associated hyponatremia. Clin J Am Soc Nephrol. 2007;2(1):151–61.
18. Chang RG, Khan JJ. Hydration Issues in the Athlete and Exercise Associated Hyponatremia – PM&R KnowledgeNow [Internet]. PM&R Knowledge Now. 2016 [cited 2019 Oct 27]. Available from: https://now.aapmr.org/hydration-issues-in-the-athlete-and-exercise-associated-hyponatremia/.

19. Howe AS, Boden BP. Heat-related illness in athletes. Am J Sports Med. 2007;35(8):1384–95.
20. Casa DJ, DeMartini JK, Bergeron MF, Csillan D, Eichner ER, Lopez RM, et al. National Athletic Trainers' Association position statement: exertional heat illnesses. J Athl Train. 2015;50(9):986–1000.
21. Navarro C, Casa D, Belval L, Nye N. Exertional heat stroke. Curr Sports Med Rep. 2017;16(5):304–5.
22. Miyake Y. Pathophysiology of heat illness: thermoregulation, risk factors, and indicators of aggravation. Jpn Med Assoc J. 2013;56(3):167–73.
23. Armstrong L, Casa D, Millard-Stafford M, Moran D, Pyne S, Roberts W. Exertional heat illness during training and competition. Med Sci Sports Exerc. 2007;39(3):556–72.
24. Casa D, Armstrong L, Kenny G, O'Connor F, Huggins R. Exertional heat stroke: new concepts regarding cause and care. Curr Sports Med Rep. 2012;11(3):115–23.
25. Gaudio FG, Grissom CK. Cooling methods in heat stroke. J Emerg Med. 2016;50(4):607–16.
26. Zhang Y, Davis J-K, Casa D, Bishop P. Optimizing cold water immersion for exercise-induced hyperthermia: a meta-analysis. Med Sci Sports Exerc. 2015;47(11):2464–72.
27. Belval LN, Casa DJ, Adams WM, Chiampas GT, Holschen JC, Hosokawa Y, et al. Consensus statement- prehospital care of exertional heat stroke. Prehosp Emerg Care. 2018;22(3):392–7.
28. Proulx CI, Ducharme MB, Kenny GP. Safe cooling limits from exercise-induced hyperthermia. Eur J Appl Physiol. 2006;96(4):434–45.
29. Hosokawa Y, Adams WM, Belval LN, Davis RJ, Huggins RA, Jardine JF, et al. Exertional heat illness incidence and on-site medical team preparedness in warm weather. Int J Biometeorol. 2018;62(7):1147–53.
30. Environmental Conditions [Internet]. Recognize to Recover. [cited 2019 Oct 28]. Available from: http://www.recognizetorecover.org/environmental.
31. Chiampas GT, Goyal AV. Innovative operations measures and nutritional support for mass endurance events. Sports Med Auckl Nz. 2015;45(Suppl 1):61–9.
32. Castellani J, Young A, Ducharme M, Giesbrecht G, Glickman E, Sallis R. Prevention of cold injuries during exercise. Med Sci Sports Exerc. 2006;38(11):2012–29.
33. Fudge J. Exercise in the cold. Sports Health. 2016;8(2):133–9.
34. Malik S, Chiampas G, Roberts WO. The collapsed athlete. In: Sports cardiology in practice: evaluation, management, and case studies. New York: Springer-Verlag; 2011.
35. Taylor EE, Carroll JP, Lovitt MA, Petrey LB, Gray PE, Mastropieri CJ, et al. Active intravascular rewarming for hypothermia associated with traumatic injury: early experience with a new technique. Proc Bayl Univ Med Cent. 2008;21(2):120–6.
36. McMahon J, Howe A. Cold weather issues in sideline and event management. Curr Sports Med Rep. 2012;11(3):135–41.
37. Darocha T, Kosiński S, Jarosz A, Drwila R. Extracorporeal rewarming from accidental hypothermia of patient with suspected trauma. Medicine (Baltimore). 2015;94(27)
38. Hilmo J, Naesheim T, Gilbert M. "Nobody is dead until warm and dead": prolonged resuscitation is warranted in arrested hypothermic victims also in remote areas – a retrospective study from northern Norway. Resuscitation. 2014;85(9):1204–11.
39. Cappaert TA, Stone JA, Castellani JW, Krause BA, Smith D, Stephens BA. National Athletic Trainers' Association Position Statement: Environmental Cold Injuries. J Athl Train. 2008;43(6):640–58.
40. Poowuttikul P, Saini S, Seth D. Anaphylaxis in children and adolescents. Pediatr Clin N Am. 2019;66(5):995–1005.
41. Hull JH, Ansley L, Robson-Ansley P, Parsons JP. Managing respiratory problems in athletes. Clin Med. 2012;12(4):351–6.
42. Bussotti M, Di Marco S, Marchese G. Respiratory disorders in endurance athletes – how much do they really have to endure? Open Access J Sports Med. 2014;5:47–63.
43. Weder MM, Truwit JD. Pulmonary disorders in athletes- ClinicalKey. Clin Sports Med. 2011;30:525–36.

44. Manwani D, Frenette PS. Vaso-occlusion in sickle cell disease: pathophysiology and novel targeted therapies. Blood. 2013;122(24):3892–8.
45. Blinder MA, Russel S. Exertional sickling: questions and controversy. Hematol Rep. 2014;6(4):66–70.
46. Mitchell BL. Sickle cell trait and sudden death. Sports Med - Open. 2018;4(19)
47. Loosemore M, Walsh SB, Morris E, Stewart G, Porter JB, Montgomery H. Sudden exertional death in sickle cell trait. Br J Sports Med. 2012;46(5):312–4.
48. Casa DJ, Guskiewicz KM, Anderson SA, Courson RW, Heck JF, Jimenez CC, et al. National Athletic Trainers' Association position statement: preventing sudden death in sports. J Athl Train. 2012;47(1):96–118.
49. Tarini BA, Brooks MA, Bundy DG. A policy impact analysis of the mandatory NCAA sickle cell trait screening program. Health Serv Res. 2012;47(1 Pt 2):446–61.
50. Eichner ER. Sickle cell considerations in athletes. Clin Sports Med. 2011;30:537–49.
51. Asplund CA, O'Connor FG, Noakes TD. Exercise-associated collapse: an evidence-based review and primer for clinicians. Br J Sports Med. 2011;45(14):1157–62.
52. Wen DY. Collapsed athlete – atraumatic. Curr Rev Musculoskelet Med. 2014;7(4):348–54.
53. Bromfield EB, Cavazos JE. Sirven JI. American Epilepsy Society: Basic mechanisms underlying seizures and epilepsy; 2006.
54. Zupanc ML, Otallah SJ, Goodkin HP. Sports and epilepsy. In: DeLee, Drez, & Miller's Orthopaedic sports medicine. 5th ed. Philadelphia: Elsevier; 2020. p. 230–4.
55. Silverman EC, Sporer KA, Lemieux JM, Brown JF, Koenig KL, Gausche-Hill M, et al. Prehospital care for the adult and pediatric seizure patient: current evidence-based recommendations. West J Emerg Med. 2017;18(3):419–36.
56. Josephson CB, Rahey S, Sadler RM. Neurocardiogenic syncope: frequency and consequences of its misdiagnosis as epilepsy. Can J Neurol Sci. 2007;34:221–4.
57. Maron BJ, Doerer JJ, Haas TS, Tierney DM, Mueller FO. Sudden deaths in young competitive athletes. Circulation. 2009;119(8):1085–92.
58. Drezner JA, Courson RW, Roberts WO, Mosesso VN, Link MS, Maron BJ. Inter-association task force recommendations on emergency preparedness and management of sudden cardiac arrest in high school and college athletic programs: a consensus statement. J Athl Train. 2007;42(1):143–58.

Chapter 21
Cardiac Arrest in Athletes

Brian J. Cross, Shayna Weinshel, and Marc Estes

> *Till in he broke: 'Rejoice, we conquer!' Like wine thro' clay,*
> *Joy in his blood bursting his heart, he died – the bliss!*
>
> —Robert Browning, "Pheidippides" (1879)

Introduction

Sudden cardiac death (SCD) in an athlete brings a paradox of competitive sports sharply into focus. Athletics, which typically enhances strength and survivability [1], may also be the cause of seemingly unexplainable death. The popular consciousness is often confused by this paradox. Widely reported sports-related deaths, from the fabled collapse of Pheidippides in Athens to more recent deaths of sports stars such as Reggie Lewis and Hank Gathers, as well as the extremely tragic, unexpected losses of athletic children, have led to often sensational and misleading headlines in the popular media, such as, "Too much exercise can kill you, scientists have revealed" [2].

The medical science at the foundation of this paradox is detailed and complex. This chapter will review the incidence and causes of sudden cardiac death in

B. J. Cross
Division of Cardiology, VA Pittsburgh Health System, Pittsburgh, PA, USA
e-mail: Brian.Cross6@va.gov

S. Weinshel
Department of Medicine, University of Central Florida, Orlando, FL, USA

M. Estes (✉)
Heart and Vascular Institute, University of Pittsburgh Medical Center, Pittsburgh, PA, USA
e-mail: Estesna@upmc.edu

© Springer Nature Switzerland AG 2021
D. J. Engel, D. M. Phelan (eds.), *Sports Cardiology*,
https://doi.org/10.1007/978-3-030-69384-8_21

361

athletes along geographic, racial, gender, and age spectra, as well as the evidence regarding the benefits of risk factor screening to prevent sudden cardiac death in athletes and the role of emergency response systems and rapid external defibrillation to abort sudden cardiac arrests.

Incidence of Sudden Cardiac Death in Athletes

The incidence of sudden death in athletes is an area of some uncertainty, as it has been reported to be both higher and lower than the non-athlete population, and estimates of incidence have historically differed geographically and as a function of method of research [3]. One constant remains, however, and that is that SCD in athletes is a very rare phenomenon globally. Using prospectively acquired data of all individuals aged 12–35 years in the Veneto Region of Italy from 1979 through 1999, Corrado et al. identified a 2.1:100,000 person-year event rate of SCD among athletes [4]. Using retrospective data, the incidence often appears lower. A study of sudden death in high school and college athletes participating in competitive, organized sports from data collected by the National Center for Catastrophic Sports Injury Research identified an incidence of 0.7 deaths per 100,000 person-years among male high school and college athletes and 0.1 deaths per 100,000 person-years among female high school and college athletes in the USA [5]. Death due to cardiac causes among high school students in Minnesota competing in organized sports was identified by Maron et al. as 0.5:100,000 person-years [6]. This assessment made use of data acquired retrospectively from catastrophic insurance claims. Other retrospective studies from Denmark, using death certificate and hospital record reviews, and from Israel, using media accounts, have shown incidences of 1.2:100,000 and 2.6:100,000 athlete-years, respectively [7, 8].

These differences among SCD incidence assessments using retrospectively and prospectively acquired data may be partly explained by study methodology. Retrospective studies based on commonly-used sources of SCD data, including media reports of SCD events and catastrophic insurance claims, miss 5–56% and 80–90% of SCD occurrences, respectively [9]. Estimating the incidence of sports-related SCD is further complicated by the evidence that within the same nationality and age range, differences exist related to gender, race, and sport. A retrospective study of National Collegiate Athletic Association (NCAA) athlete deaths, using data from NCAA and Parent Heart Watch databases, media reports, and catastrophic insurance claims, identified an overall incidence of SCD of 2.3:100,000 athlete-years. However, higher incidences were seen in male and African-American athletes, competitors in Division I play, and among basketball players, swimmers, lacrosse players, and cross-country runners. In this study, the highest risk was seen in Division I male basketball players, who had a 32:100,000 athlete-year SCD incidence, while female NCAA athletes in total had a SCD incidence that was more than 95% lower (1.2:100,000 athlete-year) [10].

There is conflicting evidence regarding the risk of SCD in athletes compared to non-athletic cohorts. Multiple studies have shown that, compared to the 0.5 to 2 per

100,000 person-year incidence range of SCD in athletes in the USA, non-athletes in populations that include American military recruits [11] and individuals under the age of 35 in Denmark [7], Norway [12], and the USA and Canada [13], among others, showed higher SCD incidences, ranging from 0.9 to 10 per 100,000 person-years [14]. Conversely, in the Veneto Region of Italy, the incidence of SCD among competitive athletes was observed to be higher (2.1:100,000 person-years) compared with non-athletes (0.7:100,000 person-years). As seen in other studies, there was a higher incidence of sudden death in males than females, both for athletes (2.6 vs. 1.1 per 100,000 person-years, respectively) and non-athletes (1.3 vs. 0.5 per 100,000 person-years, respectively), while the non-athlete population overall had a lower incidence of SCD than reported in other studies [4].

Given the range of incidences of SCD identified in these epidemiological studies and the allusiveness of a single, identifiable rate of occurrence, it may be helpful to put all of these data into a larger social and clinical context of risk. Maron et al. reviewed the US National Registry of Sudden Death in Athletes and databases of NCAA athlete deaths from 2002 to 2011. Among the young athletes who died suddenly, a majority (65%) died due to non-cardiovascular causes, including suicide (17%) and drug use (12%), and all of these causes were vastly less frequent than deaths causes by motor vehicle accidents in the same age group. While this does not disguise the importance of understanding the risk of SCD in athletes, it reveals the spectrum of risks to the safety of athletes, of which athletic competition itself occupies a relatively small space [15]. Note should be made of older athletes (age over 35 years), who are rarely included in SCD incidence studies. Prospectively acquired data from the Oregon Sudden Unexpected Death Study identified an SCD incidence of 2.2:100,000 person-years among athletes aged 35–65. While this incidence does not markedly exceed most assessments of SCD in younger athletes, the incidence of SCD in men exceeded that of women to a greater extent than seen in younger populations, with a relative risk 18.68 (95% CI, 2.50–139.56) [16].

Causes of Sudden Cardiac Death in Athletes

The majority of athletes who die suddenly of suspected cardiovascular causes show evidence of structural heart or arterial disease on postmortem analysis. Autopsy-based studies of the US athletes who died suddenly have noted hypertrophic cardiomyopathy (26.4% of cases) and anomalous coronary anatomy (13.7% of cases) to be the most common causes of SCD due to structural heart disease, along with nonspecific left ventricular hypertrophy, myocarditis, ruptured aortic aneurysm due to Marfan syndrome, arrhythmogenic right ventricular cardiomyopathy, tunneled coronary artery anatomy, aortic valve stenosis, and atherosclerotic coronary artery disease, among others. A notable exception to the presence of underlying structural heart disease is commotio cordis, identified as the second most common cardiac cause of sudden death in athletes [17].

Hypertrophic Cardiomyopathy

Hypertrophic cardiomyopathy (HCM) is a heritable, mainly autosomal dominant, and relatively common structural cardiac disease with an estimated prevalence of at least 1 in 500 people [18]. Phenotypically, HCM is characterized on a cellular level by cardiac myocyte disarray, resulting in asymmetric hypertrophy of the left ventricle (commonly at the ventricular septum) with occasional LV outflow tract obstruction and a predisposition for unstable ventricular arrhythmias and SCD. Evidence of HCM may appear on an electrocardiogram (ECG) nonspecifically as left ventricular hypertrophy (LVH), though non-pathologic or fully normal ECGs have been acquired in 10% of patients with known diagnoses of HCM [19].

While major risk markers help to identify patients with HCM at increased risk of ventricular arrhythmias and SCD and guide appropriateness of primary prevention implantable cardioverter-defibrillators (ICDs) [20–22], rigorous physical activity may promote unstable ventricular arrhythmias even in the absence of these major risk factors [23]. For this reason, current American College of Cardiology (ACC)/ American Heart Association (AHA) guidelines state that all patients with HCM, regardless of SCD risk factors, should not participate in competitive sports, with the exception of "low-static/low-dynamic" sports classified as 1A, such as billiards, bowling, and golf. It should be noted that this recommendation is independent of most demographic or clinical features including age, gender, magnitude of LVH, history of LV septal surgical myectomy or alcohol ablation, presence or absence of LV outflow obstructive physiology, cardiac symptoms, or intramural myocardial fibrosis as evidenced by late-gadolinium enhancement on cardiac magnetic resonance imaging. It is additionally not recommended to introduce therapies such as anti-arrhythmic medicines or primary prevention ICDs for the sole or primary purpose of permitting participation in competitive athletics [24].

Anomalous Aortic Origin of a Coronary Artery

Anomalous aortic origin of a coronary artery (AAOCA) occurs when, during embryologic development, coronary arteries originate abnormally from the wrong sinus of Valsalva. The most concerning of these anatomic anomalies is the left main coronary artery (LMCA) or left anterior descending artery (LAD) originating from the right sinus of Valsalva, and the right coronary artery (RCA) originating from the left sinus of Valsalva or the LAD. Pathologic studies of these hearts show acute-angle arterial take-offs resulting in "slit-like" coronary lumens. In addition, the proximal segment of the arteries often courses between the great vessels of the aorta and the pulmonary trunk. These anatomic characteristics can allow the anomalous arteries to be kinked or compressed, particularly during times of increased cardiac output, with resulting distal myocardial ischemia. Ventricular arrhythmias and sudden death in association with AAOCA may be due to an acute ischemic episode as well as, or in addition to, chronic ischemia with patchy, arrhythmogenic myocardial scarring [25].

Of note, pre-SCD exertional symptoms including angina and syncope may occur in some patients with AAOCA, specifically those with anomalous LMCA origins. Baseline ECGs acquired during both rest and stress are unreliable for detecting anomalous coronary anatomy. Suspicion for AAOCA based on prior symptoms should favor noninvasive imaging or coronary angiography to guide both diagnosis and possible cardiac surgical correction. All athletes with LMCAs originating from the right sinus of Valsalva and athletes with RCAs originating from the left sinus of Valsalva who have symptoms, arrhythmias, or ischemic findings on stress myocardial perfusion imaging should be restricted from athletic competition before surgical repair. After 3 months following surgical repair, athletes may return to competition if they are free of symptoms, arrhythmias, or ischemia on stress imaging [26].

Arrhythmogenic Right Ventricular Cardiomyopathy

The regional disparity of cardiovascular etiology of sudden death in athletes was made clear by a prospective study of all young athletes (age 12–35 years) participating in organized sports requiring regular training and competition in the Veneto Region of Italy from 1979 to 1999. In this study, the most common cause of SCD in athletes was arrhythmogenic right ventricular cardiomyopathy (ARVC), followed by atherosclerotic coronary artery disease, myocarditis, and mitral valve prolapse. HCM, the most common cause of SCD in American athletes, was the attributable cause in only 1 of 55 SCD cases in an Italian study. Hypotheses to explain the higher incidence of ARVC and lower incidence of HCM as the cause of SCD in athletes in northern Italy include regional genetic factors and the possible exclusion of individuals with HCM from competitive athletics as a product of mandatory pre-participation screening (discussed further below), as well as the influence of prospective data acquisition in the Italian study compared to retrospective data acquisition in the US. studies [4].

ARVC is a genetic disease characterized phenotypically by fibrofatty replacement of cardiac myocytes in both right ventricular (typically inferior, apical, and infundibular) and left ventricular (typically posterolateral subepicardial) myocardium, due to abnormal cell adhesion proteins, leading to wall thinning and aneurysm formation. Manifestations of ARVC on resting ECG include right bundle branch block, QRS duration >110 ms in the right precordial leads (V1-V3), T-wave inversions or epsilon waves in the right precordial leads, and left-bundle-type ventricular premature depolarizations (VPDs). Ambulatory cardiac monitoring or stress ECG may show left-bundle-type ventricular tachycardia or VPDs (more than 500 in a 24-hour period) [27]. Clinical manifestations of ARVC include palpitations, syncope, and cardiac arrest, and less commonly symptoms of clinical heart failure [28]. Additionally, ARVC can be familial, following a mainly autosomal dominant inheritance pattern, and syncope or sudden death in a family member may also be an alerting signal to the presence of ARVC [29]. Clinical or ECG findings concerning for ARVC should favor further evaluation with echocardiogram and cardiac magnetic resonance imaging. Criteria for the diagnosis of ARVC are based on quantitative variables from the clinical, family, ECG, and imaging data [30].

Athletes identified as having definitive, borderline, and possible diagnoses of ARVC should not participate in competitive sports, with the possible exception of low-static, low-dynamic class 1A sports. As in the case of HCM, prophylactic ICD placement for the sole or primary purpose of allowing competitive sports participation is not recommended [24]. In addition to the increased risk of ventricular arrhythmias and sudden death during exercise in ARVC patients, evidence from both a murine model [31] and retrospective human data [32] indicate that the cumulative amount and intensity of exercise over time increase the likelihood of ARVC genotype-positive patients developing phenotypic ARVC and its manifestations, including ventricular arrhythmias and heart failure.

Atherosclerotic Coronary Artery Disease

Advancing athlete age is an important factor in the cause of sudden death. The prevalence of coronary artery disease (CAD) increases in both athlete and non-athlete populations with advancing age, and CAD is the overwhelmingly most common cause of sudden cardiac arrest (SCA) in older athletes. Among athletes over the age of 35, atherosclerotic coronary artery disease was identified as an attributable cause of SCA in 84% of cases. Acute myocardial infarction was identified in 33% of these cases of CAD-associated SCA [16].

Commotio Cordis

Sudden cardiac death in athletes without structural heart disease occurs most commonly in cases of commotio cordis, the second most common cause of sudden death in young athletes in the USA, as well as, much less commonly, long QT syndrome. Commotio cordis (CC) describes an episode of immediate conversion from a stable cardiac rhythm to ventricular fibrillation (VF) that occurs due to chest wall impact. Specific features of chest wall impact are required for this phenomenon to occur; these include highly compliant chest walls, impact with the chest within a 20 ms window during the upslope of the T wave, and items of impact of particular size, hardness, density, and velocity of travel at the time of impact [33]. Small and hard objects [34, 35] traveling at 40 miles per hour [36] are the most likely to cause VF.

Historically, athletes sustaining cardiac arrest due to CC had only a 10–15% likelihood of survival despite administration of cardiopulmonary resuscitation (CPR) within 3 min in most cases [37], though experimental evidence reveals that automated external defibrillators (AEDs) identify CC-related VF with very high sensitivity (98%) and specificity (100%) and are efficacious in terminating VF [38]. Accordingly, in more recent years and as AED availability and use has increased, survival from CC has increased to 58%. Unfortunately, however, these improvements in survival are not uniform across races. African-American victims of CC have <5% survival, possibly due to longer rescue response time and decreased availability of AEDs at sites of athletic practice and competition [39].

Pre-competition Screening of Athletes to Prevent Sudden Cardiac Death

While there is not conclusive evidence that athletic competition increases the risk of sudden cardiac death above the risk in the non-athlete population, there are structural cardiac diseases that are clearly associated with exercise-associated cardiac arrest and sudden death. This fact can very reasonably lead to a directive to identify potential athletes with these conditions prior to participation and, when appropriate, to prohibit higher-risk individuals from participation as a means of primary prevention of sudden death. Despite the soundness of this logic in theory, available evidence has fomented debate internationally about the practical appropriateness of specific screening approaches to identify higher-risk cardiac conditions in athletes, as well as the effectiveness of any pre-participation screening at various levels of competition [40].

Three countries – the USA, Italy, and Israel – have instituted some form of pre-participation screening at all levels of competition, though the approaches among the countries differ. In the USA, practice guidelines recommend screening of all high school and college athletes with the AHA 14-point history and physical examination screening guidelines in the primary care setting, but without noninvasive testing in the absence of detected abnormalities [41]. In Italy [42] (where pre-participation screening is enforced by law) and Israel [8], routine screening ECGs are added to history and physical examinations. The European Society of Cardiology recommends routine pre-participation ECG screening as well [43], though in many European countries, it is only Olympic, professional, and other elite athletes who are routinely screened.

While clearly no one argues over the individual and societal benefits of preventing cardiovascular deaths, the disparity of approaches to pre-participation screening and the debate over the appropriateness of routine ECGs, in particular, stem largely from differing interpretations of the available data on sensitivity, specificity, and cost-effectiveness of these diagnostic modalities. In Denmark, for example, policy makers point to a review of all deaths over a 7-year period, which showed that SCD in athletes was not only very rare (1.21:100,000 person-years) but also lower than the non-athlete population (3.76:100,000 person-years), and that wide-scale cardiovascular screening of any manner prior to athletic participation would not have sufficiently high value and is not recommended [7]. Italian officials have taken a very different view of the evidence. Prospectively collected data starting in 1979 showed a 3.6:100,000 person-year incidence of SCD in athletes. After mandatory nation-wide pre-participation screening based on 12-lead ECG assessment was initiated in 1982, the incidence of SCD in athletes was seen to decrease to 0.4:100,000 person-years. An interpretation of this data in favor of the role of ECG screening can point to the 2% of potential athletes who were excluded from athletic competition based on their screening and the subsequent (and possibly consequential) absence of HCM as a leading cause of SCD in contemporary Italian athletes [42].

Opponents of routine widespread ECG screening identify several areas of clinical and practical limitations of ECG screening, including false-positive results ranging from 5% to 20% [44] and a lack of human and financial resources available in large population countries such as the USA to screen millions of ECGs annually, among others [45]. Additionally, there is the potential for deleterious effects on the long-term health of younger individuals prevented from participating in physical activity due to false-positive screening, as well as the potential for adverse consequences to athletes with false-negative ECGs, who might be persuaded to ignore subsequent warning symptoms of cardiovascular disease in the wake of a falsely reassuring non-pathologic screening ECG.

The results of a recent meta-analysis of studies on the efficacy of screening with both history and physical exam and ECG identified clear strengths of ECG as a screening tool, favoring the use of ECGs in pre-participation screening. In this study, the sensitivity of ECGs was found to be 94%, compared to 20% for clinical history and 9% for physical exam, and the false-positive rate of ECGs was found to be lower than both history and physical exam [46]. The clinical impact of these findings, though, is not clear. The most commonly identified ECG abnormality in this meta-analysis was ventricular pre-excitation, or Wolff-Parkinson-White (WPW) pattern (42%), to which only 1% of SCD cases in athletes have been attributed [47], while HCM, which has been reported to be the leading cause of SCD in athletes in the USA, was detected in only 2 of 11,104 American athletes.

Targeted, non-universal ECG screening in demographically higher-risk athletes, such as male basketball players and African-American athletes, has been proposed as an alternate approach to systematic exclusion of ECGs in the screening process. Further, improved athlete-specific ECG interpretation criteria, such as the International Recommendations, may improve sensitivity to further favor the use of the ECG as a screening tool [48].

Management of Sudden Cardiac Arrest in Athletes

Rapid identification of cardiac arrest and initiation of an emergency response system that includes early CPR and external defibrillation are the central components of decreasing mortality from sudden cardiac arrest (Fig. 21.1). Athlete victims of sudden cardiac arrest therefore have an invaluable feature favoring their survival, which is that sports-related episodes of cardiac arrest are often witnessed, such as by team

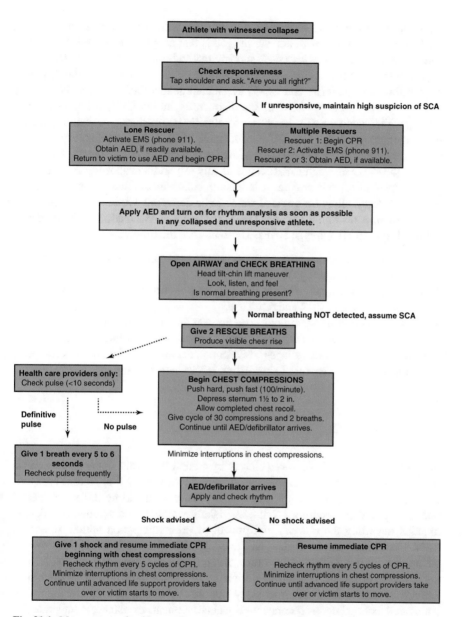

Fig. 21.1 Management of sudden cardiac arrest. (Reproduced with permission from Elsevier [56])

members, trainers, medical staff, and spectators, some of whom may have training in basic life support (BLS) and any of whom are likely to be able to contact emergency medical services (EMS). Despite this, data from several studies have shown that athlete victims of sudden cardiac arrests have poor survival outcomes, which, at an average survival rate of 11%, is only marginally better than out-of-hospital cardiac arrests in the general population [49–51]. Athletes with cardiac arrests occurring in the facilities of schools with athletic programs that adopted on-site AED programs had far better outcomes, with a 64% survival rate to hospital discharge [52].

The Inter-Association Task Force sponsored by the National Athletic Trainers' Association and the AHA and ACC have recommended that coaches and athletic trainers receive training to recognize cardiac arrests, initiate CPR, and apply and use AEDs, while schools and other hosts of athletic competitions or training should have emergency action plans (EAPs) inclusive of BLS, AED availability and use, and EMS activation. While the use of AEDs has shown mixed results for young athletes [53–55], early defibrillation is critically important in aborting cardiac arrest physiology, and for this reason, it is recommended that athletic programs design EAPs that would allow for an AED shock to be delivered within 3–5 min from the time of an athlete's initial collapse [56–58]. The Inter-Association Task Force recommends specific features of EAPs. These include the following:

1. Establishing communication systems (such as with cellular telephones or other readily usable technology)
2. Training of individuals who are likely to become first responders, such as trainers and coaches, in CPR and AED use
3. Acquiring necessary resuscitation equipment, including the AED
4. Planning and practicing the emergency response and coordination with EMS to ensure that time from collapse to EMS contact and CPR initiation is less than 1 min and time to external defibrillation is less than 3–5 min [56, 57]

Conclusion

Structural heart disease, followed closely by commotio cordis, is the leading cause of sports-related cardiac arrest among athletes. At the present time, there is not uniform agreement on the optimal strategy or tools that should be utilized to detect underlying cardiac conditions that pose risks for athletic individuals, and debate remains regarding the efficacy and impact of pre-participation athlete screening itself. Further refinement of data on the epidemiology of sudden cardiac death in athlete cohorts will influence the future role and practice of pre-participation screening. In spite of its rarity, rapid identification of cardiac arrest, implementation of emergency action plans and emergency response system protocols, and the use of automated external defibrillators are critical components of management strategies to improve survival and outcomes from such events.

References

1. Lee I-M, Skerritt PJ. Physical activity and all-cause mortality: what is the dose-response relation? Med Sci Sports Exerc. 2001;33(Suppl. 6):S459–71.
2. Southwest News Service, reported in New York Post, 17 Oct 2017.

3. Maron BJ, et al. Incidence and causes of sudden death in U.S. college athletes. J Am Coll Cardiol. 2014;63:1636–43.
4. Corrado D, Basso C, Rizzoli G, et al. Does sports activity enhance the risk of sudden death in adolescents and young adults? J Am Coll Cardiol. 2003;42:1959–63.
5. Van Camp SP, Bloor CM, Mueller FO, et al. Nontraumatic sports death in high school and college athletes. Med Sci Sports Exerc. 1995;27(5):641–7.
6. Maron BJ, Gorman TE, Aeppli D. Prevalence of sudden cardiac death during competitive sports activities in Minnesota high school athletes. J Am Coll Cardiol. 1998;32:1881–4.
7. Holst AG, Winkel BG, Theilade J, et al. Incidence and etiology of sports-related sudden cardiac death in Denmark - implications for preparticipation screening. Heart Rhythm. 2010;7:1365–71.
8. Steinvil A, Chundadze T, Zelster D, et al. Mandatory electrocardiographic screening of athletes to reduce their risk of sudden death proven fact or wishful thinking? J Am Coll Cardiol. 2011;57:1291–6.
9. Drezner JA, Harmon KG. Incidence of cardiac death in athletes. In: Pellicia A, et al., editors. The ESC textbook of sports cardiology. Oxford: Oxford University Press; 2019. p. 299.
10. Harmon KG, Asif IM, Klossner D, et al. Incidence of sudden cardiac death in National Collegiate Athletic Association Athletes. Circulation. 2011;123:1594–600.
11. Eckart RE, Scoville SL, Campbell CL, et al. Sudden death in young adults: a 25-year review of autopsies in military recruits. Ann Intern Med. 2004;141:829–34.
12. Solberg EE, Gjersten F, Haugstad E, et al. Sudden death in sports among young adults in Norway. Eur J Cardiovasc Prev Rehabil. 2010;17:337–41.
13. Atkins DL, Everson-Stewart S, Sears GK, et al. Epidemiology and outcomes from out-of-hospital cardiac arrest in children: the Resuscitation Outcomes Consortium Epistry-Cardiac Arrest. Circulation. 2009;119:1484–91.
14. Harmon KG, Drezner JA, Milson MG, et al. Incidence of sudden cardiac death in athletes: a state of the art review. Br J Sports Med published online first: June 24, 2014 as https://doi.org/10.1136/bjsports-2014-093872.
15. Maron BJ, Haas TS, Murphy CJ, et al. Incidence and causes of sudden death in U.S. College Athletes. J Am Coll Cardiol. 2014;63:1636–43.
16. Marijon E, Uy-Evanado A, Reinier, et al. Sudden cardiac arrest during sports activity in middle age. Circulation. 2015;131:1384–91.
17. Maron BJ, Shirani J, Poliac LC, et al. Sudden death in young competitive athletes: clinical, demographic, and pathological profiles. JAMA. 1996;276:199–204.
18. Semsarian C, Ingles J, Maron MS, Maron BJ. New perspectives on the prevalence of hypertrophic cardiomyopathy. J Am Coll Cardiol. 2015;65:1249–54.
19. Rowin EJ, Maron BJ, Appelbaum E, et al. Significance of false negative electrocardiograms in preparticipation screening of athletes for hypertrophic cardiomyopathy. Am J Cardiol. 2012;110:1027–32.
20. Elliott PM, Poloniecki J, Dickie S, et al. Sudden death in hypertrophic cardiomyopathy: identification of high risk patients. J Am Coll Cardiol. 2000;36(7):2212–8.
21. Monserrat L, Elliott PM, Gimeno JR, et al. Non-sustained ventricular tachycardia in hypertrophic cardiomyopathy: an independent marker of sudden death risk in young patients. J Am Coll Cardiol. 2003;42(5):873–9.
22. Maron BJ, Spirito B, Shen WK, et al. Implantable cardioverter-defibrillators and prevention of sudden cardiac death in hypertrophic cardiomyopathy. JAMA. 2007;298(4):405–12.
23. Gimeno JR, Tome-Esteban M, Lofiego C, et al. Exercise-induced ventricular arrhythmias and risk of sudden cardiac death in patients with hypertrophic cardiomyopathy. Eur Heart J. 2009;30(21):2599–605.
24. Maron BJ, Udelson JE, Bonow RO, et al. Eligibility and disqualification recommendations for competitive athletes with cardiovascular abnormalities: task force 3: hypertrophic cardiomyopathy, arrhythmogenic right ventricular cardiomyopathy and other cardiomyopathies, and myocarditis. J Am Coll Cardiol. 2015;66(21):2362–71.

25. Basso C, Maron BJ, Corrado D, Thiene G. Clinical profile of congenital coronary artery anomalies with origin from the wrong aortic sinus leading to sudden death in young competitive athletes. J Am Coll Cardiol. 2000;35:1493–501.
26. Van Hare GF, Ackerman MJ, Evangelista JK, et al. Eligibility and disqualification recommendations for competitive athletes with cardiovascular abnormalities: task force 4: congenital heart disease. Circulation. 2015;132:e281–91.
27. Basso C, Corrado D, Marcus FI, et al. Arrhythmogenic right ventricular cardiomyopathy. Lancet. 2009;373:1289–300.
28. Hulot JS, Jouven X, Empana JP, et al. Natural history and risk stratification of arrhythmogenic right ventricular dysplasia/cardiomyopathy. Circulation. 2004;110(14):1879–84.
29. Hermida JS, Minassian A, Jarry G, et al. Familial incidence of late ventricular potentials and electrocardiographic abnormalities in arrhythmogenic right ventricular dysplasia. Am J Cardiol. 1997;79(10):1375–80.
30. Marcus FI, McKenna WJ, Sherill D, et al. Diagnosis of arrhythmogenic right ventricular cardiomyopathy/dysplasia: proposed modification of the task force criteria. Eur Heart J. 2010;31:806–14.
31. Kirchof P, Fabritz L, Ziener M, et al. Age- and training-dependent development of arrhythmogenic right ventricular cardiomyopathy in heterozygous plakoglobin-deficient mice. Circulation. 2006;114:1799–806.
32. James CA, Bhonsale A, Tichnell C, et al. Exercise increases age-related penetrance and arrhythmic risk in arrhythmogenic right ventricular dysplasia/cardiomyopathy-associated desmosomal mutation carriers. J Am Coll Cardiol. 2013;62:1290–7.
33. Link MS. Commotio cordis: ventricular fibrillation triggered by chest impact-induced abnormalities in repolarization. Cir Arrhythm Electrophysiol. 2012;5:425–32.
34. Kalin J, Madias C, Alskeikh-Ali AA, et al. Reduced diameter spheres increases the risk of chest blow-induced ventricular fibrillation (commotio cordis). Heart Rhythm. 2011;8:1578–81.
35. Link MS, Maron BJ, Wang PJ, et al. Reduced risk of sudden death from chest wall blows (commotio cordis) with safety baseballs. Pediatrics. 2002;109:873–7.
36. Link MS, Maron BJ, Wang PJ, et al. Upper and lower limits of vulnerability to sudden arrhythmic death with chest-wall impact (commotio cordis). J Am Coll Cardiol. 2003;41:99–104.
37. Maron BJ, Poliac L, Kaplan JA, et al. Blunt impact to the chest leading to sudden death from cardiac arrest during sports activities. N Engl J Med. 1995;333:337–42.
38. Link MS, Maron BJ, Stickney RE, et al. Automated external defibrillator arrhythmia detection in a model of cardiac arrest due to commotio cordis. J Cardiovasc Electrophysiol. 2003;14(1):83–7.
39. Maron BJ, Haas TS, Ahluwalia A, et al. Increasing survival rate from commotio cordis. Heart Rhythm. 2013;10:219–23.
40. Maron BJ. Diversity of views from Europe on national preparticipation screening for competitive athletes. Heart Rhythm. 2010;10:1372–3.
41. Maron BJ, Thompson PD, Puffer JC, et al. Cardiovascular preparticipation screening of competitive athletes: a statement for health professionals from the Sudden Death Committee (Clinical Cardiology) and Congenital Cardiac Defects Committee (Cardiovascular Disease in the Young), American Heart Association. Circulation. 1996;94:850–6.
42. Corrado D, Basso C, Pavei A, et al. Trends in sudden cardiovascular death in young competitive athletes after implementation of a preparticipation screening program. JAMA. 2006;296:1593–601.
43. Corrado D, Pelliccia A, Bjørnstad HH, et al. Cardiovascular pre-participation screening of young competitive athletes for prevention of sudden death: proposal for a common European protocol. Consensus Statement of the Study Group of Sport Cardiology of the Working Group of Cardiac Rehabilitation and Exercise Physiology and the Working Group of Myocardial and Pericardial Diseases of the European Society of Cardiology. Eur Heart J. 2005;26(5):516–24.
44. Maron BJ, Friedman RA, Kligfield P, et al. Assessment of the 12-lead electrocardiogram as a screening test for detection of cardiovascular disease in healthy general populations of young people (12-25 years of age). J Am Coll Cardiol. 2014;64(14):1479–514.

45. Maron BJ, Levine BD, Washington RL, et al. Eligibility and disqualification recommendations for competitive athletes with cardiovascular abnormalities: Task Force 2: Preparticipation screening for cardiovascular disease in competitive athletes. J Am Coll Cardiol. 2015;66(21):2356–61.
46. Harmon KG, Zigman M, Dezner JA. The effectiveness of screening history, physical exam, and ECG to detect potentially lethal cardiac disorders in athletes: a systematic review/meta-analysis. J Electrocardiol. 2015;48:329–38.
47. Rai AL, Salerno JC, Asif IM, et al. Evaluation and management of Wolff-Parkinson-White in athletes. Sports Health. 2014;6(4):326–32.
48. Sharma S, Drezner JA, Baggish A, et al. International recommendations for electrocardiographic interpretation in athletes. J Am Coll Cardiol. 2017;69(8):1057–75.
49. Drezner JA, Rogers KJ. Sudden cardiac arrest in intercollegiate athletes: detailed analysis and outcomes of resuscitation in 9 cases. Heart Rhythm. 2006;3:755–9.
50. Maron BJ, Gohman TE, Kyle SB, et al. Clinical profile and spectrum of commotio cordis. JAMA. 2002;287:1142–6.
51. Drezner JA, Chun JS, Harmon KG, Derminer L. Survival trends in the United States following exercise-related sudden cardiac arrest in the youth: 2000-2006. Heart Rhythm. 2008;5:794–9.
52. Drezner JA, Rao AL, Heistand J, et al. Effectiveness of emergency response planning for sudden cardiac arrest in United States high schools with automated external defibrillators. Circulation. 2009;120:518–25.
53. Drezner JA, Rogers KJ, Horneff JG. Automated external defibrillator use at NCAA Division II and III universities. Br J Sports Med. 2011;45:1174–8.
54. Drezner JA, et al. Use of automated external defibrillators at NCAA Division I Universities. Med Sci Sports Exerc. 2005;37(9):1487–92.
55. Drezner JA, Toresdahl BG, Rao AL, et al. Outcomes from sudden cardiac arrest in US high schools: a 2-year prospective study from the National Registry for AED Use in Sports. Br J Sports Med. 2013;47:1179–83.
56. Drezner JA, Courson RW, Roberts WO, Mosesso VN Jr, Link MS, Maron BJ. Inter-association task force recommendations on emergency preparedness and management of sudden cardiac arrest in high school and college athletic programs: a consensus statement. Heart Rhythm. 2007;4(4):549–65. https://doi.org/10.1016/j.hrthm.2007.02.019.
57. Schwellnus M, Kipps C, Roberts WO, et al. Medical encounters (including injury and illness) at mass community-based endurance sports events: an international consensus statement on definitions and methods of data recording and reporting. Br J Sports Med. 2019; https://doi.org/10.1136/bjsports-2018-100092.
58. Link MS, Myerburg RJ, Estes NA. Eligibility and disqualification recommendations for competitive athletes with cardiovascular abnormalities: Task Force 12: emergency action plans, resuscitation, cardiopulmonary resuscitation, and automated external defibrillators. J Am Coll Cardiol. 2015;66(21):2434–8.

Chapter 22
Commotio Cordis in Athletes

Mohita Singh and Mark S. Link

Introduction

Blunt, non-penetrating chest trauma can trigger ventricular fibrillation (VF) that is unassociated with structural damage to the sternum or heart itself and cause sudden cardiac death [1]. This condition is known as commotio cordis and it has been associated with up to 3% of deaths in young athletes in the United States [2]. Commotio cordis primarily occurs in children, adolescents, and young adults and is most common during participation in sports [3].

Epidemiology

Although described as far back as the eighteenth century [4], the first series reporting 25 cases of commotio cordis was published in 1995 [5]. Since then, over 200 cases in the United States and 60 international cases of commotion cordis have been described [6]. Commotio cordis occurs predominantly in young people, with a typical age of 15–19 years, and almost exclusively (up to 95%) in male subjects. The majority of the victims are white [1]. Very few cases have been described in patients over the age of 20 years [7]. Although observed most commonly during baseball, followed by soccer, cricket, and hockey, deaths by sudden blow to the chest have been described during a variety of many recreational and competitive sports. About 25% of cases have been reported to occur during routine activities unassociated with sports [6].

M. Singh (✉) · M. S. Link
Department of Medicine, Cardiology Division, Cardiac Electrophysiology,
UT Southwestern Medical Center, Dallas, TX, USA
e-mail: Mohita.singh@phhs.org; mark.link@utsouthwestern.edu

© Springer Nature Switzerland AG 2021
D. J. Engel, D. M. Phelan (eds.), *Sports Cardiology*,
https://doi.org/10.1007/978-3-030-69384-8_22

Proposed Mechanism of Action

Insights into the proposed mechanisms of commotio cordis came from an experimental swine model developed at Tufts Medical Center [8]. Investigators induced instantaneous ventricular fibrillation (Fig. 22.1) with low impact blows to the chest when the impact occurred in a narrow 20-msec window during cardiac repolarization (immediately prior to the peak of the T wave) (Fig. 22.2). When the trauma was delivered during ventricular depolarization (QRS complex), no ventricular fibrillation was observed, but subjects were occasionally noted to have transient complete heart block followed by ST-segment elevation and, in some, left bundle-branch block [8].

Another study with the same model noted that impacts directly over the cardiac silhouette were necessary to induce ventricular fibrillation [9] and impacts directly over the center of the heart (over the left ventricular anterolateral papillary muscle) were the most lethal. Furthermore, chest blows at a speed of 40 mph were most likely to induce VF (~ 70% of the time) versus lower or higher impact velocities. Blows of less than 20 mph did not produce VF, suggesting a minimal threshold of

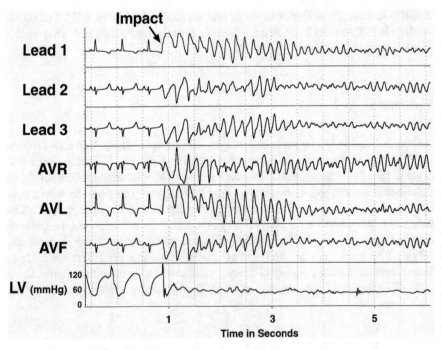

Fig. 22.1 Six-lead electrocardiogram showing the electrophysiologic and hemodynamic consequences of an impact to the chest by an object at 30 miles per hour, timed to occur 16 msec before the peak of the T wave in a 9-kg pig. Ventricular fibrillation began immediately (within one cardiac cycle) after the chest impact, which was associated with instant loss of effective left ventricular (LV) pressure. (Reprinted with permission from Link et al. [8], Massachusetts Medical Society)

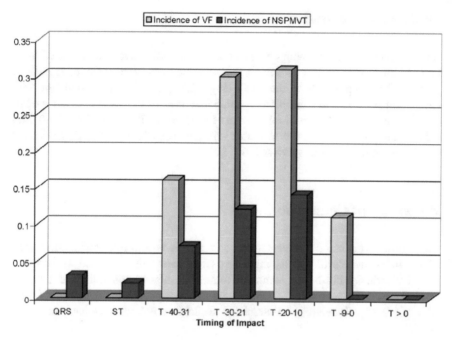

Fig. 22.2 Incidence of ventricular fibrillation (VF) and nonsustained polymorphic ventricular tachycardia (NSPMVT) relative to the timing of the cardiac cycle. Impacts were at 30 and 40 mph. VF was observed in approximately 30% of impacts that occurred in cardiac repolarization 30 to 10 ms before the T-wave peak. Nonsustained polymorphic ventricular tachycardia was predominantly observed during this time window but occasionally was seen with strikes during the QRS and ST segments. (Reprinted with permission from Link and Estes [19], Elsevier)

25–30 mph. Paradoxically, higher impact velocities of 50–70 mph caused less VF than 40-mph blows and more mechanical trauma, arguing that the model at these velocities was not consistent with commotio cordis [10, 11]. The shape of the object also contributes to the likelihood of inducing VF with smaller diameter objects being more likely to cause ventricular fibrillation [12]. In another study, smaller animals (weights < 40 kg) were more susceptible to ventricular fibrillation than their larger counterparts [7].

On a cellular level, it is hypothesized that the chest wall impact likely triggers activation of mechanosensitive K_{ATP}^+ channel during a vulnerable time window which in turn leads to inhomogeneous depolarization, thereby creating an arrhythmogenic substrate. In the experimental model, inhibition of the K_{ATP}^+ channel led to a reduction in the incidence of VF and the magnitude of ST elevation [13]. There is marked variability in individual susceptibility to ventricular fibrillation. In a study of 1274 total impacts in 139 swine, 360 impacts (28%) resulted in ventricular fibrillation; however, in 38 animals, none of the impacts resulted in ventricular fibrillation, and only 7 swine (5%) had >80% occurrence of ventricular fibrillation with chest impacts [14]. This variability may be explained by individual differences in repolarization reserve or distribution of ion channels susceptible to wall stretch/ventricular pressures, but definitive answers are pending.

Outcome/Resuscitation

Survival rates in patients with commotio cordis initially have been reported to be low, although over the last decade, the survival numbers have improved from 15% in the 1990s to up to 35% in the 2000s (Fig. 22.3) [1, 3]. Early resuscitation with chest compressions and defibrillators within 3 minutes of the event has been associated with a statistically significant increase in survival (25% versus 3%, $P = 0.007$) [15]. Standard, commercially available chest barriers have not been associated within an improvement in survival [16, 17].

Prevention of Commotio Cordis

Commotio cordis can be prevented to some degree with the following strategies. More pliable and elastic T-balls, known as safety balls, are associated with a lower risk of ventricular fibrillation compared to regulation baseballs in the swine model [7% versus 35% at 30 mph ($P < 0.0001$) and 11% versus 69% at 40 mph ($P < 0.01$)] (Fig. 22.4) [8]. Standard, commercially available chest barriers have not been

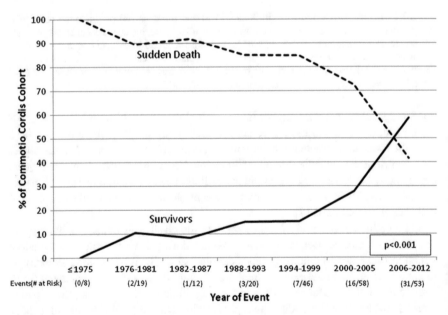

Fig. 22.3 Commotio cordis-related survival and mortality over time in the US Commotio Cordis Registry. (Reprinted with permission from Maron et al. [3], Elsevier)

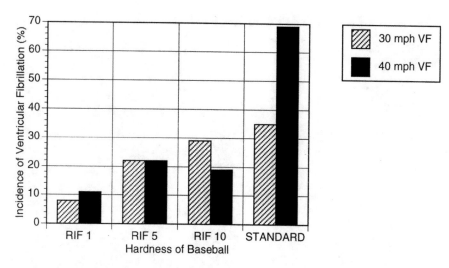

Fig. 22.4 Incidence of ventricular fibrillation (VF) in % with chest wall impacts to 8- to 12-kg swine by baseballs differing in hardness. RIF 1 are safety T-balls meant for use by youth under age 7. RIF 5 is a slightly harder ball mean for use by youth 8–10 years old and RIF 10 is even harder, but not as hard as a standard baseball, mean for use in youth 11–13 years old. (Reprinted with permission from Link et al. [20], American Academy of Pediatrics)

associated with a decrease in commotio cordis [16, 17]. Experimental models demonstrate that thicker chest protectors composed of less compressible and denser materials are able to provide increased protection against development of ventricular fibrillation than some of the commercially available chest protectors [18]. A mechanical surrogate composed of a chest model and sensors (similar to the 3-rib dummy model used for testing in automobile accidents) is now available to access the ability of chest wall protectors to lower the risk of commotio cordis (https://nocsae.org/wp-content/uploads/2018/05/1521576393ND20018CommotioCordisTestMethod.pdf).

Conclusion

Commotio cordis is a rare but tragic event that typically occurs in adolescent boys when they are struck in the chest. An experimental model has provided us with increased understanding of the factors required to induce ventricular fibrillation and the cellular mechanisms behind sudden cardiac death in commotion cordis (Fig. 22.5). Timely cardiac resuscitation remains the cornerstone of therapy. Improved recognition of the disease appears to have aided in the survival rate, but mortality associated with commotion cordis remains unacceptably high in otherwise young healthy adolescents.

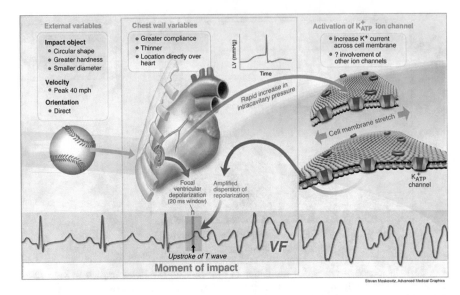

Fig. 22.5 The confluence of variables and a proposed mechanism necessary for commotio cordis to occur. Important impact-object variables are shape, hardness, diameter, and velocity. Human characteristics are the pliability of the chest wall, impact timing, location and orientation of blow, and individual susceptibility, likely carried in ion channels involved in repolarization. LV indicates left ventricle. (Reprinted with permission, Link and Estes [21], John Wiley and Sons)

References

1. Maron BJ, Estes NA 3rd. Commotio cordis. N Engl J Med. 2010;362(10):917–27.
2. Maron BJ, Doerer JJ, Haas TS, Tierney DM, Mueller FO. Sudden deaths in young competitive athletes: analysis of 1866 deaths in the United States, 1980–2006. Circulation. 2009;119(8):1085–92.
3. Maron BJ, Haas TS, Ahluwalia A, Garberich RF, Estes NA 3rd, Link MS. Increasing survival rate from commotio cordis. Heart Rhythm. 2013;10(2):219–23.
4. Nesbitt AD, Cooper PJ, Kohl P. Rediscovering commotio cordis. Lancet. 2001;357(9263):1195–7.
5. Maron BJ, Poliac LC, Kaplan JA, Mueller FO. Blunt impact to the chest leading to sudden death from cardiac arrest during sports activities. N Engl J Med. 1995;333(6):337–42.
6. Maron BJ, Ahluwalia A, Haas TS, Semsarian C, Link MS, Estes NA 3rd. Global epidemiology and demographics of commotio cordis. Heart Rhythm. 2011;8(12):1969–71.
7. Link MS. Commotio cordis: ventricular fibrillation triggered by chest impact-induced abnormalities in repolarization. Circ Arrhythm Electrophysiol. 2012;5(2):425–32.
8. Link MS, Wang PJ, Pandian NG, et al. An experimental model of sudden death due to low-energy chest-wall impact (commotio cordis). N Engl J Med. 1998;338(25):1805–11.
9. Link MS, Maron BJ, VanderBrink BA, et al. Impact directly over the cardiac silhouette is necessary to produce ventricular fibrillation in an experimental model of commotio cordis. J Am Coll Cardiol. 2001;37(2):649–54.
10. Link MS, Maron BJ, Stickney RE, et al. Automated external defibrillator arrhythmia detection in a model of cardiac arrest due to commotio cordis. J Cardiovasc Electrophysiol. 2003;14(1):83–7.
11. Link MS. Mechanically induced sudden death in chest wall impact (commotio cordis). Prog Biophys Mol Biol. 2003;82(1–3):175–86.

12. Kalin J, Madias C, Alsheikh-Ali AA, Link MS. Reduced diameter spheres increases the risk of chest blow-induced ventricular fibrillation (commotio cordis). Heart Rhythm. 2011;8(10):1578–81.
13. Link MS, Wang PJ, VanderBrink BA, et al. Selective activation of the K(+)(ATP) channel is a mechanism by which sudden death is produced by low-energy chest-wall impact (Commotio cordis). Circulation. 1999;100(4):413–8.
14. Alsheikh-Ali AA, Madias C, Supran S, Link MS. Marked variability in susceptibility to ventricular fibrillation in an experimental commotio cordis model. Circulation. 2010;122(24):2499–504.
15. Maron BJ, Gohman TE, Kyle SB, Estes NA 3rd, Link MS. Clinical profile and spectrum of commotio cordis. JAMA. 2002;287(9):1142–6.
16. Doerer JJ, Haas TS, Estes NA 3rd, Link MS, Maron BJ. Evaluation of chest barriers for protection against sudden death due to commotio cordis. Am J Cardiol. 2007;99(6):857–9.
17. Weinstock J, Maron BJ, Song C, Mane PP, Estes NA 3rd, Link MS. Failure of commercially available chest wall protectors to prevent sudden cardiac death induced by chest wall blows in an experimental model of commotio cordis. Pediatrics. 2006;117(4):e656–62.
18. Kumar K, Mandleywala SN, Gannon MP, Estes NA 3rd, Weinstock J, Link MS. Development of a chest wall protector effective in preventing sudden cardiac death by chest wall impact (commotio cordis). Clin J Sport Med. 2017;27(1):26–30.
19. Link MS, Estes NA 3rd. Mechanically induced ventricular fibrillation (commotio cordis). Heart Rhythm. 2007;4:529–32.
20. Link MS, Maron BJ, Wang PJ, Pandian NG, VanderBrink BA, Estes NAM. Reduced risk of sudden death from chest wall blows (commotio cordis) with safety baseballs. Pediatrics. 2002;109:873–7.
21. Link MS, Estes NAM. Athletes and arrhythmias. J Cardiovasc Electrophysiol. 2010;21:1184–9.

Chapter 23
The Impact of COVID-19 on Sports Cardiology

Bradley Lander, David J. Engel, and Dermot M. Phelan

Background

The coronavirus disease-19 (COVID-19) is caused by the severe acute respiratory syndrome coronavirus 2 (SARS-CoV-2) and spread predominantly by respiratory droplets. COVID-19 garnered international attention as it rapidly developed into a global pandemic in early 2020 and its dramatic morbidity and mortality necessitated the implementation of public health measures designed to limit close contact and large public gatherings. To achieve that goal, organized sports from the recreational level to the Olympic Games were postponed, altered, or canceled altogether. As we gradually make progress in the fight against COVID-19 and our society focuses on the means to restore and restart all facets of normal life, including the resumption of organized athletics, sport and health organizations continue to face significant challenges designing and implementing safe return-to-play (RTP) strategies.

B. Lander · D. J. Engel (✉)
Division of Cardiology, Columbia University Irving Medical Center, New York, NY, USA
e-mail: bl2276@cumc.columbia.edu; de165@cumc.columbia.edu

D. M. Phelan
Sport Cardiology Center, Hypertrophic Cardiomyopathy Center, Atrium Health Sanger Heart & Vascular Institute, Charlotte, NC, USA
e-mail: dermot.phelan@atriumhealth.org

© Springer Nature Switzerland AG 2021
D. J. Engel, D. M. Phelan (eds.), *Sports Cardiology*,
https://doi.org/10.1007/978-3-030-69384-8_23

Cardiac Considerations

Early data from critically ill and hospitalized COVID-19 patients demonstrate the common association between COVID-19 and myocardial injury, defined as a cardiac troponin level greater than the 99th percentile upper reference limit [1–4]. Several mechanisms of myocardial injury have been proposed and include direct viral myocardial injury, microvascular injury, cytokine and stress mediated cardiomyopathies, acute coronary syndromes, pulmonary emboli, and systemic hyperinflammatory responses [5, 6] (Fig. 23.1). SARS-CoV-2 is thought to enter the body through the angiotensin-converting enzyme 2 (ACE2) receptor, a receptor present in the lungs, myocardium, and on vascular endothelial cells [5, 7]. As such, direct viral myocardial injury is a potential mechanism for myocarditis and has been supported by autopsy data demonstrating viral presence, progeny, and shedding in cardiac tissue [6]. Other theoretical mechanisms of direct viral injury include infection-mediated vasculitis, as the ACE2 receptor is expressed in arterial and venous endothelial cells, or an indirect immunological response and resultant hypersensitivity reaction [5, 8]. Microvascular injury is also a proposed mechanism for

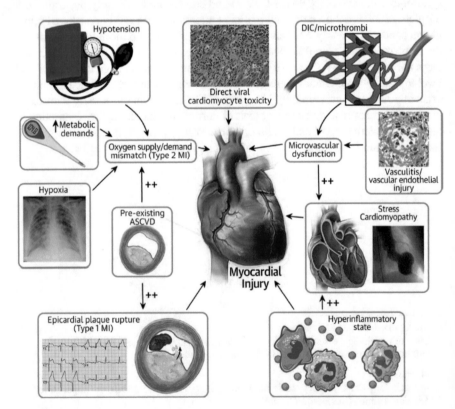

Fig. 23.1 Potential mechanisms of myocardial injury in COVID-19. (Reprinted with permission from Atri et al. [5] (Elsevier))

myocardial injury given the significant proportion of patients with severe COVID-19 meeting criteria for disseminated intravascular coagulation (DIC) [9]. Immune activation as a result of severe COVID-19 is thought to trigger DIC, microvascular dysfunction, and subsequent myocardial injury [5].

COVID-19 myocarditis has emerged as a critical issue in the discussions regarding RTP strategies for athletes [3, 10, 11]. Because myocarditis is a prominent etiology of sudden cardiac death (SCD) among athletes, accounting for approximately 4–7.5% of SCD in athletes [12], current guidelines addressing myocarditis recommend against competition or strenuous training for 3–6 months after diagnosis [12–16]. Recent studies of cardiac magnetic resonance imaging (CMR) in patients recovering from COVID-19 have demonstrated findings suggestive of residual myocardial inflammation, and as such, highlighted concerns about COVID-19-related myocarditis [17, 18]. Additionally, after several media reports of athletes diagnosed with presumed COVID-19 myocarditis, widely publicized discussions arose regarding the feasibility of continuing or resuming athletic training and competition in the midst of the pandemic [19].

While inflammatory heart disease, including pericarditis and myocarditis, poses an enhanced risk to athletes on resumption of training and competition, the true incidence and prevalence of COVID-19-related subclinical inflammatory heart disease, particularly among athletes who were asymptomatic or mildly symptomatic, remain unknown and existing data are limited to small observational case series [18, 20–22]. Current studies evaluating the incidence of myocardial injury in asymptomatic or mildly symptomatic athletes provide highly variable findings [18, 21, 22, 23]. Adding to the diagnostic difficulty in detecting potential subclinical COVID-19 cardiac injury in athletes is the fact that certain abnormalities described in association with myocarditis, such as troponin elevation, ECG abnormalities and imaging findings including increased left ventricular (LV) wall thickness, increased chamber size, and mild reduction in ventricular ejection fraction, can be seen as attributes of the athlete's heart [24–26].

Recognizing these challenges, the American College of Cardiology Sports and Exercise Cardiology Council, and other organizations, generated RTP recommendations for athletes recovering from COVID-19 [10, 20, 27–31]. While many athletes will be asymptomatic or minimally symptomatic, some may have experienced more pronounced viral symptoms such as prolonged fever with myalgias, chest pain, reduced exercise tolerance, or shortness of breath. Ascertained symptom burden should guide the next steps in the evaluation of the athlete, with an assumption of a correlation of potential risk of cardiac sequelae of COVID-19 with the severity of initial COVID-19 viral illness [31]. Although there has been some variation between published RTP cardiovascular screening recommendations, a conservative approach consisting of the combination of an electrocardiogram (ECG), transthoracic echocardiogram (TTE), and cardiac biomarker evaluation (troponin evaluation) was initially put forth by the ACC Sports and Exercise Cardiology Council in May 2020 for all athletes with prior mild to severe COVID-19 viral illness [10, 20, 27–29, 31, 32]. RTP without additional cardiovascular risk stratification was deemed reasonable in asymptomatic athletes who test positive for COVID-19, as long as clinical observation is available and there is stepwise and pragmatic training intensification [31].

The decision to pursue additional downstream testing, including CMR, should be based on concerns raised on the initial screening exams. The widespread use of advanced imaging methods, such as CMR, as part of the initial pre-participation screening process of athletes has not been recommended. There remain valid concerns that increased testing will lead to increased sensitivity, but will invariably decrease specificity for detecting clinically relevant cardiac pathology, especially given the challenges in distinguishing potential COVID-19 cardiac pathology from adaptive remodeling in athletes [31]. The initial RTP recommendations were put forth with the understanding that the screening approach will evolve as more data on the prevalence of COVID-19 cardiac involvement and the diagnostic performance of screening measures become available.

Practical Use of Cardiac Testing for COVID-19 Myocarditis

In the assessment for potential COVID-19 cardiac pathology, it is important to understand the strengths and limitations of the cardiac tests currently recommended in RTP cardiac screening algorithms. Appropriate use and interpretation of the results will help enhance detection of disease and athlete protection while minimizing false-positive results that could adversely affect athletes by causing unnecessary delays in RTP or disqualification. The four tests that have been addressed in the most detail in the evaluation of athletes in the RTP screening algorithm include cardiac biomarkers (troponin), ECG, echocardiography, and CMR.

Troponin

Several COVID-19 RTP documents have recommended measuring high-sensitivity cardiac troponin (hs-cTn) levels to assess for the biochemical presence of myocardial injury and diagnose subclinical myocarditis [20, 27, 31, 32]. However, strenuous exercise may also cause an elevation in troponin that peaks and returns to baseline approximately 24–48 hours after exercise [26, 31, 33, 34]. As such, hs-cTn testing should not be done within this timeframe and testing should be repeated following an isolated abnormal result [10]. Persistently elevated troponin levels should prompt characterization of the myocardium with echocardiography and CMR [10]. It is important to note that the data linking elevated hs-cTn to worse outcomes in COVID-19 was derived from hospitalized patients. The full implications of elevated hs-cTn among younger, asymptomatic, or mildly symptomatic athletes is currently not known [10, 35]. Because there are no established reference ranges for hs-cTn in athletes, results need to be incorporated with other clinical data obtained in the screening process to properly interpret and act on the result.

Electrocardiography

The 12-lead ECG is simple, inexpensive, and useful in detecting conditions associated with SCD. While myocarditis, or myopericarditis, may manifest on an ECG in the form of premature ventricular contractions, arrhythmias, ST and T wave abnormalities, pseudoinfarction pattern (Q waves and ST elevation), bundle branch and atrioventricular (AV) blocks, the sensitivity of the ECG for detecting myopericarditis remains less than 50% [31, 36]. Moreover, many of the physiological, adaptive electrical changes commonly seen on athletes' ECGs, such as repolarization abnormalities and tall T waves, could be misinterpreted as myopericarditis [31] (Fig. 23.2). The specificity of ECG changes for diagnosing myocarditis is expected to be low but comparison with previous ECGs is of paramount importance [31].

Echocardiography

Given their relative accessibility compared with other forms of advanced cardiac imaging, and excellent diagnostic capabilities, echocardiograms have been recommended as first-line imaging exams in several RTP strategies for symptomatic COVID-19-positive athletes [27–29, 31, 32]. The presence of left or right ventricular systolic or diastolic dysfunction, or more than a trivial pericardial effusion, are important findings on echocardiography, especially if the findings are new in comparison with available prior studies. These abnormalities should prompt consideration of additional imaging to exclude COVID-19-related inflammatory heart disease. Occasionally, elite endurance athletes may demonstrate a low normal to mildly reduced resting left and right ventricular systolic function [37–39]. In this

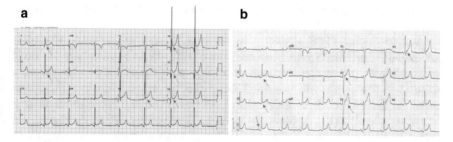

Fig. 23.2 Challenges with ECG screening in athletes post COVID-19. ECGs performed on two athletes highlighting challenges with differentiating normal changes associated with athletic training and pathology. Panel A is a normal healthy endurance athlete's ECG showing diffuse ST segment elevation due to early repolarization (arrows). Panel B is an ECG from a 23-year-old soccer player presenting with positional pleuritic chest pain, elevated high-sensitivity troponin (> 5000 ng/l) with confirmed myopericarditis on MRI; the ECG also shows diffuse ST segment elevation (blue arrows) but also subtle PR depression (red arrows). (Reprinted with permission from Phelan et al. [11], Elsevier)

instance, stress echocardiography demonstrating normal augmentation of left ventricular wall segments and normal exercise hemodynamics is a useful tool to help distinguish features of the athlete's heart from potential cardiac pathology. However, in the context of concern for COVID-19 myocarditis, this should only be undertaken after a CMR has ruled out active myocardial inflammation. Implementation of echocardiography may be limited by cost and access in areas of high disease prevalence [31].

Cardiac Magnetic Resonance Imaging

The important diagnostic role of CMR for the detection myocarditis and pericarditis in patients with high clinical suspicion is well established. CMR should only be performed during the acute illness if needed for immediate patient management decisions, otherwise, it should be performed >10 days after initial diagnosis in order to limit exposure to hospital and MRI staff [31, 40]. Some small CMR-specific studies demonstrated a significant prevalence of cardiac involvement in patients who recovered from COVID-19. In a cohort of 26 patients in Wuhan, China, recovering from moderate to severe COVID-19 pneumonia, 31% had late gadolinium enhancement (LGE), and there were additional markers of myocardial inflammation in a high prevalence of patients including increased global native T1, T2, and extracellular volume [41]. Puntmann et al. studied a German cohort of 100 middle-age patients recovering from COVID-19 illness and reported that 78% of this cohort had evidence of myocardial injury on CMR (median 71 days post-diagnosis) [17]. Importantly, the cohort had a mean (SD) age of 49 (14) years and a clinically significant burden of preexisting conditions (hypertension 22%; diabetes 18%; intrinsic lung disease 21%), and 36% had ongoing symptoms at the time of CMR. It is evident that this cohort may not be generalizable to younger, healthier athletes. Notably, a revised manuscript was ultimately published because of inaccurate data analysis and inconsistencies within the data.

Athlete-specific CMR studies have reported highly variable rates of cardiac abnormalities in athletes who recovered from COVID-19. In one single-center study of 26 athletes (mean age 19) with prior asymptomatic or mildly symptomatic COVID-19 illness, and with normal ECG, hs-cTn, and echocardiogram, CMR demonstrated that 46% of these athletes had LGE and 15% had CMR findings suggestive of myocarditis [18]. Another observational case series of 46 collegiate athletes (mean age 19) who recovered from COVID-19 and underwent a screening CMR demonstrated 41% of athletes had pericardial hyperenhancement, suggesting pericarditis. Only 1 athlete had myocardial LGE and no athletes had abnormal native T2 values [22]. In contrast to these studies, a third CMR study evaluating 12 Hungarian athletes recovering from COVID-19 (median age 23) showed no evidence of myocardial or injury [21], and a CMR-based study of 145 collegiate athletes recovered from COVID-19 showed that the prevalence of detected myocarditis was 1.4% [43].

Given the variability associated with the results of these three small-cohort studies, it is clear that large, multicenter, controlled, and blinded CMR studies are needed.

At present, there are insufficient data to recommend CMR for all athletes with confirmed or suspected COVID-19 or for those without clinical suspicion for myocarditis [10]. As learned during the introduction of ECG screening for athletes, widespread CMR-based screening without standardized measurements and normative data may lead to high false-positive rates, unnecessary subsequent testing, and needless medical disqualifications [10, 42].

Clinical Experience

Clinical experience gained in 2020 through widespread performance of COVID-19 RTP cardiac testing and gradual return of organized sports has fortunately yielded very few cases of relevant cardiac pathology in young athletes thus far. The major US professional sporting leagues were among the first sporting organizations to return to full-scale sport activity in the setting of the COVID-19 pandemic, with provision of extensive health and safety measures as recommended by public health, infectious disease, and cardiac consultants. A program for pre-participation RTP cardiac testing, in alignment with the initial May 2020 ACC recommendations, was implemented by each of these leagues for all athletes that tested positive for COVID-19. A study of the collective results of the systematic cardiac RTP COVID-19 screening program utilized by these professional leagues demonstrated that the prevalence of clincally detectable inflammatory heart disease in professional athletes who underwent RTP cardiac screening was 0.6% [43]. Safe return to professional sporting activity has been achieved thus far with no cardiovascular events occurring within these professional leagues during and on completion of competitive play in 2020. The implementation of RTP cardiac screening by the professional leagues has provided a large-scale practical paradigm demonstrating the clinical efficacy of the ACC expert consensus-generated screening recommendations in achieving safe return to intensive sport activity. In parallel to the experience with professional athletes, a registry of National Collegiate Athletic Association (NCAA) athletes is planned to assess the impact of COVID-19 on cardiovascular pathology and the risk of myocardial injury for collegiate athletes afflicted with COVID-19.

Updated Expert Consensus Recommendations

Based on the data and clinical experience generated after publication and practice of the initial RTP screening algorithm, members of the American College of Cardiology's Sports and Exercise Cardiology Council published updated RTP screening recommendations in October 2020. These recommendations do not advocate for cardiovascular (CV) risk stratification among athletes with prior asymptomatic or mild COVID-19 viral illness (defined as nonspecific and self-limited fatigue, anosmia or ageusia, nausea, vomiting, diarrhea, headache, cough, sore throat, and nasopharyngeal congestion), who remain asymptomatic after completion of appropriate self-isolation [10].

For high school athletes younger than 15 years recovering from moderate to severe COVID-19 illness (defined as persistent fever [temperature 100.4 °F] or chills, myalgias, severe lethargy, and hypoxia or pneumonia and/or CV symptoms such as dyspnea and chest pain, tightness, or pressure at rest or during exertion), evaluation by a pediatrician or pediatric cardiologist has been recommended to determine the need for further CV risk stratification [10]. For high school athletes older than 15 years following asymptomatic to mildly symptomatic COVID-19 illness, the updated ACC recommendations do not advocate for CV risk stratification. However, for high school athletes who had systemic or CV specific symptoms, a similar approach to symptomatic older athletes is recommended [10].

For masters-level athletes, routine RTP CV assessment is not recommended considering the logistics required for widespread screening and the low risk of clinically significant cardiac injury after mild infection. However, risk stratification may benefit master's athletes older than 65 years, particularly individuals with preexisting CV disease and those with moderate to severe prior COVID-19 infection (Fig. 23.3).

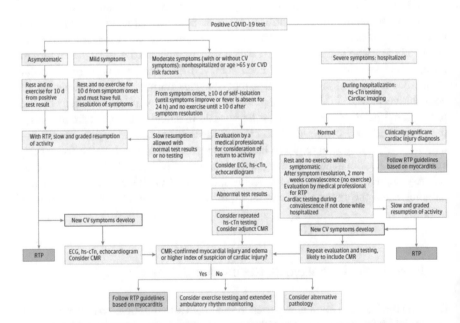

Fig. 23.3 American College of Cardiology October 2020 COVID-19 Return-to-Play Algorithm for recreational masters athletes. (Reprinted with permission from Kim et al. [10], American Medical Association)

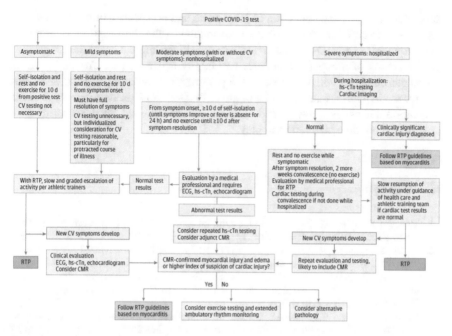

Fig. 23.4 American College of Cardiology October 2020 COVID-19 Return-to-Play Algorithm for adult athletes in competitive sports. (Reprinted with permission from Kim et al. [10], American Medical Association)

In line with the Centers for Disease Control and Prevention (CDC) recommendation to reduce self-isolation from 14 to 10 days from the time of documented infection, the updated RTP algorithm reduced the time period recommended for complete exercise abstinence from 14 days to 10 days from the date of the positive test result for asymptomatic COVID-19 infection [10]. A graded resumption of exercise remains recommended after this 10 day period. Furthermore, given the available data suggesting that RTP CV risk stratification appears to be low yield in competitive athletes with mild, self-limited disease, competitive athletes with mild COVID-19 illness may resume training in a graded fashion without pre-participation RTP testing after 10 days of symptom resolution. However, CV risk stratification is appropriate for competitive athletes with prior moderate or severe COVID-19 illness [10] (Fig. 23.4).

Conclusions

The sporting world has been heavily impacted by the COVID-19 pandemic. Concerns of potential COVID-19 cardiac pathology have driven the formation of expert consensus RTP algorithms designed to protect the athletic heart. While early experience suggests that implementation of targeted cardiac screening can promote safe return to sport, the collection of large-scale and prospective clinical and imaging data is essential to enhance our understanding of the short- and long-term cardiac sequelae of COVID-19, and to provide data-driven approaches to the counseling and screening of competitive athletes and highly active people. The inclusion of sports cardiologists with expertise in the performance and interpretation of athlete cardiac testing will remain essential in the COVID-19 RTP process to optimize and streamline downstream testing and to minimize the potential for unnecessary disqualification or delays in return to play.

Bibliography

1. Thygesen K, Alpert JS, Jaffe AS, et al. Fourth universal definition of myocardial infarction (2018). J Am Coll Cardiol. 2018;72(18):2231–64. https://doi.org/10.1016/j.jacc.2018.08.1038.
2. Clerkin KJ, Fried JA, Raikhelkar J, et al. COVID-19 and cardiovascular disease. Circulation. 2020;141(20):1648–55. https://doi.org/10.1161/CIRCULATIONAHA.120.046941.
3. Fried JA, Ramasubbu K, Bhatt R, et al. The variety of cardiovascular presentations of COVID-19. Circulation. 2020;141(23):1930–6. https://doi.org/10.1161/CIRCULATIONAHA.120.047164.
4. Sandoval Y, Januzzi JLJ, Jaffe AS. Cardiac troponin for assessment of myocardial injury in COVID-19: JACC review topic of the week. J Am Coll Cardiol. 2020;76(10):1244–58. https://doi.org/10.1016/j.jacc.2020.06.068.
5. Atri D, Siddiqi HK, Lang JP, Nauffal V, Morrow DA, Bohula EA. COVID-19 for the cardiologist: basic virology, epidemiology, cardiac manifestations, and potential therapeutic strategies. JACC Basic Transl Sci. 2020;5(5):518–36. https://doi.org/10.1016/j.jacbts.2020.04.002.
6. Lindner D, Fitzek A, Bräuninger H, et al. Association of cardiac infection with SARS-CoV-2 in confirmed COVID-19 autopsy cases. JAMA Cardiol. 2020. https://doi.org/10.1001/jamacardio.2020.3551.
7. Libby P. The heart in COVID-19: primary target or secondary bystander? JACC Basic Transl Sci. 2020;5(5):537–42. https://doi.org/10.1016/j.jacbts.2020.04.001.
8. Hamming I, Timens W, Bulthuis MLC, Lely AT, Navis GJ, van Goor H. Tissue distribution of ACE2 protein, the functional receptor for SARS coronavirus. A first step in understanding SARS pathogenesis. J Pathol. 2004;203(2):631–7. https://doi.org/10.1002/path.1570.
9. Tang N, Li D, Wang X, Sun Z. Abnormal coagulation parameters are associated with poor prognosis in patients with novel coronavirus pneumonia. J Thromb Haemost. 2020;18(4):844–7. https://doi.org/10.1111/jth.14768.
10. Kim JH, Levine BD, Phelan D, et al. COVID-19 and the athletic heart: emerging perspectives on pathology, risks, and return-to-play. JAMA Cardiol. 2021;6(2):219–27. https://doi.org/10.1001/jamacardio.2020.5890.
11. Phelan D, Kim JH, Elliott MD, et al. Screening of potential cardiac involvement in competitive athletes recovering from COVID-19: an expert consensus statement. JACC Cardiovasc Imaging. 2020;13:2635–52. https://doi.org/10.1016/j.jcmg.2020.10.005.
12. Maron BJ, Udelson JE, Bonow RO, et al. Eligibility and disqualification recommendations for competitive athletes with cardiovascular abnormalities: task force 3: hypertrophic cardiomyopathy, arrhythmogenic right ventricular cardiomyopathy and other cardiomyopathies, and myocarditis: a scientific statement From the American Heart Association and American College of Cardiology. Circulation. 2015;132(22):e273–80. https://doi.org/10.1161/CIR.0000000000000239.
13. Maron BJ, Doerer JJ, Haas TS, Tierney DM, Mueller FO. Sudden deaths in young competitive athletes: analysis of 1866 deaths in the United States, 1980–2006. Circulation. 2009;119(8):1085–92. https://doi.org/10.1161/CIRCULATIONAHA.108.804617.

14. Pelliccia A, Solberg EE, Papadakis M, et al. Recommendations for participation in competitive and leisure time sport in athletes with cardiomyopathies, myocarditis, and pericarditis: position statement of the Sport Cardiology Section of the European Association of Preventive Cardiology (EAPC). Eur Heart J. 2019;40(1):19–33. https://doi.org/10.1093/eurheartj/ehy730.
15. Phillips M, Robinowitz M, Higgins JR, Boran KJ, Reed T, Virmani R. Sudden cardiac death in Air Force recruits. A 20-year review. JAMA. 1986;256(19):2696–9.
16. Kiel RJ, Smith FE, Chason J, Khatib R, Reyes MP. Coxsackievirus B3 myocarditis in C3H/HeJ mice: description of an inbred model and the effect of exercise on virulence. Eur J Epidemiol. 1989;5(3):348–50. https://doi.org/10.1007/BF00144836.
17. Puntmann VO, Carerj ML, Wieters I, et al. Outcomes of cardiovascular magnetic resonance imaging in patients recently recovered from coronavirus disease 2019 (COVID-19). JAMA Cardiol. 2020. https://doi.org/10.1001/jamacardio.2020.3557.
18. Rajpal S, Tong MS, Borchers J, et al. Cardiovascular magnetic resonance findings in competitive athletes recovering from COVID-19 infection. JAMA Cardiol. 2020; https://doi.org/10.1001/jamacardio.2020.4916.
19. Heart condition linked with COVID-19 fuels Power 5 concern about season's viability. https://www.espn.com/college-football/story/_/id/29633697/heart-condition-linked-covid-19-fuels-power-5-concern-season-viability.
20. Baggish A, Drezner JA, Kim J, Martinez M, Prutkin JM. Resurgence of sport in the wake of COVID-19: cardiac considerations in competitive athletes. Br J Sports Med. 2020. https://doi.org/10.1136/bjsports-2020-102516.
21. Vago H, Dohy Z, Merkely B. Cardiac magnetic resonance findings in patients recovered from COVID-19: initial experiences in elite athletes. JACC Cardiovasc Imaging. 2020;S1936-878X:31021–4.
22. Brito DM, Yanamala N, Heenaben P, et al. High prevalence of pericardial involvement in college student-athletes recovering from COVID-19. JACC Cardiovasc Imaging. 2020;S1936-878X:30946–3.
23. Starekova J, Bluemke DA, William S Bradham WS, et al. Evaluation for Myocarditis in Competitive Student Athletes Recovering From Coronavirus Disease 2019 With Cardiac Magnetic Resonance Imaging. JAMA Cardiol. 2021;14:e207444. https://doi.org/10.1001/jamacardio.2020.7444. Online ahead of print.
24. Baggish AL, Battle RW, Beaver TA, et al. Recommendations on the use of multimodality cardiovascular imaging in young adult competitive athletes: a report from the American Society of Echocardiography in collaboration with the Society of Cardiovascular Computed Tomography and the Society for Car. J Am Soc Echocardiogr Off Publ Am Soc Echocardiogr. 2020;33(5):523–49. https://doi.org/10.1016/j.echo.2020.02.009.
25. Shave R, Baggish A, George K, et al. Exercise-induced cardiac troponin elevation: evidence, mechanisms, and implications. J Am Coll Cardiol. 2010;56(3):169–76. https://doi.org/10.1016/j.jacc.2010.03.037.
26. La Gerche A, Burns AT, Mooney DJ, et al. Exercise-induced right ventricular dysfunction and structural remodelling in endurance athletes. Eur Heart J. 2012;33(8):998–1006. https://doi.org/10.1093/eurheartj/ehr397.
27. Phelan D, Kim JH, Chung EH. A game plan for the resumption of sport and exercise after coronavirus disease 2019 (COVID-19) infection. JAMA Cardiol. 2020. https://doi.org/10.1001/jamacardio.2020.2136.
28. Schellhorn P, Klingel K, Burgstahler C. Return to sports after COVID-19 infection: do we have to worry about myocarditis? Eur Heart J. 2020. https://doi.org/10.1093/eurheartj/ehaa448.
29. Wilson MG, Hull JH, Rogers J, et al. Cardiorespiratory considerations for return-to-play in elite athletes after COVID-19 infection: a practical guide for sport and exercise medicine physicians. Br J Sports Med. 2020;54(19):1157–61. https://doi.org/10.1136/bjsports-2020-102710.
30. Bhatia RT, Marwaha S, Malhotra A, et al. Exercise in the severe acute respiratory syndrome coronavirus-2 (SARS-CoV-2) era: a question and answer session with the experts endorsed by the section of sports cardiology & exercise of the European Association of Preventive Cardiology (EAPC). Eur J Prev Cardiol. 2020;27(12):1242–51. https://doi.org/10.1177/2047487320930596.

31. Phelan D, Kim JH, Elliot MD, et al. Screening of potential cardiac involvement in competitive athletes recovering from COVID-19: an expert consensus statement, vol. 13; 2020. p. 2635–52.
32. Baggish AL, Levine BD. Icarus and sports after COVID 19: too close to the Sun? Circulation. 2020. https://doi.org/10.1161/CIRCULATIONAHA.120.048335.
33. Donnellan E, Phelan D. Biomarkers of cardiac stress and injury in athletes: what do they mean? Curr Heart Fail Rep. 2018;15(2):116–22. https://doi.org/10.1007/s11897-018-0385-9.
34. Kleiven Ø, Omland T, Skadberg Ø, et al. Race duration and blood pressure are major predictors of exercise-induced cardiac troponin elevation. Int J Cardiol. 2019;283:1–8. https://doi.org/10.1016/j.ijcard.2019.02.044.
35. Shi S, Qin M, Shen B, et al. Association of cardiac injury with mortality in hospitalized patients with COVID-19 in Wuhan, China. JAMA Cardiol. 2020;5(7):802–10. https://doi.org/10.1001/jamacardio.2020.0950.
36. Morgera T, Di Lenarda A, Dreas L, et al. Electrocardiography of myocarditis revisited: clinical and prognostic significance of electrocardiographic changes. Am Heart J. 1992;124(2):455–67. https://doi.org/10.1016/0002-8703(92)90613-z.
37. Engel DJ, Schwartz A, Homma S. Athletic cardiac remodeling in US professional basketball players. JAMA Cardiol. 2016;1(1):80–7. https://doi.org/10.1001/jamacardio.2015.0252.
38. Abergel E, Chatellier G, Hagege AA, et al. Serial left ventricular adaptations in world-class professional cyclists: implications for disease screening and follow-up. J Am Coll Cardiol. 2004;44(1):144–9. https://doi.org/10.1016/j.jacc.2004.02.057.
39. Teske AJ, Prakken NH, De Boeck BW, et al. Echocardiographic tissue deformation imaging of right ventricular systolic function in endurance athletes. Eur Heart J. 2009;30(8):969–77. https://doi.org/10.1093/eurheartj/ehp040.
40. Han Y, Chen T, Bryant J, et al. Society for Cardiovascular Magnetic Resonance (SCMR) guidance for the practice of cardiovascular magnetic resonance during the COVID-19 pandemic. J Cardiovasc Magn Reson. 2020;22(1):26. https://doi.org/10.1186/s12968-020-00628-w.
41. Huang L, Zhao P, Tang D, et al. Cardiac involvement in patients recovered from COVID-2019 identified using magnetic resonance imaging. JACC Cardiovasc Imaging. 2020:3427. https://doi.org/10.1016/j.jcmg.2020.05.004.
42. Sharma S, Drezner JA, Baggish A, et al. International recommendations for electrocardiographic interpretation in athletes. J Am Coll Cardiol. 2017;69(8):1057–75. https://doi.org/10.1016/j.jacc.2017.01.015.
43. Martinez MW, Tucker AM, OJ Bloom, et al. Prevalence of Inflammatory Heart Disease Among Professional Athletes with Prior COVID-19 Infection Who Received Systematic Return-to-Play Cardiac Screening. JAMA Cardiol. 2021;4. https://doi.org/10.1001/jamacardio.2021.0565.

Index

© Springer Nature Switzerland AG 2021
D. J. Engel, D. M. Phelan (eds.), *Sports Cardiology*,
https://doi.org/10.1007/978-3-030-69384-8

Printed in the United States
by Baker & Taylor Publisher Services